KW-045-807

# The neurobiology of the cardiorespiratory system

# Studies in neuroscience

*Series editor*: William Winlow, *Lecturer in Physiology, The University, Leeds LS2 9NQ, UK*

Titles in this series:

**The neurobiology of pain**
*Editors*: A. V. Holden and W. Winlow

**The neurobiology of dopamine systems**
*Editors*: W. Winlow and R. Markstein

**Working methods in neuropsychopharmacology**
*Editors*: M. Joseph and J. Waddington

**The neurobiology of the cardiorespiratory system**
*Editor*: E. W. Taylor

**Growth and plasticity of neural connections**
*Editors*: W. Winlow and C. R. McCrohan

**Aims and methods in neuroethology**
*Editor*: D. M. Guthrie

3 0073442 7U

MAGDALEN COLLEGE LIBRARY
SHELF No. TAY
591.11

£44,50
2552

# The neurobiology of the cardiorespiratory system

*edited by*   E. W. Taylor

MAGDALEN COLLEGE LIBRARY

Manchester University Press

Copyright © Manchester University Press 1987

Whilst copyright in the volume as a whole is vested in Manchester University Press,
copyright in the individual chapters belongs to their respective authors,
and no chapter may be reproduced wholly or in part without the express
permission in writing of both author and publisher.

*Published by* Manchester University Press,
Oxford Road, Manchester M13 9PL, UK

*Distributed exclusively in the USA and Canada*
*by* St. Martin's Press, Inc., 175 Fifth Avenue, New York, NY 10010, USA

*British Library Cataloguing in publication data*
The Neurobiology of the cardiorespiratory system. —(Studies in neuroscience).
  1. Cardiovascular system   2. Neurophysiology   3. Respiratory organs
  I. Taylor, E. W.   II. Series
  591.1'1        QP102

*Library of Congress cataloging in publication data*

The Neurobiology of the cardiorespiratory system/edited by E. W.
  Taylor
      p.    cm. — (Studies in neuroscience)
  Includes bibliographies and index.
  ISBN 0-7190-2452-8.
    1. Respiration—Regulation.   2. Blood—Circulation—Regulation.
  3. Nervous system, Autonomic.   I. Taylor, E. W.   II. Series.
    [DNLM:   1. Cardiovascular System—physiology.   2. Central Nervous
  System—physiology.   3. Respiration.   WL 300 N49375]
  QP123.N47 1988
  591.1'2—dc19
  DNLM/DLC

ISBN 0 7190 2452 8 *hardback*


*Printed in Great Britain by Biddles Ltd., Guildford and King's Lynn*

# Contents

# Preface

In the vertebrates and larger, more highly organised invertebrates rhythmical mechanical movements of the ventilatory and circulatory systems combine to provide oxygen to metabolising tissues and to remove the waste products of metabolism to the environment. The central nervous system is typically a highly aerobic organ, requiring a good blood supply for effective function, and it also largely determines the co-ordinated action of the respiratory and circulatory pumps.

Regular ventilatory movements originate in a central respiratory rhythm generator consisting, in crustaceans, of paired non-spiking oscillator interneurones and in vertebrates of a pool of inspiratory neurones in the medulla, which are self-contained, autorhythmic but not independent. The rhythm from these primary pattern generators is modulated by inputs from a wide range of peripheral mechanoreceptors and chemoreceptors. These may sustain or even generate the rhythm (e.g. lung stretch receptors in mammals terminate the inspiring burst, and rhythmical stimulation of the oval organ in crustaceans can entrain the central oscillator neurones). Inputs from different receptors may have interactive effects (e.g. chemoreceptor stimulation in mammals modulates baroreceptor responses), and this is achieved by their convergence upon central integration sites in the CNS such as the nucleus tractus solitarius in the mammalian brainstem. This also receives inputs from higher centres such as the hypothalamus where overriding physiological responses such as the defence or visceral alerting response may be initiated, following consciousness of an environmental threat such as the appearance of a predator or loss of contact with the water surface during a dive. Behavioural responses vary and the cardiovascular components of the fright or flight response are susceptible to habituation, if the appropriate stimulus is presented repeatedly.

These and other pieces of this four-dimensional (topographical and temporal) jigsaw of interactive controls are examined in detail, and often from more than one viewpoint, in this book. It is not a textbook as it does not attempt to present a generalised overview of the subject. Rather, it is a collection of independent but related chapters, each produced by research workers in the relevant field. The predominance of biomedical research in this area has resulted in over half the chapters being concerned with mammalian systems. Other chapters consider the evolution in vertebrates, from fish to mammals, of the control of ventilation, the distribution of preganglionic vagal motoneurones and the renin-angiotensin system. The control of ventilation in birds and crustaceans and the cardiovascular system in fish are also described.

Some chapters are highly specific, considering in detail the central roles of GABA, noradrenaline and 5HT; the central and peripheral influence of vasopressin and angiotensin; the role of the atrial receptors in the heart, the carotid sinus baroreceptors and carotid body chemoreceptors. The integration of these various influences by the CNS and the overriding effect of changes at higher levels such as induction of the defence response, sleep, and a decision to initiate or terminate a dive are considered in detail. Other chapters concern the human cardiac response to psychological challenge and the central control of fetal breathing. The practical experience of the authors in their chosen areas of the subject often shows in their emphasis of the techniques and progression of ideas which result in their interpretation of their data.

What I hope we have produced is an authoritative and broadly based overview of current work of use of researchers, teachers and students, both postgraduate and advanced undergraduate, interested in the control of the respiratory and cardiovascular systems of animals. The blend of mammalian, lower vertebrate and invertebrate physiology arose indirectly from two meetings of the Society for Experimental Biology, the first in 1984 in Birmingham, the second in 1985 in Leeds. From the stimulating discussions which took place at these meetings came the realisation that these often separate disciplines have much to learn from one another. Whilst the relatively sophisticated mammalian studies often provide useful methodology for the comparative physiologist, the study of lower vertebrate and invertebrate preparations can help us to interpret how the more complex mammalian systems function and may have evolved. The chapters have accumulated over the last two years and during this period they were passed to other appropriate authors, often on a reciprocal basis, or to external referees, for comment. Some editorial cross-referencing and a final revision brought the recent literature cited to its publication date in 1987, thus minimising reference to work 'in press' which so often frustrates the reader of timely reviews. The index is an important part of this volume because it attempts to draw together the different approaches and methods described in each chapter. The reader can explore the coverage offered by this volume by tracing a typical item from the index such as 'heart rate', 'hypothalamus' or 'sinus arrhythima'. Finally, because the comparative approach introduces exotic animals into the text and comparative physiologists will wish to locate them, I have added an index of animals.

I wish to acknowledge the effort and dedication of all the authors and their co-workers in providing manuscripts and updating and reviewing chapters.

One author in particular, Coen Ballintijn, who supplied our stimulating first chapter and whose career has been interrupted by early retirement following a traffic accident, deserves special mention.

On a personal level I wish to thank Mrs Jean Hill for her tireless processing of manuscripts and to dedicate my own work on the book to my family, namely: Ann, Annie, Ann-Marie, Elizabeth, Ted (Snr.), Ted (Jnr.), Patrick and Daniel for their support.

E.W.T.

# Part I

# Control of ventilation

# 1

# Evolution of central nervous control of ventilation in vertebrates

**C. M. Ballintijn†**

*Department of Animal Physiology, Neurophysiology Section, Biological Centre, 9751 NN Haren, The Netherlands*

## 1.1. Introduction

In vertebrates fundamental changes in respiratory apparatus accompanied the transition from water to air breathing. In water-breathers such as fishes, the gas exchangers are the gills, contained in the branchial cavities. The actual gas exchange takes place at the surface of numerous secondary lamellae, protruding from gill filaments which are implanted in double rows on the gill arches. In air-breathers respiratory gases are exchanged through a very thin epithelium which (except in birds) lines the folded internal surfaces of sac-like lungs, contained in the thoracic cavity.

For the renewal of the respiratory medium three major types of respiratory pumping system were developed in the course of evolution: one for water breathing and, at a later stage, two for air breathing. These three pumps are vastly different in construction and in operation. It is therefore interesting to pose the question as to the extent to which the ancestral neural control system has been retained while the respiratory apparatus has been subjected to such drastic modifications. Unfortunately, only for the two ends of the evolutionary scale, fishes and mammals, is a reasonable amount of information available on the nervous circuits engaged in the control of ventilation. For other animal groups data are, if present at all, extremely scarce. The neurophysiological part of the present chapter will therefore be devoted to fishes and mammals alone. However, the evolution of the respiratory pumps will first be described for vertebrates in general, because it is a good basis for interpretation of the development of the associated neural control circuits.

## 1.2. The respiratory pumps

Fishes possess a dual-action, suction–pressure pump which generates a practically continuous, unidirectional water current over the gills in the

† *Present address: B. Boermalaan 7, 9765 AP. Paterswolde, Netherlands.*

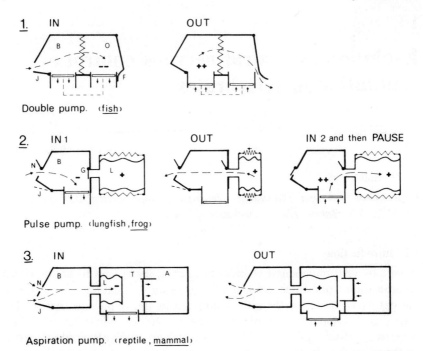

1. IN      OUT

Double pump. ⟨fish⟩

2. IN 1      OUT      IN 2 and then PAUSE

Pulse pump. ⟨lungfish, frog⟩

3. IN      OUT

Aspiration pump. ⟨reptile, mammal⟩

Fig. 1.1. Diagrams of the main respiratory pumps of vertebrates (except birds). **(1)** Unidirectional flow, constant current, double pump of fishes. **(2)** Bidirectional flow, interrupted current, positive-pressure pump of lungfishes and amphibians. **(3)** Tidal aspiration pump of reptiles and mammals. (In birds the pumping system is comparable, but thoracic volume changes affect air sacs rather than lungs. Aerodynamic properties result in unidirectional gas flow across the respiratory epithelium.) In the diagrams pistons represent active volume changes. Positive and negative pressures with respect to ambient are denoted by $+$ and $-$. A, Abdominal cavity; B, buccal cavity; F, flexible opercular rim; G, glottis; J, lower jaw; L, lung; N, nares; O, opercular cavity; T, thoracic cavity.

following way (Fig. 1.1). The buccal and opercular cavities, which are separated by the gill curtain, contract and expand synchronously. During expansion ('inspiration', Fig. 1.1(1): IN) the mouth is open but a flexible rim around the operculum seals the opercular slits against the body of the fish. Consequently a considerable negative (i.e. subambient) pressure is built up in the opercular cavities and water is sucked in through the mouth and over the gills. During contraction ('expiration', Fig. 1.1(1): OUT) the mouth is closed, and as a result the buccal cavity pressure becomes strongly positive. This forces water over the gills, which then can leave freely through the opercular slits because the opercular rim is blown away from the body. The lower jaw, as is apparent from the above description, plays the role of an actively controlled inlet valve. The opercular rim in teleosts, and probably also the posterior border of the elasmobranch gill slits, acts as a passive outlet valve.

The pump is powered by cranial muscles. In teleosts both respiratory phases are active. In elasmobranchs the contraction phase is active but the expansion phase is passive during normal respiration, using the elastic forces built up in the branchial skeleton (Ballintijn & Hughes, 1965; Hughes & Ballintijn, 1965; Ballintijn, 1969a, b, c, 1985b; Osse, 1969; Ballintijn & Punt, 1985).

The simplest and earliest transitions to air breathing occurring in fish employed extensively vascularised cavities which could be filled with air. In the examples of such primitive air-breathers that are still living, air pumping movements are derivations of the normal teleostean respiratory movements or the cough. An example of the first kind is *Helostoma*, which fills its air sac through the mouth with fresh air and expels used air via the opercular slits. Liem (1980) compares the movement to 'preparatory feeding', but in our opinion a comparison to normal respiratory movements is better. *Channa*, and sometimes also *Helostoma*, according to Liem (1980), display a respiratory pattern which closely resembles the coughing movement observed in many water-breathing teleosts (Ballintijn, 1969b, c; Holeton & Jones, 1975; Hughes, 1975; Ballintijn & Jüch, 1984). Expansion of the respiratory cavities with mouth closed flushes the spent air forward into the buccal cavity, from where it is released through the mouth (Liem, 1980). This simple form of air breathing has to be essentially arrhythmic, as the fish spends most of the time under water (McMahon, 1969; Gans, 1970a, b, 1974; Liem, 1980).

Other primitive air-breathers use the walls of the gut for respiratory gas exchange (e.g. *Cobitis*), and some have evolved blind sacs from the gut wall which function as primordial lungs (the lungfishes). The lungs of lungfishes and of amphibians are ventilated by a 'pulse pump' or 'buccal pressure' pump (Fig. 1.1(2). The overall principle is that air is first taken into the buccal cavity and subsequently, by muscular force generating a positive pressure, it is transferred to the lungs, where it is kept for some time. Respiration is therefore discontinuous, with an interrupted, bidirectional flow instead of being continuously rhythmic. The frog provides a good example of a well developed pulse-pump system (Figs 1.1(2) and 1.10(1)) (de Jongh & Gans, 1969; Gans *et al.*, 1969; Gans, 1970a, b, 1974). Inspiration occurs in two parts, separated by an expiration. In the first part of inspiration (Fig. 1.1(2): IN 1) air is sucked through the nares into the mouth by buccal expansion, while the lungs are closed by a valve in the trachea. Then there is an expiratory phase (Fig. 1.1(2): OUT) during which the tracheal valve opens and stale air from the lungs is expelled through the nares. It passes over the fresh air taken in before, which is located behind the tongue so that hardly any mixing takes place. In the second inspiratory part (Fig. 1.1(2): IN 2) the nares, which are also valved, close and air is transferred to the lungs by buccal-cavity compression. Then the tracheal valve closes again and gases are exchanged with the air trapped in the lungs during the respiratory pause that follows.

Both the valves, in the nares and at the entrance of the lungs, are actively controlled. Inspiration is powered by buccal musculature. Expiration depends a great deal on tension developed by smooth muscles. Thus a large proportion of the work of breathing is not recoverable as elastic energy, and this, together with the fact that lung pressures are above ambient, results in a fairly low efficiency in terms of energy consumption (Gans, 1970a, b).

In reptiles and mammals, with the advent of aspiration or suction respiration, the power consumption of the system is appreciably reduced. The reason is that in these systems elasticity of the lungs and rib cage allows partial recovery of the work of breathing, and the contents of the lungs are always near ambient pressure (Gans, 1970a, b). (The same holds true, of course, for birds.) In suction-breathers the lungs are included in a thoracic cavity surrounded by ribs. Expansion of this cavity produces a slight negative pressure around the lungs which, as a consequence, fill themselves with fresh air (Fig. 1.1(3): IN). Contraction of the chest results in expiration (Fig. 1.1(3): OUT). Valves are not necessary and, at least in the higher forms, are not present.

Thorax cavity volume changes are brought about in a number of ways, depending on animal species. In lower reptiles it is only a matter of abduction and adduction of the ribs, but in turtles and tortoises, with their inflexible carapace, volume changes result from pectoral and pelvic-girdle movements (Hughes & Gans, 1965; Gans & Hughes, 1967; Gaunt & Gans, 1969; Gans, 1970a, b, 1974). In crocodiles, muscles pull the liver backwards during inspiration, thus giving an additional increase in thoracic volume (Gans, 1970a, b). This system is further refined in mammals, where the diaphragm which separates the thoracic from the intestinal cavity fulfils a comparable function. The way in which aspiration respiration is powered depends very much on the species in question and on the circumstances. In some animals inspiration is brought about by muscle contraction and expiration passively, under the influence of elastic recoil and/or gravitational forces. In other animals it is just the other way round. In some species the pattern even depends on the position of the animal (lying or standing), which changes the influence of gravity (Gans, 1970a, b). Sometimes, during quiet respiration, one phase is active and the other passive, whereas at high-intensity ventilation both phases are the result of muscle contraction.

Thus, in summary, in addition to an appreciable difference in gas-exchange organs for water and air breathing, there is an extensive variation in respiratory motor apparatus between vertebrates. Moreover, even within one animal species, there can be a considerable difference in breathing movements under various circumstances. As a result respiration ranges from the rhythmic, continuous, unidirectional flow pattern of fishes via the intermittent multiphasic respiration of amphibia to the rhythmic tidal ventilation of mammals.

## 1.3. **The central nervous control mechanism**

As has been mentioned in the introduction, a reasonable amount of data for a comparison of the central nervous circuits engaged in the control of vertebrate respiration is only available for the lowest group (fishes) and the highest group (mammals). A comparison of these will be the topic of this section.

Transection experiments have shown that both in mammals and fishes the primary respiratory rhythm generator is located in the brainstem. Because its neurones continue firing rhythmically during paralysis with muscle relaxants (curare, flaxedyl, succinylcholine, etc.), it can be concluded that the generators are autorhythmic and do not need peripheral feedback. Important structures are:

(a) the reticular formation, in both mammals and fishes;
(b) the vagus nerve, which in mammals innervates the lungs and in fishes supplies the motor and sensory innervation of the gill arch system;
(c) the pneumotaxic centre in the pons, which only occurs in mammals because fishes occupy a position on the evolutionary scale where a pons has not yet evolved;
(d) several mesencephalic neurone groups, again in both mammals and fishes.


### 1.3.1. *Teleost respiratory centres*

(a) *Rhythm generation.* In the medulla oblongata of fishes, respiratory rhythmic neurones occur in the reticular formation, in the trigeminal, facial, glossopharyngeal and vagal motor nuclei which drive the respiratory muscles, and in the descending trigeminal nucleus and the intermediate facial nucleus, which process sensory information (Shelton, 1959, 1961; von Baumgarten & Salmoiraghi, 1962; Waldron, 1972; Bamford, 1974; Ballintijn & Roberts, 1976; Ballintijn 1982, 1985a; Ballintijn *et al.*, 1983). The respiratory rhythm originates in a long strip of reticular formation tissue. The generator is diffusely organised, with a considerable amount of redundancy. This can be concluded from the fact that it is possible to lesion anywhere in the reticular formation without stopping rhythmic breathing, unless the destroyed area is too large. Obviously the amount of generator tissue rather than the exact localisation is important.

(b) *Vagus input.* The gills of fishes are extensively endowed with various receptors (Sutterlin & Saunders, 1969; Poole & Satchell, 1979) of which mechanoreceptors influence the respiratory pattern considerably (Ballintijn *et al.*, 1983). An extensive study of the properties of branchial mechanoreceptors in the carp has recently been made by de Graaf. He distinguishes

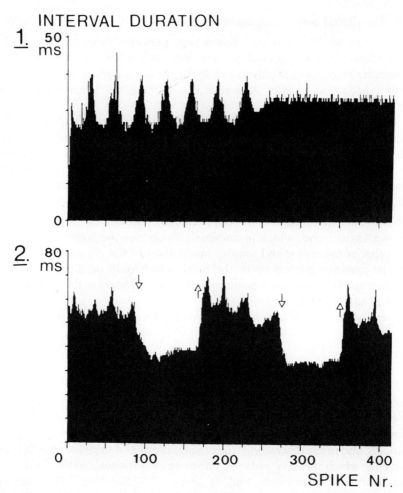

Fig. 1.2.   Interval plot of firing pattern of gill arch mechanoreceptor neurones in the carp. **(1)** During normal respiration. In the second half of the graph a respiratory pause starts, as is reflected in the steady firing level of the receptor. **(2)** During normal respiration. After about 100 and 275 spike intervals (at the arrows) the gill arch was held adducted by the experimenter for a while. Note the tonic change in firing level.

at least two types which are important in the present context. One is located in the flexible cartilaginous joint in the middle of each gill arch, and the other is in the gill filaments and the gill rakers (de Graaf & Ballintijn, 1987; de Graaf *et al.*, 1987). The first receptors, which are tonic in nature, provide detailed information on the exact position of the gill arches (Fig. 1.2) and the second, which possess a markedly phasic firing pattern with a fairly high threshold, signal sudden disturbances of the gill system. The extensive influence of vagally mediated gill mechanoreceptor information upon the

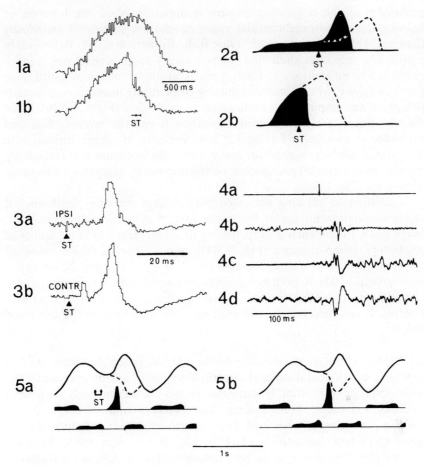

Fig. 1.3. Vagal influences upon respiration. **(1)** Inspiratory termination by cervical vagus stimulation in cat as revealed by phrenic activity. a: Normal phrenic activity; b: phrenic activity with vagal stimulation starting 1000 ms after inspiration onset, showing premature inspiratory termination. Each trace is summed over 19 respiratory cycles. **(2)** Respiratory phase switching by branchial vagal stimulation in the carp. a: Expiratory termination through stimulation during adduction as shown by the EMG of the adductor mandibulae; b: inspiratory termination through stimulation during abduction as shown by the EMG of the levator hyomandibulae. ST = stimulus. Integrated EMG: black during stimulation; broken line during normal respiration. **(3)** Short-latency phrenic motor responses to cervical vagus stimulation in the cat. a: In the ipsilateral phrenic nerve; b: in the contralateral phrenic nerve. Responses summed over 99 sweeps. **(4)** Short-latency motor responses to branchial vagus stimulation in the carp. a: Stimulus; b: adductor mandibulae EMG reaction; c: levator hyomandibulae EMG reaction; d: dilatator operculi EMG reaction. **(5)** a: Cough-like expulsion reflex elicited by branchial vagus stimulation in the carp. b: Normal, spontaneous cough in the carp. Traces are from top to buttom: movement; EMG levator hyomandibulae; EMG adductor mandibulae. (**1** and **3** from Iscoe *et al.*, 1979; **2**, **4** and **5** from Ballintijn *et al.*, 1983.)

generation of the respiratory pattern is apparent when vagal nerves or sensory neurones in epibranchial vagus ganglia are stimulated electrically (Satchell, 1959; Ballintijn *et al.*, 1983; B. L. Roberts & C. M. Ballintijn, in prep.). The responses show that the respiratory rhythm generator is influenced in two different ways. First, it reacts to single pulse stimulation with phase switching: when a stimulus pulse is given during inspiration, it curtails this phase and respiration switches over to expiration (Fig. 1.3 (2b)); when the stimulus is presented during expiration it has the reverse effect and expiration is switched off (Fig. 1.3(2a)). Secondly, rhythmic stimuli, with frequencies slightly higher or lower than the spontaneous respiratory rhythm, have a synchronising effect on the respiratory generator and entrain respiration (Fig. 1.6(3)).

In addition to affecting the respiratory rhythm generator, epibranchial vagus stimulation influences the motor system in a more direct manner. Single pulse stimuli elicit a short-latency (*c.* 20 ms) reaction in a number of respiratory pump muscles (Fig. 1.3(4)), which appears to be mediated bisynaptically. Short trains of stimuli (about five pulses, 10 to 20 ms apart) elicit a reaction which, both in muscle co-ordination and movement pattern, cannot be distinguished from a normal cough (compare Figs. 1.3(5a) with 1.3(5b)). It can therefore be regarded as a 'defence reaction' or expulsion reflex.

(c) *Higher influences; the mesencephalon.*   Although the medullary rhythm generator is self-contained and autorhythmic, it is not independent. The basic respiratory rhythm it generates is modulated by both peripheral feedback and higher brain centres. The mesencephalon of the carp, for instance, contains at least two neurone groups which influence the respiratory pattern (Ballintijn *et al.*, 1979; Jüch & Ballintijn, 1983). They are situated close together near the longitudinal medial fascicle, in the region of the oculomotor nucleus (Fig. 1.4(1) at A and B) (Jüch & Luiten, 1981). One group (A), according to horseradish peroxidase (HRP) tracer experiments, has direct connections with the medullary reticular formation. It affects the respiratory rhythm generator in two ways. In the first place it modifies the respiratory rhythm. This influence is obvious when the neurones are stimulated rhythmically with electrical pulses at a frequency slightly higher or lower than the spontaneous respiratory rhythm, when the generator is then easily entrained (Figs 1.4(5d) and (5e)). In the second place these A-neurones play a role during so-called intermittent or bout respiration. Bout respiration occurs in a number of fish species (e.g. the carp) when they are quiet and in oxygen-rich water. It consists of a regular pattern of a short series of respiratory cycles (about three to ten), separated by fairly long pauses (lasting for a period of several respiratory cycles) (Fig. 1.9(1)). The mesencephalic neurone group A always starts firing just before the beginning of a bout of respirations (Fig. 1.4(4)). In fact, they contribute to starting the rhythm generator at the end of the pause, because electrical stimulation can

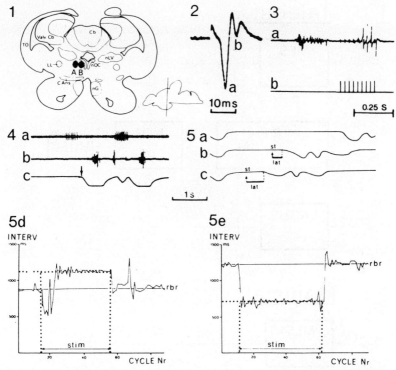

Fig. 1.4. **(1)** Cross-section of the brain of the carp showing the position of mesencephalic type A and type B neurones. (Insert indicates level of section in the sagittal plane.) CAns, commissura ansulata; Cb, corpus cerebellum; LL, lemniscus lateralis; nG, nucleus glomerulosus; nLV, nucleus lateralis valvulae; nOC, nucleus oculomotorius; TO, tectum opticum; Valv Cb = valvulae cerebelli. **(2)** Short-latency synchronous muscle-twitch response to single-shock electrical stimulation of mesencephalic group B neurones in the carp. a: First component (latency 7 ms); b: second component (latency 11.5 ms). **(3)** Muscle response to electrical stimulation of group B neurones with repetitive subthreshold stimuli. a: Levator hyomandibulae activity. The first part of the trace shows a normal muscle contraction, followed by the responses to stimulation. Notice that a reaction is not elicited by the first pulses, but gradually builds up. b: Stimulus pulses. **(4)** Respiration-starting effect of mesencephalic group A neurones during intermittent (bout) respiration. a: Neurone activity, starting in advance of a bout of respirations (at the arrow in trace c); b: EMG levator hyomandibulae; c: movement trace (respiration starts at arrow). **(5)** a to c: Electrical stimulation of mesencephalic group A neurones in the pause during intermittent respiration advances the next bout. a, Normal: b and c stimulated at different intervals after the previous bout. st, Stimulus; lat, latency of the response. d and e: Entrainment of the respiratory rhythm generator by rhythmic electrical stimulation of group A neurones; d: stimulus frequency lower than the spontaneous respiratory rhythm; e: stimulus frequency higher than the spontaneous respiratory rhythm. rbr, Spontaneous respiratory rhythm (respiratory base rate, drawn in as a horizontal line). stim, Stimulation period (between vertical broken lines). The stimulus interval is represented by a horizontal broken line. INTERV, Interval in ms between successive respiratory cycles or stimuli, plotted along the $y$ axis. CYCLE Nr, Successive respiratory cycles plotted along the $x$ axis. (All figures from Jüch & Ballintijn, 1983.)

*Control of ventilation*

**1    Teleost.**

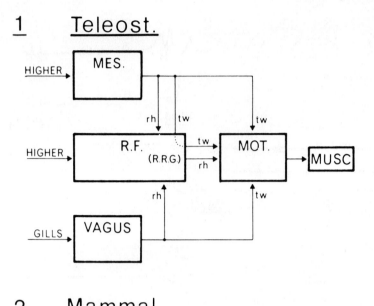

**2    Mammal.**

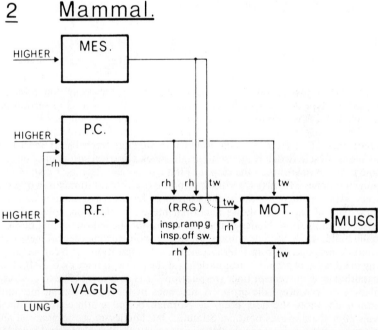

Fig. 1.5.   Summary diagrams of the central nervous respiration control circuits in teleosts **(1)** and mammals **(2)** Abbreviations: insp. off sw., inspiratory off switch; insp. ramp g., inspiratory ramp generator; MES., mesencephalon; MOT., peripheral motor control system; MUSC., muscles; P.C., pneumotaxic centre; R.F., reticular formation; rh, rhythmic influence; −rh, rhythm suppression; R.R.G., respiratory rhythm generator; tw, twitch response. Further explanation in the text.

prematurely bring a pause to an end and start a new bout (Fig. 1.4(5)a–c).

The other neurones, the B group (Fig. 1.4(1) at B), influence the motor output to respiratory muscles. Their firing frequency is proportional to EMG intensities. Electrical stimulation of these neurones elicits a reaction in a number of respiratory pump muscles (Fig. 1.4(3)). Signal averaging shows that this reaction consists of two responses with different latencies (about 7 and 11 ms) (Fig. 1.4(2)). This observation agrees well with the fact that HRP tracing reveals two different routes from the mesencephalic B cell group to the respiratory motor nuclei. There is one direct connection and one running via the medullary reticular formation, which projects on to the medullary motor nuclei secondarily. The reticular connection is probably the cause of the fact that when the mesencephalic B locus is stimulated with subliminal stimuli at 10–50 Hz, reactions which increase in size appear after a few stimuli (Fig. 1.4(3)). Obviously, somewhere a level of excitation builds up until it reaches a threshold value. The mesencephalic B-neurone group is thought to play a role in adjusting the balance of the activity of different cranial muscles, in relation to the situation and the demands on the system (Jüch & Ballintijn, 1983).

A diagram of the neural circuits engaged in the control of respiratory movements in teleosts, based on the data described above, is presented in Fig. 1.5(1). Its operation can be summarised as follows. A rhythm generator in the reticular formation generates the respiratory movements through rhythmical excitation of the respiratory motor nuclei. Mechanoreceptive signals from the gills, mediated via the glossopharyngeus and vagus system, exert a dual influence. They strongly influence the rhythm generator, modifying the respiratory frequency, and, apart from that, they elicit twitch and other motor responses via short reflex loops to the motor nuclei. Higher centres in the mesencephalon exert influences on the rhythm generator and on the motor system directly. One neurone group can both entrain the rhythm generator and start it after a pause. Another modulates the respiratory motor pattern via two pathways: through a direct projection on to the respiratory motor nuclei and through an indirect projection via reticular neurones.

### 1.3.2. *Mammalian respiratory centres*

(a) *Rhythm generation.* In mammals inspiratory neurones in the medulla oblongata appear to play a crucial role in respiratory rhythm generation. They are components of an inspiratory ramp generator which is periodically switched off for expiration. Thus inspiration is dominant. In switching between the phases, reciprocal inhibition, and possibly recurrent inhibition, plays some role (Cohen & Feldman, 1977; Cohen, 1974, 1981; Richter, 1982). The major influences that cause inspiratory off-switching originate in the brainstem reticular formation, the pulmonary vagus feedback system

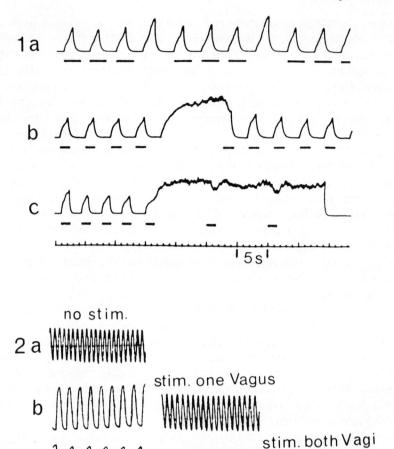

1a

b

c

|  5s  |

no stim.

2 a

stim. one Vagus

b

stim. both Vagi

c

1s

3

st
1Hz

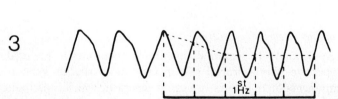

Fig. 1.6.  **(1)** Effects of changes in pulmonary afferent (vagus) and pneumotaxic
centre activity upon respiration in cat. The cats are paralysed and ventilated with a
'cycle-triggered' respiration pump which is triggered from phrenic nerve activity and
produces a single inflation of constant flow and fixed duration. The traces illustrated
are integrated phrenic records, representing central respiratory activity. Bars indicate

(Fig. 1.3(1)) and the pneumotaxic centre (nucleus parabrachialis medialis and Kölliker–Fuse nucleus in the pons). Each of these three systems is able to support rhythmic respiration in the absence of the other two, as can be concluded from the following data. In anaesthetised mammals reticular formation activity is severely depressed. Under such circumstances respiration is only maintained when either the pneumotaxic centre or the vagus is intact: lesioning of the pneumotaxic centre in combination with sectioning of the vagus (or paralysis with a muscle relaxant) during anaesthesia stops respiration at maximal inspiration (Fig. 1.6(1a–c)). In such a preparation central rhythmogenesis is only resumed in the following cases: (1) when the central stumps of the vagi are stimulated with bursts of electrical pulses; (2) when rhythmic artificial respiration is applied to paralysed animals; (3) when the animal is allowed to come round from anaesthesia, which reactivates the reticular formation (St. John *et al.*, 1972; Feldman & Gautier, 1976; D'Angelo, 1979; Hugelin, 1980). This last observation leads to the hypothesis that the reticular formation is the main source of the respiratory rhythm in the waking state (Hugelin, 1980).

Only when the vagus system is inoperative can rhythmic neurone activity be recorded in the pneumotaxic centre. Thus it appears that pulmonary feedback inhibits pneumotaxic rhythmogenesis (Feldman *et al.*, 1976; Knox & King, 1976). With intact vagus input the pneumotaxic centre is continuously active and presumably only provides a tonic drive to the respiratory rhythm generator.

Because both the pulmonary vagus feedback system and the pneumotaxic centre, apart from their influence on rhythmogenesis, play a further role in the control of respiratory movements, these systems will be treated in more detail below.

(b) *Vagus input.* The importance of vagus input for respiratory rhythmogenesis has been demonstrated clearly with rhythmic electrical stimulation

inflation by the ventilation pump. a: Intact pneumotaxic centre. Stopping the pump (no pulmonary vagus feedback) lengthens inspiration. b: Bilateral lesion in pneumotaxic centre. Stopping the pump results in inspiratory arrest. Rhythmic respiratory activity resumes after vagus feedback is restarted with a pump inflation. c: Same as **b** but pump flow is smaller and only produces partial inspiratory off-switching. (From Feldman & Gautier, 1976.) **(2)** Electrical stimulation of the central vagus stumps with frequencies proportional to transpulmonary pressure restores the original breathing pattern in vagotomised mammals. a: Spontaneous respiration of a non-vagotomised rabbit. b: After unilateral vagotomy (first column) and stimulation of the central vagus stump (second column). c: After bilateral vagotomy (first column), stimulation of one central vagus stump (second column) and bilateral stimulation of the vagus stumps (third column). (From Trenchard, 1977.) **(3)** Entrainment of the respiratory rhythm by electrical stimulation of a branchial vagus ganglion in the carp. The stimulus, which is of a higher frequency than respiration, shifts along the respiratory cycle until it locks in at a certain phase relationship.

experiments. It then appears possible to entrain the respiratory rhythm generator and drive it at both lower and higher frequencies than its spontaneous rate (Vibert *et al.*, 1981; Baconnier *et al.*, 1983). It appears to be more difficult to obtain entrainment of the respiratory rhythm generator by the stimulus when arterial carbon dioxide levels are high or the level of anaesthesia is low. These factors both lead to an increase in the general activity in the reticular formation. Vibert *et al.* (1981) therefore suppose that reticular neurones superimpose 'noise' on the vagally controlled Hering–Breuer system. There appears, however, to be another explanation. The fact that the reticular formation is able to maintain respiration in awake mammals with severed vagi and lesioned pneumotaxic centres (St. John *et al.*, 1972; Hugelin, 1980) implies that it can drive the respiratory rhythm generator. In this context it appears more reasonable to postulate that with increased reticular activity its contribution to rhythmogenesis becomes more dominant over that of other systems (e.g. vagus and pneumotaxic input).

Vagally mediated lung receptor activity also plays a role in shaping individual respiratory cycles by determining the level of inspiratory cut-off, as has been clearly demonstrated by Trenchard (1977). She showed that in mammals with uni- or bilateral vagus transection it is possible to restore the normal respiratory pattern through controlled electrical stimulation of the central nerve stumps (Fig. 1.6(2 a–c)).

Inspiratory termination by vagal afferents, together with a fairly weak phrenic motor reaction (Fig. 1.3(3)) appears to be part of an expulsion reflex which can be elicited by vagal afferent stimulation. Comparable but stronger reactions occur in response to superlaryngeal stimulation (Iscoe *et al.*, 1979), which in mammals is more suited to a 'defence reflex' that prevents foreign particles from reaching the lungs.

(c) *Pneumotaxic centre.* As mentioned above, the pneumotaxic centre is able to drive the respiratory rhythm generator on its own, in the absence of reticular and vagal input. Its powerful influence on the respiratory rhythm generator is demonstrated by the fact that electrical stimulation during inspiration induces inspiratory termination (Cohen, 1971, 1974). With continuous rhythmical electrical stimulation it is possible to obtain synchronisation between phrenic motor activity and the stimulus (Bertrand & Hugelin, 1971). Normally, in awake animals, it co-operates with the pulmonary vagus system and the reticular formation in facilitating the switch-over from inspiration to expiration and setting the volume threshold for the inspiration off-switch mechanism. Inspiratory duration in an intact, awake mammal is thus determined by tonic pneumotaxic-centre input, together with augmenting reticular formation and vagus input. It is this triple control that causes the redundancy-based plasticity of respiration control (Cohen, 1971; Feldman & Gautier, 1976; Knox & King, 1976; Hugelin, 1977, 1980; Baker *et al.*, 1981). The influences of somesthetic information, arousal, etc. on respiration are mediated in part through the pneumotaxic centre (Baker *et al.*, 1981; Caille *et al.*, 1981).

Apart from its influence on respiratory rhythm generation, the pneumotaxic centre directly influences motor activity. Electrical stimulation of the nucleus parabrachialis medialis elicits respiratory phase switching plus a short-latency response (6–12 ms) in the phrenic nerve (Fig. 1.7(1,2)) (Bertrand & Hugelin, 1971; Villard *et al.*, 1984). The latter authors also found that tegmental fields adjacent to the pneumotaxic complex directly project on to phrenic motor neurones and/or bulbospinal neurones, bypassing the phase-switching interneurones.

(d) *Mesencephalic influences.* Although not 'essential for respiratory rhythm generation, mesencephalic neurone groups influence both motor output and respiratory rhythm markedly. Neurones in the central or periaqueductal grey (Fig. 1.7(3)) (Gauthier *et al.*, 1983) and the reticular formation (Fig. 1.7(4)) (Bassal & Bianchi, 1982), when stimulated electrically, exert powerful influences. From the first location two types of motor response can be distinguished, a short-latency primary response (latency 20 ms, duration 40 ms) and a patterned response that occurs later and lasts up to 1 s (Fig. 1.7(3a, 3b)). To stimulation of the reticular area, the rhythm generator reacts with entrainment (Fig. 1.7(4a, 4b)) and on-switching of inspiration. Entrainment occurs for frequencies between 1 and 5 Hz (for higher frequencies at ratios of 1:2 or 1:3). In some areas entrainment only lasts for the first 8–10 s of a stimulation period. In general, the effect of mesencephalic stimulation upon respiration is more powerful when the basic respiratory system itself is depressed in activity. The functional significance of mesencephalic modulation of respiration is thought to be related to incorporation of a postural component in the respiratory output, the adjustment of respiration to a behavioural situation and the synchronisation of respiration with other motor outputs (Bassal & Bianchi, 1982; Gauthier *et al.*, 1983).

A generalised diagram of the neural circuits engaged in the control of respiratory movements in mammals, based on the data described above, is presented in Fig. 1.5(2). Its operation can be summarised as follows. The respiratory rhythm is generated by an inspiratory ramp generator in the medulla oblongata which is periodically switched off under the influence of three neural networks (inspiration is dominant). In the waking state the brainstem reticular formation and pulmonary vagus feedback (to a lesser extent?) fulfil this task, while the pneumotaxic centre, through tonic activity, influences the switch-off threshold level. During sleep and under anaesthesia the reticular formation is severely depressed and inspiration is switched off by augmenting vagal activity. If, in experiments, both reticular formation and vagus influences are abolished, pneumotaxic neurones develop a rhythmic firing pattern and initiate periodic switching off of inspiration. Apart from

MAGDALEN COLLEGE LIBRARY

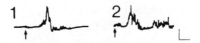

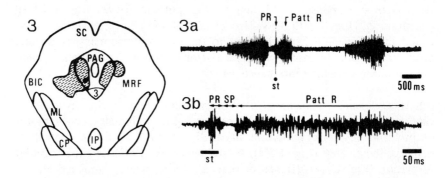

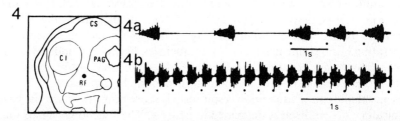

Fig. 1.7.   Influence of pneumotaxic centre stimulation upon respiration in mammals.
**(1)** and **(2)** Single shock electrical stimulation of the pneumotaxic centre in cats elicits
short-latency responses in the phrenic nerve, which are different during expiration **(1)**
and inspiration **(2)**. (From Bertrand & Hugelin, 1971.) **(3)** Electrical stimulation of
the mesencephalic periaqueductal (central) grey in cats, with trains of electrical
pulses, elicits motor responses in the phrenic nerve. In the histological cross-section
the stimulus site is indicated by a black dot; the areas which give similar responses are
hatched. BIC, Brachium of the inferior colliculus; CP, cerebral peduncle; IP,
interpeduncular nucleus; ML, medial lemniscus; MRF, mesencephalic reticular
formation; PAG, periaqueductal grey; SC, superior colliculus; 3, oculomotor nucleus.
a and b: phrenic recordings at respectively low and high speed show a short-latency
primary response (PR), a pause (SP) and a long-latency, long-duration patterned
response (Patt R). (From Gauthier *et al.*, 1983.) **(4)** Electrical stimulation with
rhythmical trains of pulses of the mesencephalic reticular formation in cats results in
entrainment of the respiratory rhythm. In the histological cross-section the stimulation site is represented as a black dot. CI, Inferior colliculus; CS, superior colliculus;
PAG, periaqueductal grey; RF, reticular formation. a and b: Phrenic activity
indicates entrainment of the respiratory rhythm generator at respectively 1 and 5 Hz.
(From Bassal & Bianchi, 1982.)

their influence upon the respiratory rhythm generator, both the pneumotaxic centre and, to a lesser extent, the vagus system can elicit short-latency responses in the muscles (motor nerves) which are the basis of expulsion reflexes. Mesencephalic neurone groups strongly influence respiratory rhythm generation, causing entrainment and inspiration on-switch effects. In addition motor responses to mesencephalic activity occur via direct short-latency pathways and also with longer latency through mediation of the reticular formation.

### 1.3.3. *Comparison of teleostean and mammalian respiratory centres*

Comparison of the neural circuits that control respiratory movements of fishes and mammals reveals a striking resemblance between the two. In both groups of animals the basic respiratory rhythm generator is situated in the medulla oblongata. In fishes it is located in the reticular formation. In mammals its structure is more complicated, there being a separate inspiratory ramp generator, but the reticular formation still plays a crucial role in rhythm generation. In the waking state it co-operates with vagal feedback from the lungs, which causes inspiratory termination, and in fact appears to be able to support rhythm generation on its own. Surprisingly, the vagus system in fishes, although it innervates completely different peripheral structures (gill arches and filaments as opposed to lungs) appears to play an identical role. Vagal input in these animals also causes switching between the respiratory phases, and although it is not known whether it can drive the respiratory rhythm generator in isolation as it does in mammals, the experimental entrainment of respiration with rhythmic vagal input demonstrates its profound influence. In mammals the pneumotaxic centre in the pons (the area in the border region of the mesencephalon and the medulla oblongata) appears to compete with the vagus in importance for the generation of the respiratory rhythm. As a result of vagal suppression, it is only tonically active in the normal situation, and thus contributes to the threshold for phase switching. In the absence of vagal and reticular formation influences, it is able to drive the rhythm generator completely. As fishes do not possess a pons, which first appears in higher evolutionary stages, direct comparison is not possible. The teleostean mesencephalon does, however, contain groups of neurones with comparable properties. Under their influence the rhythm generator can be entrained and, moreover, they contribute to the switch-on of breathing at the end of a pause during intermittent respiration. In mammals mesencephalic influences upon respiration are also present. Entraining of the rhythm generator, inspiration on-switch effects and short- to longer-latency motor responses resulting from mesencephalic stimulation have been demonstrated. It is striking that the same mesencephalic areas as described in teleosts (between the lemniscus and the ventricle, close to the oculomotor nucleus) are engaged. In both fishes and mammals vagal structures give rise to shorter- and longer-latency motor responses (in mammals this is the case for the pneumotaxic centre as well). The vagal responses appear to be related to expulsion reflexes; the reactions in the higher centres are considered to play a role in the interaction between respiration and other systems (posture, etc.).

## 1.4. Evolution of neural control of respiration

In the first part of this paper, the enormous differences between the peripheral respiratory systems of various classes of vertebrates in general and of fishes and mammals in particular have been described. In spite of the dissimilarity in gas exchange and pumping systems, there appears to be a striking resemblance in the neural control mechanisms for respiration. Even sensory vagal signals, which in mammals originate from stretch receptors and nociceptors in the lungs and in fishes from receptors in the completely different system of gill arches and filaments, have comparable central roles. Against this background it is tempting to speculate that during the evolution from water to air breathing, from fishes up to mammals, the major conversions occurred in the gas-exchange organs (gills to lungs) and the medium pumps (cranial pump, powered by cranial muscles to rib cage, powered by intercostal and diaphragmatic muscles) while the central control circuits and sensory routes to the respiratory apparatus remained basically the same. Possible support for such a hypothesis could undoubtedly be gained from knowledge of the respiratory centres of amphibians and reptiles. Unfortunately, however, such data are hardly available at all.

One observation could argue strongly against a continuity in the evolution of central nervous control systems for respiration from fishes to mammals. This is that amphibians seem to breathe in quite a different way. Whereas fishes and mammals normally ventilate their respiratory organs with a continuous rhythm, amphibians (just like lungfishes) possess arrhythmic ventilation. At long intervals their respiratory cavities are filled with air and then closed, after which respiration stops until the air is spent and has to be renewed. At first sight it looks as if there will be very few properties in common between systems that generate and control continuously rhythmic respiratory movements and systems that generate isolated, single breaths. Closer inspection of the various respiration patterns of animals belonging to the teleostean, amphibian, reptilian and mammalian groups, however, shows that the distinction between rhythmic and arrhythmic ventilation is not strict at all, as will be explained below.

Several species of fish (shark, marlin, tuna, blue bass, mackerel, herring, etc.), when swimming fast, employ so-called ram ventilation. They then stop making rhythmic respiratory movements and swim with the mouth open to irrigate their gills (Fig. 1.8). Switching over from normal to ram ventilation depends on swimming speed in a gradual manner. At a critical velocity

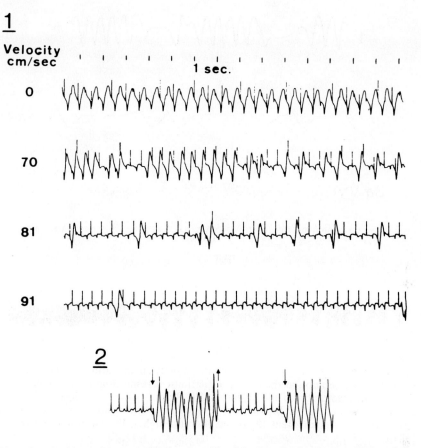

Fig. 1.8. Active and ram ventilation in a bluefish. Respiration is recorded as slow-wave EMG potentials with superimposed ECG spikes. The fishes were held in a respirometer and made to swim against a water current, generated by a pump, which imposed the swimming speed. **(1)** The transition from normal respiration to ram ventilation as a result of increasing swimming speed. At higher velocities the number of active respiratory cycles drops progressively. **(2)** Switching on and off ram ventilation by valving the water pump (at the arrows) from above to below the critical water speed and vice versa. (From Roberts, 1975.)

respiratory cycles begin to drop out, and, with increasing swimming speed, pauses get longer and bursts of rhythmic respiration shorter until finally they disappear completely (Brown & Muir, 1970; Roberts, 1975; Ballintijn & Roberts, 1976; Steffensen, 1985). Energetically it appears to be advantageous to displace the work of breathing from the respiratory muscles to the large locomotory muscles. In addition the drag characteristics are improved as well, so that a rainbow trout, for instance, saves more than 10% of potential energy expensive on ventilation and locomotion (Steffensen, 1985).

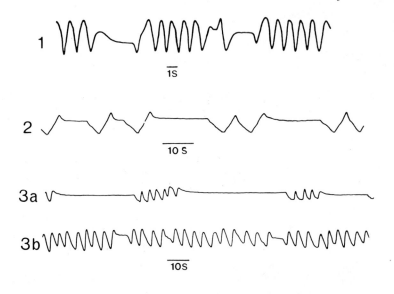

1

$\overline{1s}$

2

$\overline{10\ S}$

3a

3b

$\overline{10S}$

4

$\overline{1m}$

Fig. 1.9. Intermittent (periodic or bout) respiration in various vertebrates. **(1)** Intermittent respiration in the carp. **(2)** Intermittent respiration in the caiman. **(3a)** Intermittent respiration in the alligator. **(3b)** Respiration of an alligator during a period of excitement. **(4)** Intermittent respiration changing to normal continuous respiration in a human infant. (**2, 3a** and **3b** from Hughes, 1973; **4** from Prechtl *et al.*, 1979.)

Some fishes, such as the carp, display intermittent respiration under favourable respiratory conditions: when they are quiet and in oxygen-rich water. It is a regular pattern of a few respiratory cycles alternating with pauses of a duration of several respirations (Fig. 1.9(1)) (Jüch & Ballintijn, 1983; Ballintijn, 1985a). Apparently here also, energy is saved. The power consumption of shallow, continuously rhythmic respiration is higher than that of intermittent, medium-intensity respiration because muscle contraction efficiency is minimal under moderate load conditions.

Many reptiles, such as the crocodile and the turtle, can breathe with a more or less regular, continuous rhythm. During low oxygen consumption combined with good oxygen availability, however, they also switch over to intermittent ventilation (Fig. 1.9(2, 3a, 3b)) (Hughes, 1973). In the turtle, T. Vitalis and W. Milsom (unpublished observation) have shown that this also results in optimalisation of the work of breathing.

Although not common in higher vertebrates (except when breath-holding

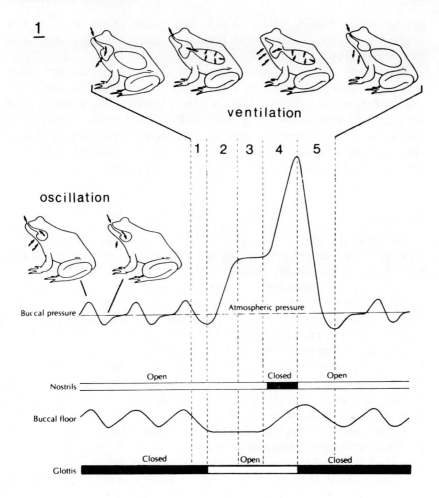

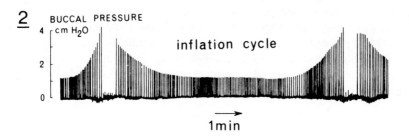

Fig. 1.10. Respiration in the frog. **(1)** Buccal movements and pressures together with opening and closing of the naral and glottal valves are shown during a ventilation cycle and oscillation cycles. **(2)** Respiratory pattern and buccal pressure during an inflation cycle. (From Gans, 1974.)

during diving), human infants in their first period of life alternate long
periods of normal ventilation with periods of clear intermittent ventilation
(Fig. 1.9(4)) (Prechtl *et al.*, 1979).

Amphibians cannot be regarded as pure intermittent breathers either.
Admittedly their lungs are filled with air at intervals. However, during so-
called inflation cycles (Gans, 1974) the bouts of respirations between pauses
are fairly rhythmic in nature (Fig. 1.10(2)). In addition to that, the air in the
buccal cavity is continuously renewed in a rhythmic fashion (oscillation
cycles) during the periods of gas exchange, when air is trapped in the lungs
(Fig. 1.10(1)) (de Jongh & Gans, 1969; Gans *et al.*, 1969).

### 1.5. Conclusion

Summarising the observations presented above, it appears that in lower,
water-breathing vertebrates such as fishes the central nervous respiratory
control system can already generate both continuous rhythmic respiration
and intermittent respiration. In amphibians (and lungfishes) arrhythmic,
intermittent respiration has been developed to a large extent. However, their
system is certainly not exclusively arrhythmic because there are definite
rhythmic components, as shown for the frog. The dominance of intermittent
respiration in these animal groups is probably related to the following two
factors. Lungfishes have to stop aerial respiration during periods of submersion. For frogs, on the other hand, filling the lungs at long intervals may well
be more economic in view of the high energy consumption of positive-
pressure buccal-pulse pumping and the severe non-elastic losses that occur.
In reptiles both the rhythmic and the arrhythmic form of breathing are
practised, and even in mammals intermittent respiration can occur. Thus, in
view of all these observations, the conclusion seems justified that the early
teleostean central nervous mechanisms for control of respiration already
incorporated both options: that of rhythmic and that of intermittent
respiration. During the evolution of vertebrates and the adaptive changes
that accompanied the changeover from aquatic to aerial respiration, various
animals have employed these options in different proportions. However,
both are still present in man. It therefore appears that, although respiratory
pumping and gas-exchange organs have been drastically altered in the course
of evolution, the principles of central nervous control of respiration have
remained basically the same.

### References

Baconnier, P., Benchetrit, G., Demongeot, J. & Pham Dinh, T. (1983). Entrainment
of the respiratory rhythm. I Experiment and physiological model. II Mathematical
models. In *Modelling and Control of Breathing* (eds B. J. Whipp & D. M. Wiberg).
Amsterdam: Elsevier.

Baker, T. L. Netick, A. & Dement, W. C. (1981). Sleep-related apneic and apneustic breathing following pneumotaxic lesion and vagotomy. *Resp. Physiol.* **46**, 271–94.

Ballintijn, C. M. (1969a). Functional anatomy and movement coordination of the respiratory pump of the carp (*Cyprinus carpio* L.). *J. Exp. Biol.* **50**, 547–67.

Ballintijn, C. M. (1969b). Muscle coordination of the respiratory pump of the carp (*Cyprinus carpio* L.). *J. Exp. Biol.* **50**, 569–91.

Ballintijn, C. M. (1969c). Movement pattern and efficiency of the respiratory pump of the carp (*Cyprinus carpio* L.). *J. Exp. Biol.* **50**, 593–613.

Ballintijn, C. M. (1982). Neural control of respiration in fishes and mammals. In *Exogenous and Endogenous Influences on Metabolic and Neural Control*, pp. 137–40 (eds A. D. F. Addink & N. Spronk). Oxford: Pergamon Press.

Ballintijn, C. M. (1985a). Neural representation of a behavioral pattern: respiration. *Neth. J. Zool.* **35**, 186–208.

Ballintijn, C. M. (1985b). The respiratory function of gill filament muscles in the carp. *Resp. Physiol.* **60**, 59–74.

Ballintijn, C. M. & Hughes, G. M. (1965). The muscular basis of the respiratory pumps in the trout. *J. Exp. Biol.* **43**, 349–62.

Ballintijn, C. M. & Jüch, P. J. W. (1984). Interaction of respiration with coughing, feeding, vision and oculomotor control in fish. In *Brainstem Organization of Interacting Behavioral Systems* (ed. J. A. W. M. Weijnen). *Brain, Behav. Evol.* **25**, 99–108.

Ballintijn, C. M., Luiten, P. G. M. & Jüch, P. J. W. (1979). Respiratory neuron activity in mesencephalon, diencephalon and cerebellum of the carp. *J. Comp. Physiol.* **133**, 131–9.

Ballintijn, C. M. & Punt, G. J. (1985). The role of gill arch movements and the function of the dorsal gill arch muscles in the carp. *Resp. Physiol.* **60**, 39–57.

Ballintijn, C. M. & Roberts, J. L. (1976). Neural control and proprioceptive load matching in reflex respiratory movements of fishes. *Fed. Proc.* 1983–91.

Ballintijn, C. M., Roberts, B. L. & Luiten, P. G. M. (1983). Respiratory responses to stimulation of branchial vagus nerve ganglia of a teleost fish. *Resp. Physiol.* **51**, 241–57.

Bamford, O. S. (1974). Respiratory neurons in the rainbow trout. *Comp. Biochem. Physiol.* **48**, 77–83.

Bassal, M. & Bianchi, A. L. (1982). Inspiratory onset or termination induced by electrical stimulation of the brain. *Resp. Physiol.* **50**, 23–40.

Baumgarten, R. von & Salmoiraghi, G. C. (1962). Respiratory neurones in the goldfish. *Arch. Ital. Biol.* **100**, 31–47.

Bertrand, F. & Hugelin, A. (1971). Respiratory synchronising function of nucleus parabrachialis medialis: pneumotaxic mechanisms. *J. Neurophysiol.* **34**, 189–207.

Brown, C. E. & Muir, B. S. (1970). Analysis of ram ventilation of fish gills with application to skipjack tuna (*Katsuwonus pelamis*). *J. Fish. Res. Bd Can.* **27**, 1637–52.

Caille, D., Vibert, J. F. & Hugelin, A. (1981). Apneusis and apnea after parabrachial or Kölliker–Fuse n. lesion; influence of wakefulness. *Resp. Physiol.* **45**, 79–95.

Cohen, M. I. (1971). Switching of the respiratory phases and evoked phrenic responses produced by rostral pontine electrical stimulation. *J. Physiol.* **217**, 133–58.

Cohen, M. I. (1974). The genesis of respiratory rhythmicity. In *Central-Rhythmic and Regulation* (eds W. Umbach & H. P. Koepchen). Stuttgart: Hippokrates Verlag.

Cohen, M. I. (1981). Central determinants of respiratory rhythm. *Ann. Rev. Physiol.* **43**, 91–104.

Cohen, M. I. & Feldman, J. L. (1977). Models of respiratory phase switching. *Fed. Proc.* **36**, 2367–74.

D'Angelo, E. (1979). Mechanisms controlling inspiration studied by electrical vagal stimulations in rabbits. *Resp. Physiol.* **38**, 185–202.

de Graaf, P. J. F. & Ballintijn, C. M. (1987). Mechanoreceptor activity in the gills of the carp. II. Gill arch proprioceptors. *Resp. Physiol.* in press.

de Graaf, P. J. F., Ballintijn, C. M. & Maes, F. W. (1987). Mechanoreceptor activity in the gills of the carp. I. Gill filament and gill raker mechanoreceptors. *Resp. Physiol.* in press.

De Jongh, H. J. & Gans, C. (1969). On the mechanism of respiration in the bullfrog, *Rana catesbeiana*: a reassessment. *J. Morin.* **127**, 259-90.

Feldman, J. L., Cohen, M. I. & Wolotsky, P. (1976). Powerful inhibition of pontine respiratory neurons by pulmonary afferent activity. *Brain Res.* **104**, 341–6.

Feldman, J. L. & Gautier, H. (1976). Interaction of pulmonary afferents and pneumotaxic centre in the control of respiratory pattern in cats. *J. Neurophysiol.* **39**, 31–44.

Gans, C. (1970a). Strategy and sequence in the evolution of the external gas exchangers of ectothermal vertebrates. *Forma et functio* **3**, 61–104.

Gans, C. (1970b). Respiration in early tetrapods–the frog is a red herring. *Evolution* **24**, 723–34.

Gans, C. (1974). *Biomechanics*. Philadelphia, PA: Lippincott.

Gans, C., de Jongh, H. J. & Farber, J. (1969). Bullfrog (*Rana catesbeiana*) ventilation. How does the frog breathe? *Science* **163**, 1223–5.

Gaunt, A. S. & Gans, C. (1969). Mechanics of respiration in the snapping turtle (*Chelidra serpentina*). *J. Morph.* **128**, 195–228.

Gans, C. & Hughes, G. M. (1967). The mechanism of lung ventilation in the tortoise (*Testudo graeca* L.). *J. Exp. Biol.* **47**, 1–20.

Gauthier, P., Monteau, R. & Dussardier, M. (1983). Inspiratory on-switch evoked by stimulation of mesencephalic structures: a patterned response. *Exp. Brain Res.* **51**, 261–70.

Holeton, G. F. & Jones, D. R. (1975). Water flow dynamics in the respiratory tract of the carp. *J. Exp. Biol.* **63**,.537–49.

Hugelin, A. (1977). Anatomical organization of bulbopontine respiratory oscillators. *Fed. Proc.* **36**, 2390–449.

Hugelin, A. (1980). Does the respiratory rhythm originate from a reticular oscillator in the waking state? In *The Reticular Formation Revisited* (eds). J. A. Hobson & M. A. B. Brazier New York: Raven Press.

Hughes, G. M. (1973). Comparative vertebrate ventilation and heterogeneity. In *Comparative Physiology*, pp. 188–220 (eds L. Bolis, K. Schmidt-Nielsen & S. H. P. Maddrell). Amsterdam: North-Holland.

Hughes, G. M. (1975). Coughing in the rainbow trout and the effect of pollutants. *Revue Suisse Zool.* **82**, 47–64.

Hughes, G. M. & Ballintijn, C. M. (1965). The muscular basis of the respiratory pumps in the dogfish (*Sciliorhinus canicula*). *J. Exp. Biol.* **43**, 363–83.

Hughes, G. M. & Gans, C. (1965). Electromyographic analysis of respiratory movements in *Testudo graeca*. *Am. Zool.* **6**, 272–3.

Iscoe, S., Feldman, J. L. & Cohen, M. I. (1979). Properties of inspiratory termination by superlaryngeal and vagal stimulation. *Resp. Physiol.* **36**, 353–66.

Jüch, P. J. W. & Ballintijn, C. M. (1983). Tegmental neurons controlling medullary respiratory centre neuron activity in the carp. *Resp. Physiol.* **51**, 95–107.

Jüch, P. J. W. & Luiten, P. G. M. (1981). Anatomy of respiratory rhythmic systems in brainstem and cerebellum of the carp. *Brain Res.* **230**, 51–64.

Knox, C. K. & King, G. W. (1976). Changes in the Hering–Breuer reflexes following rostral pontine lesion. *Resp. Physiol.* **28**, 189–206.

Liem, K. F. (1980). Air ventilation in advanced teleosts: biomechanical and evolutionary aspects. In *Environmental Physiology of Fishes*, pp. 57–91. (ed. M. A. Ali) New York: Plenum.

McMahon, B. R. (1969). A functional analysis of the aquatic and aerial respiratory movements of an African lungfish, *Protopterus aethiopicus*, with reference to the evolution of the lung ventilation mechanism in vertebrates. *J. Exp. Biol.* **51**, 407–30.

Osse, J. W. M. (1969). Functional morphology of the head of the perch: an electromyographic study. *Neth. J. Zool.* **19**, 289–392.

Poole, C. A. & Satchell, G. H. (1979). Nociceptors in the gills of the dogfish, *J. Comp. Physiol.* **130**, 1–7.

Prechtl, H. F. R., O'Brien, M. J. & van Eykern, L. A. (1979). Neonatal breathing in different states of sleep and wakefulness. In *Central Nervous Control Mechanisms in Breathing*, pp. 443–55 (eds C. von Euler & H. Lagercrantz). Oxford: Pergamon Press.

Richter, D. W. (1982). Generation and maintenance of the respiratory rhythm. *J. Exp. Biol.* **100**, 93–107.

Roberts, J. L. (1975). Active branchial and ram gill ventilation in fishes. *Biol. Bull.* **148**, 85–105.

Satchell, G. H. (1959). Respiratory reflexes in the dogfish. *J. Exp. Biol.* **36**, 62–71.

Shelton, G. (1959). The respiratory centre in the tench (*Tinca tinca* L.). I. The effects of brain transection on respiration. *J. Exp. Biol.* **36**, 191–202.

Shelton, G. (1961). The respiratory centre in the tench (*Tinca tinca* L.). II. Respiratory neuronal activity in the medulla oblongata. *J. Exp. Biol.* **38**, 79–92.

Steffensen, J. F. (1985). The transition between branchial pumping and RAM ventilation in fishes: energetic consequences and dependence on water oxygen tension. *J. Exp. Biol.* **114**, 141–50.

St. John, W. M., Glasser, R. L. & King, R. A. (1972). Rhythmic respiration in awake, vagotomised cats with chronic pneumotaxic area lesions. *Resp. Physiol.* **15**, 233–44.

Sutterlin, A. M. & Saunders, R. L. (1969). Proprioceptors in the gills of teleosts. *Can. J. Zool.* **47**, 1209–12.

Trenchard, D. (1977). Role of pulmonary stretch receptors during breathing in rabbits, cats and dogs. *Resp. Physiol.* **29**, 231–46.

Vibert, J. F., Caille, D. & Segundo, J. P. (1981). Respiratory oscillator entrainment by periodic vagal afferents: an experimental test of a model. *Biol. Cybern.* **41**, 119–30.

Villard, M. F., Caille, D. & Hugelin, A. (1984). Dissociation between respiratory phase switching and phasic phrenic response on low-intensity stimulation of pneumotaxic complex and nearby structures. *J. Physiol. Paris* **79**, 11–16.

Waldron, I. (1972). Spatial organization of respiratory neurones in the medulla of tench and goldfish. *J. Exp. Biol.* **57**, 449–59.

# 2

# Experimental studies in fetal breathing

**O. S. Bamford**

*Nuffield Institute for Medical Research, Headley Way, Headington, Oxford OX3 9DS, UK*

## 2.1. Introduction

Fetal breathing was clearly demonstrated in man nearly a hundred years ago (Ahlfeld, 1888), and observations in the early part of this century on the acutely exteriorised uterus showed that fetal rabbits also appeared to breathe *in utero*. Breathing was depressed by anaesthesia and hypoxia, and increased in hypercapnia (Rosenfeld & Snyder, 1936). Subsequently Bonar *et al.* (1938) reviewed their experimental work on rabbits, dogs and rats, and came to similar conclusions. However, Barcroft *et al.* (1936) were unable to show spontaneous breathing in fetal lambs, and Becker *et al.* (1964) obtained inconclusive results from fetal rats. Faced with the apparent failure of direct observation, many workers turned to indirect methods using contrast medium or other tracers in the amniotic fluid, though with no more conclusive results (see Wilds, 1978, for review). Although these studies mostly demonstrated that amniotic fluid could reach the lungs, they were unable to show whether this normally took place. By the end of the 1960s, Barcroft's view that fetal breathing did not occur spontaneously in the near-term fetus was generally accepted. However, Dawes *et al.* (1970) and Merlet *et al.* (1970) independently developed chronic *in utero* fetal lamb preparations and were able to demonstrate spontaneous breathing in the unanaesthetised fetus. A later report (Dawes *et al.*, 1972) described the phenomenon in detail, and since that time the occurrence of fetal breathing has been widely accepted (Fig. 2.1). Most of the work described below was on the fetal lamb, and there may be important species differences, but what little is known of other species suggests that the fetal lamb is representative.

Published descriptions of fetal breathing are consistent, and well reviewed by Jansen & Chernick (1983), Maloney (1983) and Dawes (1984). In normal conditions breathing movements are irregular in both rate and depth (Dawes *et al.*, 1982) and are driven mainly by the diaphragm so that the ribs move inwards during inspiration (Poore & Walker, 1980). Each diaphragm

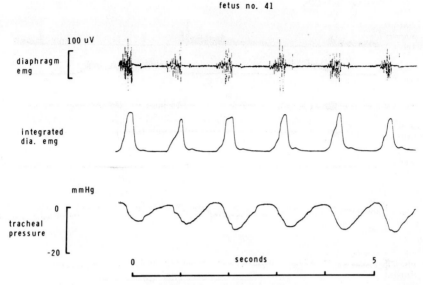

Fig. 2.1. Breathing in an intact fetal lamb near term. The upper two traces show the diaphragm emg after high-pass filtering at 30 Hz (top trace) and after processing by a leaky integrator with a 30-ms time constant (middle trace). The lower trace shows fetal tracheal pressure with respect to amniotic pressure. Variability in amplitude, breath-to-breath interval and inspiratory times and slopes is apparent even in the few seconds of recording shown here.

contraction is accompanied by a fall in tracheal pressure from a slightly positive value to up to 10 mmHg negative (Fewell & Johnson, 1983), and a small but measurable influx of fluid (Boddy *et al.*, 1974). However, the fluid originates in the lungs which secrete continuously (Kitterman *et al.*, 1979a); this is why earlier workers often failed to find amniotic fluid markers in the lungs. It is probable that amniotic fluid enters the trachea only during asphyxic gasps or powerful uterine contractions. Breathing movements in the fetal lamb are at first sporadic but later become almost continuous; after about 0.8 of term, breathing movements become organised into episodes 10–30 min long, separated by apnoeic periods of about the same duration (Fig. 2.2). The appearance of this episodic pattern is associated with the development of high-voltage slow-wave electrocortical activity (ECoG). After a few days a clear pattern of alternating low-voltage and high-voltage ECoG emerges, with only a small proportion of the time being spent in a transitional state. Breathing occurs only in low-voltage (LVECoG), and terminates abruptly on the onset of HVECoG (Dawes *et al.*, 1970). This pattern persists for the last three weeks of fetal life, though the incidence of breathing falls immediately before birth.

A number of factors are known to affect the incidence, rate and depth of

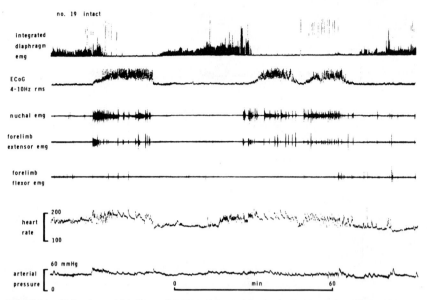

no. 19 intact

integrated
diaphragm
emg

ECoG
4-10Hz rms

nuchal emg

forelimb
extensor emg

forelimb
flexor emg

heart
rate

200

100

arterial
pressure

60 mmHg

0

0　　　　　　min　　　　　　60

Fig. 2.2.　Episodes of high- and low-voltage electrocortical activity (ECoG) in an intact fetal lamb near term. Traces show: integrated diaphragm emg (see legend to Fig. 2.1 for derivation of this signal); amplitude of the low-frequency components of ECoG; filtered emg activity in three skeletal muscles; fetal heart rate and arterial pressure. In high-voltage ECoG, the amplitude of the low-frequency components increases, and there is increased activity in nuchal and forelimb extensor muscles. Heart rate and arterial pressure may also increase. Breathing is confined to periods of low-voltage ECoG.

fetal breathing. As in adults, a rise in arterial $PCO_2$ increases rate and depth (Dawes *et al.*, 1980, 1982), and there is also an increase in incidence, though breathing is still confined to LVECoG. Fetal $P_aCO_2$ is normally in the range 40–45 mmHg. At high fetal $P_aCO_2$ (more than 50 mmHg) breathing takes up almost the whole of a low-voltage episode, while at $P_aCO_2$ below 35 mmHg breathing is rare. The amplitude and frequency of breathing are also increased in hypercapnia, and breathing becomes more regular and involves the intercostal muscles (Dawes *et al.*, 1980, 1982) and laryngeal abductors (Fewell & Johnson, 1983). Thus some aspects of the respiratory response to $CO_2$ resemble that of the adult, and the central control of this response may not change greatly between fetal and postnatal life. In contrast, fetal hypoxaemia causes respiratory arrest (Boddy *et al.*, 1974).

There is some evidence that maternal factors may affect fetal breathing: in the sheep there are regular small uterine contractions and it has been reported that these are associated with arrests of breathing (Nathanielsz *et al.*, 1980) though the effect seems smaller than at first reported (Hofmeyr *et al.*, 1985a). Such uterine contractions reduce uterine blood flow (Harding

& Poore, 1984) and this may explain the effect on fetal activity. Clearly maternal behaviour that alters the composition of the blood (e.g. consuming alcohol or nicotine) is potentially able to affect the fetus. McLeod *et al.* (1983) showed that ethanol decreased the incidence of fetal breathing for up to 3 h. Human fetal breathing is sensitive to maternal blood glucose, and increases after a meal (Natale *et al.*, 1978). This is not true for sheep, though the difference may be due to a difference in energy substrates as the sheep uses fatty acids more than the human, and usually feeds, or at least absorbs, continuously.

## 2.2. Current work on fetal breathing

There are two main areas of research in fetal breathing:

(1) What are its effects on the fetus?
(2) How is it controlled?

### 2.2.1. *Effects on the fetus*

Physiological effects of fetal breathing on lung development have been investigated by cervical cord transection (Wigglesworth & Desai, 1979), by diaphragmatic hernias (De Lorimer *et al.*, 1967), by phrenic nerve section (Alcorn *et al.*, 1980) and by thoracoplasty in which thoracic pressure changes are reduced (Liggins *et al.*, 1981). In all cases lung hypoplasia and dysplasia has been demonstrated, and clearly lung distension is important in normal lung development, though it is unclear whether tonic or phasic distension is important. Tracheostomy also leads to lung hypoplasia, indicating a role for the upper airways in maintaining positive lung fluid pressure (Fewell *et al.*, 1983). Presumably motor activity is also important in the maturation of the neuromuscular pathways needed for breathing, though this idea has not been investigated. Fetal lung development has recently been reviewed by Kitterman (1984) and will not be considered further here. It is likely that fetal breathing also affects cardiovascular, muscular and skeletal development, but no studies have been made.

### 2.2.2. *Control of breathing*

The control of fetal breathing has received extensive study, perhaps because of its clinical significance in neonatal respiratory pathology. Most efforts have been concentrated on the two most obvious differences between fetal and adult respiratory responses: the lack of breathing in HVECoG, and the suppression of breathing by hypoxia.

The HVECoG is dominated by frequencies below 5 Hz, and the overall amplitude near term is about four times that of LVECoG, which has a flat power spectrum. HVECoG is accompanied in the fetus by a reduction in eye movements, an increased incidence of skeletal muscle activity, and a slightly raised arterial pressure and heart rate (Fig. 2.2). There are also minor differences between high- and low-voltage ECoG in blood flow to the gastro intestinal tract and parts of the brain (Jensen *et al.*, 1985). Fetal breathing is absent in this state, which appears to correspond to slow-wave sleep in the adult. HVECoG first appears in the fetal lamb at about 120 days and is organised into distinct episodes by 125 days. After this the pattern remains unchanged to term, though the amplitude increases with gestational age.

Isocapnic hypoxia can be produced experimentally by careful adjustment of the inspired gas mixture. Boddy *et al.* (1974) first showed that in late-gestation fetal lambs, breathing stopped when the $P_aO_2$ fell by about 8 mmHg from its normal 20–22 mmHg, and this has since been confirmed by all investigators. In the intact hypoxic fetus near term, the arterial pressure rises and the heart rate falls at first, though there is a later rise in heart rate to control values.

The lack of breathing in HVECoG and hypoxia could, *a priori*, be due to a lack of sufficient stimulation of the respiratory neurones in these states, or to increased inhibition. The electrocorticogram appears to be a property of the forebrain, and it could therefore be expected that transecting the brainstem, thus separating the forebrain from the respiratory neurones in the pons and medulla, would help to resolve this question. Dawes *et al.* (1983) performed a series of brainstem transections on the brains of fetal lambs at about 120 days, and found that if the section was sufficiently caudal, passing through or slightly rostral to the pons, the incidence of fetal breathing increased until it was almost continuous. The relation between ECoG and breathing was of course lost. The frequency distribution of respiratory intervals and ampli-tudes remained unaltered, so there was no reason to believe that breathing was neurologically different in the brain-transected fetuses; only the control was affected. The effects of hypoxia on these preparations were also studied, and it was found that there was an increase in the amplitude of breathing which continued at $P_aO_2$ levels well below those found to arrest breathing in the intact fetus.

These results led to the conclusion that fetal brething is under a predomi-nantly inhibitory control from some area or areas above the pons, and that the incidence of breathing observed depends partly on activity in those areas. It is possible that the pneumotaxic centre described for the adult is anatomically related to this area which has not yet been identified. Since this observation efforts have been made to locate the inhibitory mechanisms and to identify the neurotransmitters involved. Two approaches have been used. Attempts have been made to interrupt CNS pathways by lesioning either mechanically or using RF current, or in some studies by chemical lesioning with specific neurotoxins. The other approach has been to use neurotrans-mitter agonists and antagonists with central actions to mimic or block endogenous neurotransmission, in an attempt to induce fetal breathing which continues through hypoxia or through high-voltage electrocortical activity.

## 2.3. Lesioning experiments

Surgical intervention in the brain has become more sophisticated since the pioneering transection studies of Dawes *et al.* (1983). Gluckman & Parsons (1984) have recently produced a stereotaxic atlas for the fetal lamb brain which should make further studies of this type easier to standardise, and Johnston *et al.* (1985) have described hypothalamic lesions that allow breathing during hypoxia. At present there appears to be a contradiction between their results and those of Dawes *et al.* (1983), who reported that brainstem transection at the level of the hypothalamus did not affect the hypoxic arrest of breathing. Walker *et al.* (1985) have recently reported that selective pituitary destruction had only minor effects on fetal breathing. Publication of more detailed descriptions of the lesions may clarify this point. Selective lesioning in this laboratory without the benefit of stereotaxic technique has shown that the ventrolateral rostral pons appears to be important for respiratory inhibition during both HVECoG and hypoxia. These lesions are not at present sufficiently well defined for precise identification of the structures damaged, though this region includes the substantia nigra, which is particularly rich in dopaminergic neurones: recent findings on dopaminergic pathways will be discussed below. One important finding is that the inhibitions occurring during HVECoG and during hypoxia can be separated by lesions, and it is possible to produce a fetal lamb which breathes in HVECoG but whose breathing is suppressed by hypoxia. There must therefore be two anatomically distinct pathways involved in the suppression of breathing by hypoxia or by high-voltage activity. The breathing that occurs during HVECoG after such lesions is often of a different pattern from that normally seen (Fig. 2.3). The significance of this will be discussed later.

## 2.4. Drug experiments

Although some promising lines of enquiry have appeared as a result of lesioning experiments, the results to date tell us little about the mechanism of respiratory inhibition. Experiments with drugs have produced equally interesting data but have not yet identified which neurotransmitters are involved.

The obvious first step has been to mimic or block common neurotransmitters and to observe the effect on breathing. This approach has been tried for serotonin and adrenergic agents, muscarinic cholinergic agents, GABA, and most recently dopamine.

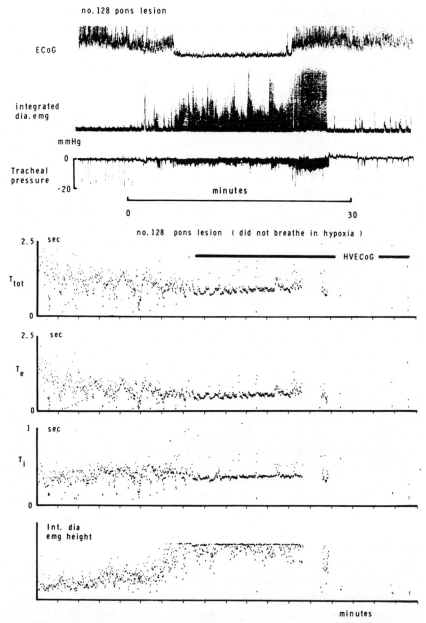

Fig. 2.3. (i) Electrocortical activity and breathing in a fetal lamb with bilateral pontine lesions. Breathing occurs occasionally in high-voltage ECoG episodes, and this breathing is more regular and of higher amplitude than normal. (ii) Computer analysis of part of the diaphragm emg signal above. Note the expanded time scale. Each point represents a measurement made from a single breath. Plots show breath–breath interval, expiratory time, inspiratory time and peak height of the integrated diaphragm emg.

(a) *Serotonin*.  The interest in serotonin arises from the possible role of serotinergic raphe neurones in the genesis of sleep states (Yamasaki & Lico, 1981), together with more recent findings implicating it in central control of ventilation (Millhorn *et al.*, 1980, 1983; McCrimmon & Lalley, 1982). All this work is on adults, and evidence for its effects on the fetus is limited. Serotonin does not cross the blood–brain barrier, but 5-hydroxytryptophan (5HTP), a serotonin precursor, does so readily, and can be converted to serotonin centrally. Quilligan *et al.* (1981) infused 5HTP into fetal lambs and reported sustained HVECoG and prolonged intense regular breathing. This could be interpreted as showing a serotonin-induced slow-wave sleep together with a stimulation of breathing by a central mechanism normally masked by another inhibitory control. However, the doses of 5HTP needed to produce such responses are very high, typically 100–150 mg, and the effects may not be primary or central. 5HT causes constriction of the umbilical vessels (McGrath & Stuart-Smith, 1982), and 5HTP infusions are often followed by a fall in $P_aO_2$ to as low as 12–15 mmHg (O. S. Bamford, G. I. Dawes & R. A. Ward, unpublished observations). Recently the centrally acting serotonin agonist 5MDMT has been shown to stimulate breathing and to induce a period of HVECoG. These effects occur in intact and brainstem-transected fetal lambs, but the breathing response is more intense and lasts longer after transection (Ward *et al.*, in preparation). These observations support the concept of separate central serotonergic pathways that stimulate fetal breathing and induce HVECoG, but tell us little about active inhibitory mechanisms. Until recently the only centrally acting 5HT antagonist generally available has been methysergide, a drug with some non-specific antagonist and agonist properties. Pilot studies in this laboratory with methysergide have shown prolonged HVECoG and hypertension with hypoxaemia but no consistent effects on fetal breathing.

Attempts have also been made to lesion fetal serotonergic neurones chemically. Johnston *et al.* (1984) gave parachlorophenylalanine (PCPA) systemically to fetal lambs. PCPA causes long-term depletion of serotonin in adults by inhibiting tryptophan hydroxylase and so blocking synthesis. They found their injections had acute effects but were unable to detect any long-term changes in fetal breathing, and 5HT assay of brain regions showed no significant changes from control animals. More recently another attempt using the irreversible neurotoxin 5,7-dihydroxytryptamine given via the cisterna magna also failed to produce detectable changes in either brain serotonin concentrations or fetal breathing (A. W. Quail, unpublished observations). It may be that the fetal brain is resistant to this type of damage, or is sufficiently plastic to recover after damage that would be permanent postnatally; in either case, the technique does not appear very promising.

(b) *Acetylcholine*.  Acetylcholine does not cross the blood–brain barrier readily, and so cannot be given systemically to study central effects. Two tools have been used for studying central cholinergic effects on fetal breathing. The muscarinic antagonists atropine and hyoscine and the cholinesterase inhibitor physostigmine (eserine) have been given systemically.

Van der Wildt (1982) first reported that atropine sulphate given intra-arterially to fetal lambs induced prolonged HVECoG but did not appear to affect breathing, which continued episodically. This work was repeated and extended by Bamford *et al.* (1984), who analysed the post-atropine HVECoG and breathing in detail and concluded that the patterns of both were indistinguishable from normal. The effect was shown to be central by the lack of effect of atropine methyl nitrate, which does not cross the blood–brain barrier. They concluded that HVECoG does not cause apnoea, but that both phenomena have a common cause. It can also be concluded that there are no significant central muscarinic effects on fetal breathing, which was unaffected by either atropine or the pharmacologically similar hyoscine.

The mode or site of action of atropine or fetal electrocortical activity is not known. Scremin *et al.* (1983) demonstrated a cholinergic cerebral vasodilatation which could be elicited independently of cerebral metabolic changes. If atropine blocked tonic vasodilator activity, it would cause a reduction in cerebral blood flow. Milligan (1979) reported that total cerebral blood flow in newborn babies was lower in slow-wave sleep than in REM sleep. It therefore seemed possible that an atropine-induced fall in blood flow might be responsible for the observed HVECoG, but evidence against this proposal is provided by the study of Jensen *et al.* (1985) who showed that cortical blood flow, as distinct from total cerebral flow, changed very little between LVECoG and HVECoG in the fetal lamb. The effect of atropine on ECoG is therefore probably direct and not mediated by circulatory changes.

It is unfortunate that the action of nicotinic blocking agents cannot be so easily investigated. Few cross the blood–brain barrier and in any case they would block the neuromuscular junctions of the diaphragm, so no response would be seen. It would be possible to give such drugs by cerebroventricular perfusion, or to record respiratory motor output from the phrenic nerves instead of the diaphragm, but these techniques have not yet been applied to this problem. However, some information can be gained by increasing acetylcholine levels using a cholinesterase inhibitor such as physostigmine. This has both central and peripheral effects at all types of cholinergic synapse, but in small doses (100 μg, i.a.) peripheral effects seem to be minor. The effect of physostigmine given in HVECoG is an immediate shift to LVECoG and (usually) an onset of breathing at high amplitude for a few minutes (Bamford *et al.*, in preparation). Responses to both atropine and physostigmine have been studied after brainstem transection. The effects of atropine on ECoG, and of physostigmine on ECoG and breathing, are still present following brainstem transection (Bamford *et al.*, in preparation). These observations suggest that these actions of acetylcholine take place at two sites, a nicotinic site in the brainstem affecting breathing, and a muscarinic suprapontine site affecting electrocortical activity. Neither site can be identified at present, though the medulla may be the site of action for the effect on breathing. Haxhiu *et al.* (1984) showed that cholinergic agonists, applied to the ventral medulla of cats in the area reported by Mitchell *et al.* (1963) to show respiratory chemosensitivity, caused an increase in amplitude of phrenic and hypoglossal motor activity, and Metz (1966) showed that the release of acetylcholine by the medulla of anaesthetised dogs was increased in hypercapnia and hypoxia, and was greatest in the areas with respiratory sensitivity to $CO_2$. There is therefore some evidence to link acetylcholine with the stimulation of breathing in hypercapnia, suggesting that the observed effects of physostigmine could work by the same mechanism. However, Haxhiu *et al.* (1984) also found that their effects of acetylcholine on breathing were blocked by atropine, suggesting they were muscarinic. Atropine does not affect fetal breathing, and it seems likely therefore that the nicotinic effects of physostigmine on the fetus are unrelated to the central chemoreceptors. The location of the sites of action of physostigmine in the fetus will have to await more specific drugs and better methods of administration.

(c) *Noradrenaline.* Catecholamines cross the blood–brain barrier only slowly and have powerful cardiovascular effects via peripheral α- and β-adrenergic receptors, so they are not ideal agonists for systemic administration. Murata *et al.* (1981), working on fetal monkeys, gave infusions of noradrenaline, which is mainly an α-agonist, isoproterenol (mainly a β-agonist) and adrenaline (a mixed α- and β-agonist) and reported that noradrenaline decreased and isoproterenol increased the incidence of fetal breathing, while adrenaline had no overall effect. They were understandably cautious in interpreting these results, which appear to demonstrate α-adrenergic inhibition and β-adrenergic excitation of breathing. ECoG activity was not recorded, so it is not clear how far these changes in incidence of breathing reflect changes in ECoG pattern, nor is it known whether the drugs were affecting primarily peripheral or central sites. Jones & Ritchie (1978) reported a significant increase in the incidence of breathing in fetal lambs after adrenaline infusion, but none after noradrenaline, or adrenaline plus the α-antagonist phentolamine or the β-antagonist propranolol.

Recently, actions of the presynaptic $α_2$-adrenergic agonist clonidine and the $α_2$ antagonist idazoxan have been investigated in this laboratory (Bamford *et al.*, 1986b). Both these drugs cross the blood–brain barrier readily. In intact animals, clonidine (10–20 μg, i.a.) given in LVECoG was followed within a few seconds by an episode of HVECoG, a cessation of breathing and other skeletal muscle activity, and a loss of heart-rate variability (Fig. 2.4). Idazoxan (100 μg, i.a.) reversed the effects of clonidine. When given alone, idazoxan injections were followed by an episode of LVECoG, and breathing and skeletal muscle activity started. Since the

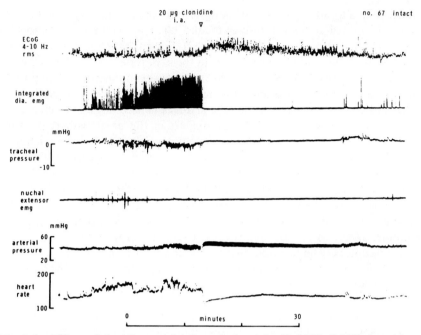

Fig. 2.4. Effects of clonidine on electrocortical activity (4–10 Hz RMS), breathing, nuchal extensor activity,arterial pressure and heart rate in an intact fetus. Note the absence of skeletal muscle activity during the clonidine-induced high-voltage ECoG (cf. Fig. 2.2) and the loss of variability in heart rate and arterial pressure.

normal association of ECoG and breathing was still present, it was not clear from these results alone whether $\alpha_2$-adrenergic effects on fetal breathing were mediated directly or via effects of ECoG. In an attempt to clarify this, the experiments were repeated on fetuses after brainstem transection. The effects of clonidine and idazoxan on breathing and ECoG were still present, so it appears that the effects on ECoG and breathing are independent. Clonidine is believed to reduce the release of noradrenaline at nerve terminals, and idazoxan to increase it, so these results appear to conflict with those of Murata *et al.* (1981) who reported a decrease in incidence of fetal breathing during noradrenaline infusion. However, the two studies are not strictly comparable, and it is possible that their infused catecholamines did not cross the blood–brain barrier and hence had no direct effect.

An unexpected finding from the clonidine injections was a long-term disruption of electrocortical activity cycling. Normally ECoG cycles regularly between distinct high- and low-voltage states, but after 10–20 µg of clonidine the regular cycling was replaced by erratic, rapidly changing activity with a high proportion of intermediate voltage. This type of activity continued for 2–3 h before regular cycling resumed, and far outlasted the initial episode of HVECoG which followed clonidine injection. The significance of the long-term disruption is not known, but the immediate production of HVECoG is consistent with the findings of Keanne *et al.* (1976) who showed that noradrenaline release is necessary for low-voltage ECoG in *encephale isole* cats, though Hilakivi (1983) found that clonidine depressed both slow-wave and REM sleep in intact cats. The cycling of fetal ECoG activity is at present poorly understood; these observations may give some insight into its control.

(d) *Dopamine.* Dopamine and the dopamine agonist apomorphine depress ventilation in most adult mammals by an action on the carotid body (Bisgard *et al.*, 1980; Lahiri *et al.*, 1980; Mayock *et al.*, 1983), but there is some evidence for a central effect. Hedner *et al.* (1982) reported increases in breathing rate after central administration of apomorphine in adult rats. Dopamine has powerful vasoconstrictor actions on the fetus, is rapidly metabolised in the circulation and probably crosses the blood–brain barrier slowly if at all, so is not a good agonist for investigating central effects. Apomorphine, a fairly specific dopamine agonist, crosses the blood–brain barrier readily. In a recent study (Bamford *et al.*, 1985), small doses of apomorphine were given as i.a. injections to fetal lambs *in utero* and the effects on breathing and electrocortical activity were monitored. In intact and chemodenervated fetuses, apomorphine (100 µg–1 mg) was almost always followed by an episode of intense breathing lasting anywhere between 1 and 20 min, often accompanied by a burst of skeletal muscle activity lasting 1 or 2 min, and if the injection was given in HVECoG, there was an immediate shift to LVECoG. These effects occurred in hypoxia as well as in normoxia (Fig. 2.5). There were no consistent effects on arterial pressure or heart rate. The effects of apomorphine were blocked by the dopamine antagonist haloperidol.

Apomorphine is a powerful emetic in man, in the doses used in this study. However, it is unlikely that the observed response was a vomiting fit as there were none of the stereotyped characteristics of vomiting, tracheal pressure rarely became positive, and breath time intervals were within the normal range. Thus although the amplitude of the breathing was often high, in other respects it appeared to be normal (Fig. 2.6).

As the fetus was always in low-voltage ECoG just after an injection of apomorphine, it was not clear whether the effect on breathing was direct or secondary to the onset of the low-voltage episode. After pontine brainstem transection (Bamford *et al.*, 1986a) the same dose of apomorphine did not stimulate breathing or skeletal muscle activity, and the effect on electrocortical activity was reduced to below the level of significance. In brainstem-transected fetuses that breathed almost continuously, apomorphine often depressed the amplitude of breathing for up to 10 min. Haloperidol, which had no effect on spontaneous breathing in the intact fetus, produced a

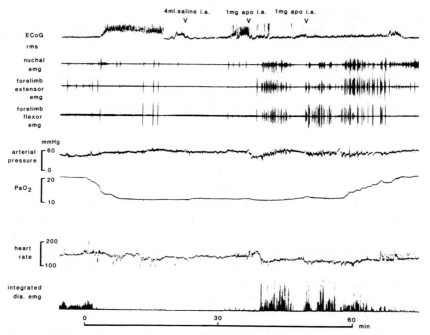

Fig. 2.5. Effects of apomorphine on fetal ECoG, movements and breathing during isocapnic hypoxia induced by making the ewe breathe a hypoxic gas mixture. Traces show the low-frequency power in the ECoG signal; emgs in three skeletal muscles; fetal arterial pressure; fetal arterial $PO_2$ measured by an indwelling electrode in the ascending aorta; fetal heart rate; and integrated diaphragm emg. Apomorphine stimulates movements and breathing, even when they are inhibited by hypoxia.

long-lasting apnoea after brainstem transection, with the incidence of breathing reduced for up to 4 h. These results suggest that there is a central dopaminergic pathway which can stimulate breathing and skeletal muscle activity, and which is located (at least partly) above the level of the pons, but which is not tonically active in the intact fetus under our experimental conditions. Its function is at present unknown, but stimulation of breathing induced by dopamine is strong enough to break through the inhibition of breathing and skeletal muscle activity caused by hypoxia.

The effects of apomorphine and haloperidol after brainstem transection are harder to interpret. Haloperidol reduced the incidence of breathing for several hours. While this could be taken as evidence for a dopaminergic drive to breathe, perhaps released by the transection, apomorphine failed to stimulate, and sometimes depressed, the amplitude of breathing movements. Haloperidol, though most effective at dopaminergic synapses, also has actions on noradrenergic transmission, so it is possible that this effect of haloperidol is unrelated to the dopaminergic pathway discussed above. Clearly there is a need for more study, using a wider range of antagonists.

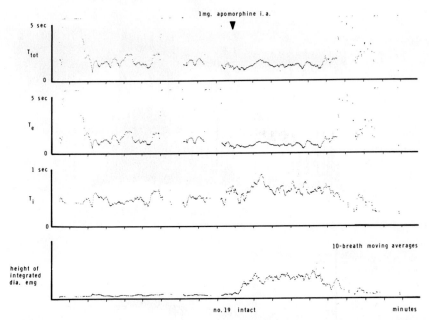

Fig. 2.6. Computer analysis and plots showing changes in the breathing pattern after apomorphine injection. The points were calculated as in Fig. 2.3a, but the plots have been smoothed by plotting each point as a running average of the 10 adjacent points. After apomorphine the height of the integrated diaphragm emg increases but the inspiratory and expiratory times do not alter significantly.

In some fetuses that were breathing continuously, apomorphine reduced the amplitude of breathing for a few minutes. It is possible that this response was the same as that shown in adults and was mediated by a depression of carotid-body chemoreceptor activity. Little is known of the role of the carotid chemoreceptors in fetal breathing, as access is difficult, and the standard experiments such as single breaths of oxygen or nitrogen cannot be done on a fetus *in utero*. However, it is known from acute experiments (Blanco *et al.*, 1984a) that the chemoreceptors discharge slowly at normal fetal blood gas levels, and respond to hypoxia by increasing their discharge rates, so at least the afferent limb of a respiratory chemoreflex exists. The respiratory stimulant doxapram, which is thought to work chiefly via the carotid-body receptors in adults (Mitchell & Herbert, 1975; Nishino *et al.*, 1982), stimulates breathing in fetal lambs, both when intact (Hogg *et al.*, 1977; Piercy *et al.*, 1977) and after brainstem transection. However, the action of doxapram on fetal breathing is still present after carotid-body denervation and bilateral vagotomy (Bamford *et al.*, in preparation) (Fig. 2.7), so it is unlikely to be mediated by any peripheral chemoreceptors and is presumably a central action on the respiratory neurones. Doxapram and

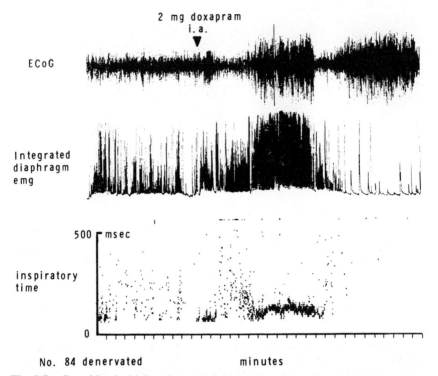

Fig. 2.7. Breathing in high-voltage electrocortical activity after doxapram administration to a chemodenervated fetal lamb with an intact brain. Traces show: unprocessed ECoG; integrated diaphragm emg; and a computer plot of inspiratory time, measured from the diaphragm emg signal. The time scale is common to all three traces. Note the increased amplitude and decreased variability of breathing in high-voltage ECoG.

almitrine both stimulate fetal carotid body chemoreceptors in acute preparations but the effect is not reproducible (M. A. Hanson, personal communication.) At present no reliable test exists for fetal carotid chemosensitivity in the chronic preparation.

(e) *Gamma-amino butyric acid (GABA)*.   Yamada *et al.* (1982) showed that GABA applied to some areas of the ventral medulla in cats reduced tidal volume, heart rate and blood pressure, and that these effects were reversed by the GABA antagonist bicuculline. GABA itself cannot be administered systemically but several drugs are available that interact with GABA receptors. Johnston & Gluckman (1983) used the GABA agonist muscimol and the antagonist picrotoxin, and reported a depression of breathing after muscimol and continuous breathing after picrotoxin. Hypoxia reduced but did not abolish the continuous breathing. Picrotoxin also induced prolonged high-voltage electrocortical activity. These authors concluded that GABA might be involved in the inhibitory control of breathing, though as picrotoxin is not a very specific GABA antagonist the findings do not form conclusive proof. Piercy *et al.* (1977) have shown that diazepam inhibits fetal breathing. The mechanism and site of action are not known, but diazepam is known to form a complex with a GABA receptor and may partly mimic the action of GABA. Thus there is some evidence for an inhibitory effect of GABA on fetal breathing, but it is not clear whether it is physiologically important.

(f) *Other drugs.* The same statement could be made for a number of other drugs whose effects on fetal breathing have been studied. Adenosine depresses fetal breathing and heart rate (Szeto & Umans, 1985) as does methionine–enkephalin (Hofmeyr *et al.*, 1985b). The opiates generally are antagonised by naloxone, which has been shown to have little or no effect on fetal breathing in either normoxia or hypoxia (Adamson *et al.*, 1984), so it is unlikely that opiates are important in controlling fetal breathing under normal conditions. Prostaglandin synthetase inhibitors such as meclofenamate and indomethacin induce continuous breathing, after a delay of several minutes (Kitterman *et al.*, 1979b). This could be interpreted as evidence for a tonic inhibitory control of breathing by endogenous prostaglandins, and $PGE_2$ has been shown to inhibit fetal breathing (Kitterman *et al.*, 1983). It should be remembered that prostaglandin synthetase inhibitors are often toxic and have side effects unrelated to inhibition of central PG synthesis. Among these effects are vasoconstriction, and it is likely that placental blood flow is reduced during these experiments. In our hands the systemic use of mefanemate results in a severe fetal acidosis and hypoxaemia. However, Koos (1982) and Bissonnette *et al.* (1981) gave prostaglandin synthetase inhibitors by intracerebral perfusion through the CSF and repeated these effects, so they are probably centrally mediated, though their mechanism is not known. Koos (1982) also found that pontine brainstem transection did not abolish the effects, so the site of action is presumably in the pons or medulla.

## 2.5. Other aspects of the control of fetal breathing
Most of the work described above is concerned with the relationships between breathing and ECoG, and breathing and $P_aO_2$. There have also been a few studies on the effects of somatic sensory inflow on fetal breathing. Gluckman *et al.* (1983) cooled fetal lambs *in utero* and found that when the skin was cooled, the fetus shivered (as shown by skeletal muscle emg activity), went into high-voltage ECoG, and started continuous breathing. Internal cooling by a gastric tube also induced shivering but not continuous breathing. It is not clear whether the breathing response was specific to cold,

or was a non-specific response to increased sensory input. Ioffe *et al.* (1980)
electrically stimulated the sciatic nerve, nasal septum and tail in chronically
prepared fetal lambs, and found that stimulation increased breathing in low-
voltage ECoG but had little effect in high voltage. The effects of such neural
stimulation differ from those of skin cooling, but as neural stimulation
mimicked a range of different modalities this is perhaps not surprising. The
effects of fetal heating have also been studied. Robinson (unpublished:
quoted by Dawes, 1973) warmed exteriorised fetal lambs and reported rapid
breathing movements described as panting. Recently Walker *et al.* (1985)
found that raising the maternal temperature of pregnant ewes to 43°C for 8 h
did not affect fetal breathing until 1–2 h after the heating period, when an
episode of high-intensity breathing started, lasting up to 12 h and continuing
through high-voltage ECoG and hypoxia. The significance of this extraordinary finding is not clear, but it cannot be a direct response to warming. The
delayed onset and prolonged effect are reminiscent of the response to 5-
hydroxytryptophan infusions (Quilligan *et al.*, 1981) and may reflect long-
term biochemical effects of the severe heating.

## 2.6. **Directions of future research**

The last decade has seen an increased interest in, and understanding of, the
control of fetal breathing, but many intriguing puzzles remain. The episodic
nature of fetal breathing has not been explained. There are two separate
problems to consider: breathing is absent for all of the time in HVECoG, and
for much of LVECoG. These two states appear to correspond to postnatal
slow-wave sleep and REM sleep respectively, and breathing patterns in the
two sleep states postnatally are different. In REM sleep breathing is shallow,
does not involve the intercostal muscles (so the thorax collapses in inspiration) and is irregular in rate and depth, whereas in slow-wave sleep breathing
is deeper, more regular, and the thorax expands on inspiration. It has been
argued that these two distinct patterns of breathing reflect two separate
control systems (Coote, 1982), or that part of the control system is inactive in
REM sleep (Philipson, 1978; Parmeggiani, 1979). The pattern of fetal
breathing is usually characteristic only of REM sleep, but the regular pattern
characteristic of slow-wave sleep can occasionally occur after brain lesions
(e.g. Fig. 2.3) or even in the intact fetus, particularly in the presence of drugs
that stimulate breathing. Figure 2.7 shows an unusual episode of fetal
breathing following a doxapram injection. Breathing continued into an
episode of HVECoG when the pattern changed and became more regular, as
well as faster and deeper.

   It appears therefore that the breathing patterns characteristic of different
sleep states are both potentially present in the fetus, but that one is entirely
suppressed and the other is suppressed episodically. The significance of this
difference is unknown, though it is of interest that postnatally the regular

type of breathing is more sensitive to reflex control, particularly from chemoreceptors (Coote, 1982). Fetal breathing has little effect on blood gases, and so this high-gain respiratory-control system in the fetus would be operating under open-loop conditions, possibly leading to instability and excessive breathing efforts and made worse by the probable inactivity of the Hering–Breuer reflex. This is of course pure speculation, and until high-voltage ECoG breathing can be induced in a repeatable preparation the phenomenon cannot be studied. One research objective should be to explore ways of stimulating breathing in HVECoG, either through brain lesioning to interrupt inhibitory control, or the use of drugs to antagonise the presumed central inhibition, and to study the development of respiratory reflex sensitivity in this state.

Another unsolved problem is the change in respiratory reflex sensitivity at birth. The neonate must breathe continuously, despite a large decrease in $P_a CO_2$ which would be expected to reduce respiratory drive. It seems unlikely that the sudden increase in somatic afferent activity alone can account for the onset and maintenance of breathing, and other changes occurring at birth have been invoked to explain the phenomenon. Lung inflation and a rise in $P_A O_2$ are apparently both ruled out by the work of Blanco *et al.* (1984b) who ventilated fetal lambs *in utero* and showed that neither lung inflation *per se*, nor changing fetal blood gases to neonatal levels, permanently affects fetal respiratory responses. While asphyxia and cold may be vital for the onset of breathing, its maintenance demands the removal or overriding of inhibition, by some means not yet explained. Berger *et al.* (1985) reported marked changes in breathing pattern and ECoG in the hour before birth, so postnatal peripheral stimulation may be only partly responsible for the change.

The central inhibitory control of fetal breathing in hypoxia is a third major area of controversy, but considerable progress has been made towards understanding this mechanism, and new techniques may soon allow a full explanation. It is now possible to place small brain lesions stereotaxically, and to microinject neurotransmitter agonists, antagonists and depletors. Recent developments in histochemistry using monoclonal antibodies make it possible to stain cells containing selected neurotransmitters with a high degree of specificity, and it should soon be possible to block or stimulate identified brainstem pathways without causing generalised damage. These new methods should allow complete mapping of descending inhibitory pathways projecting on to respiratory neurones and to measure their activity before and after birth. Findings from this work could eventually lead to improved therapy for central apnoeic disorders of breathing as well as providing a better understanding of the development of respiratory control.

**References**

Adamson, S. L., Patrick, J. E. & Challis, J. R. G. (1984). Effects of naloxone on the breathing, electrocortical, heart rate, glucose and cortisol responses to hypoxia in the sheep fetus. *J. Dev. Physiol.* **6**, 495–507.

Ahlfeld, F. (1888). Uber bisher noch nicht beschriebene intrauterine Bewegungen des Kindes. *Verh. Dtsch. Ges. Gynaecol.* **2**, 203.

Alcorn, D., Adamson, T. M., Maloney, J. E. & Robinson, P. M. (1980). Morphological effects of chronic bilateral phrenectomy or vagotomy in the fetal lamb lung. *J. Anat.* **130**, 683–95.

Bamford, O. S., Dawes, G. S., Parkes, M. J. & Quail, A. W. (1984). Atropine, electrocortical activity and breathing in fetal lambs. *J. Physiol.* **349**, 59P.

Bamford, O. S., Dawes, G. S. & Ward, R. A. (1985). A possible dopaminergic pathway stimulating breathing in fetal lambs. *J. Physiol.* **365**, 105P.

Bamford, O. S., Dawes, G. S. & Ward, R. A. (1986a). Effects of apomorphine and haloperidol in fetal lambs. *J. Physiol.* **377**, 37–47.

Bamford, O. S., Dawes, R. & Ward, R. A. (1986b). Effects of the $\alpha_2$ adrenergic agonist clonidine and its antagonist idazoxan on the fetal lamb. *J. Physiol.* **381**, 29–37.

Barcroft, J., Barron, D. H. & Windle, W. F. (1936). Some observations on genesis of somatic movements in sheep embryos. *J. Physiol.* **87**, 73–8.

Becker, R. F., King, J. E., Marsh, R. H. & Wyrick A. D. (1964). Intrauterine respiration in the rat fetus. I. Direct observations — comparison with the guinea pig. *Am. J. Obs. Gynecol.* **90**, 236–46.

Berger, P. J., Walker, A. M., Horne, R., Brodecky, V., Wilkinson, M. H., Wilson, F. & Maloney, J. E. (1985). Perinatal respiratory activity in the lamb. In *Physiological Development of the Fetus and Newborn* (eds C. T. Jones & P. W. Nathanielsz). London: Academic Press.

Bisgard, G. E., Forster, H. V., Klein, J. P., Manohar, M. & Bullard, V. A. (1980). Depression of ventilation by dopamine in goats — effects of carotid body excision. *Resp. Physiol.* **41**, 379–92.

Bissonnette, J. M., Hohimer, A. R. & Richardson, B. S. (1981). Ventriculocisternal cerebrospinal perfusion in unanaesthetized fetal lambs. *J. Appl. Physiol.* **50**, 880–3.

Blanco, C. E., Dawes, G. S., Hanson, M. A. & McCooke, H. B. (1984a). The response to hypoxia of arterial chemoreceptors in fetal sheep and newborn lambs. *J. Physiol.* **351**, 25–38.

Blanco, C. E., Martin, C. B., Crevels, A. J. & Arts, T. H. M. (1984b). Electrocortical activity, breathing and body movements, heart rate and blood pressure during mechanical pulmonary ventilation in fetal sheep. *Proceedings of XIth Annual Meeting, Society for the Study of Fetal Physiology*, July 1984, Oxford, England.

Boddy, K., Dawes, G. S., Fisher, R., Pinter, S. & Robinson, J. S. (1974). Fetal respiratory movements, electrocortical and cardiovascular responses to hypoxaemia and hypercapnia in sheep. *J. Physiol.* **243**, 599–618.

Bonar, B. E., Blumenfeld, C. M. & Fenning, C. (1938). Studies of fetal respiratory movements: historical and present day observations. *Am. J. Dis. Child.* **55**, 1–11.

Coote, J. H. (1982). Respiratory and circulatory control during sleep. *J. Exp. Biol.* **100**, 223–44.

Dawes, G. S. (1973). Breathing and rapid-eye-movement sleep before birth. In: *Foetal and Neonatal Physiology: Sir Joseph Barcroft Centenary Symposium*. Cambridge: Cambridge University Press.

Dawes, G. S. (1984). The central control of fetal breathing and skeletal muscle movements. *J. Physiol.* **346**, 1–18.

Dawes, G. S., Fox, H. E., Leduc, B. M., Liggins, G. C. & Richards, R. T. (1970). Respiratory movements and paradoxical sleep in the foetal lamb. *J. Physiol.* **210**, 47–8P.

Dawes, G. S., Fox, H. E., Leduc, B. M., Liggins, G. C. & Richards, R. T. (1972). Respiratory movements and rapid eye movement sleep in the fetal lamb. *J. Physiol.* **220**, 119–43.

Dawes, G. S., Gardner, W. N., Johnston, B. M. & Walker, D. W. (1980). Activity of intercostal muscles in relation to breathing movements, electrocortical activity and gestational age in fetal lambs. *J. Physiol.* **307**, 47–8P.

Dawes, G. S., Gardner, W. N., Johnston, B. M. & Walker, D. W. (1982). Effects of hypercapnia on tracheal pressure, diaphragm and intercostal electromyograms in unanaesthetized fetal lambs. *J. Physiol.* **326**, 461–74.

Dawes, G. S., Gardner, W. N., Johnston, B. M. & Walker, D. W. (1983). Breathing in fetal lambs: the effects of brain stem section. *J. Physiol.* **335**, 535–53.

De Lorimer, A. A., Tierney, O. F. & Parker, H. B. (1967). Hypoplastic lungs in fetal lambs with surgically produced congenital hernia. *Surgery* **62**, 12–17.

Fewell, J. E. & Johnson, P. (1983). Upper airway dynamics during breathing and during apnea in fetal lambs. *J. Physiol.* **339**, 495–504.

Fewell, J. E., Hislop, A., Kitterman, J. A. & Johnson, P. (1983). Effect of tracheostomy on lung development in fetal lambs. *J. Appl. Physiol.* **55**, 1103–8.

Gluckman, P. D., Gunn, T. R. & Johnston, B. M. (1983). The effect of cooling on breathing and shivering in unanaesthetized fetal lambs *in utero. J. Physiol.* **343**, 495–506.

Gluckman, P. D. & Parsons, Y. (1984). Stereotaxic neurosurgery on the ovine fetus. In *Animal Models in Fetal Medicine* (ed. P. W. Nathanielsz), Perinatology Press.

Harding, R. & Poore, E. R. (1984). The effect of myometrial activity on fetal thoracic dimensions and uterine blood flow during late gestation in the sheep. *Biol. Neonate* **45**, 244–51.

Haxhiu, M. A., Mitra, J., van Lunteru, E., Bruce, E. N. & Cherniak, N. S. (1984). Hypoglossal and phrenic responses to cholinergic agents applied to ventral medullary surface. *Am. J. Physiol.* **247**, R939–44.

Hedner, J., Hedner, T., Jonason, J. & Lundberg, D. (1982). Evidence for a dopamine interaction with the central respiratory control system in the rat. *Eur. J. Pharmacol.* **81** 603–15.

Hilakivi, I. (1983). The role of $\alpha$- and $\beta$-adrenoreceptors in the regulation of the stages of the sleep–waking cycle in the cat. *Brain Res.* **277**, 109–18.

Hofmeyr, G. J., Bamford, O. S., Gianopoulos, J., Parkes, M. J. & Dawes, G. S. (1985a). The partial association of uterine contractions with electrocortical activity, breathing and $PaO_2$ in the fetal lamb: effects of brain stem section. *Am. J. Obs. Gynecol.* **152**, 905–10.

Hofmeyr, G. J., Bamford, O. S., Howlett, T. & Parkes, M. J. (1985b). Methionine–enkephalin and the arrest of breathing. In *Physiological Development of the Fetus and Newborn* (eds C. T. Jones & P. W. Nathanielsz). London: Academic Press.

Hogg, M. I. J., Golding, R. H. & Rosen, M. (1977). The effect of doxapram on fetal breathing in the sheep. *Br. J. Obs. Gynaecol.* **84**, 48–50.

Ioffe, S., Jansen, A. J., Russell, B. J. & Chernick, V. (1980). Respiratory response to somatic stimulation in fetal lambs during sleep and wakefulness. *Pflügers Arch.* **388**, 143–8.

Jansen A. H. & Chernick V. (1983). Development of respiratory control. *Physiol. Rev.* **63**, 437–83.

Jensen, A., Bamford, O. S., Dawes, G. S., Hofmeyr, G. J. & Parkes, M. J. (1985). Changes in organ blood flow between high and low voltage electrocortical activity and during isocapnic hypoxia in intact and brain stem transected fetal lambs. In *Physiological Development of the Fetus and Newborn* (eds C. T. Jones & P. W. Nathanielsz). London: Academic Press.

Johnston, B. M. & Gluckman, P. D. (1983). GABA-mediated inhibition of breathing in the late gestation sheep fetus. *J. Dev. Physiol.* **5**, 353–60.

Johnston, B. M., Gluckman, P. D.& Parsons, Y. (1985). The effect of mid-brain lesions on breathing in fetal lambs. In *Physiological Development of the Fetus and Newborn* (Eds C. T. Jones & P. W. Nathanielsz), London: Academic Press.

Johnston, B. M., Walker, D. W. & Green, A. R. (1984). Lack of long term effect of *p*-chlorophenylalanine on brain 5-hydroxytryptamine and electrocortical activity in conscious fetal sheep. *Experientia* **40**, 291–4.

Jones, C. T. & Ritchie, J. W. K. (1978). The cardiovascular effects of circulating catecholamines in fetal sheep. *J. Physiol.* **285**, 381–93.

Keanne, P. E., Candy, J. M. & Bradley, P. B. (1976). The role of endogenous catecholamines in the regulation of electrocortical activity in the encephale isole cat. *EEG Clin. Neurol.* **41**, 561–70.

Kitterman, J. A. (1984). Fetal lung development. *J. Dev. Physiol.* **6**, 67–82.

Kitterman, J. A., Ballard, P. L., Clements, J. A., Mescher, E. J. & Tooley, W. H. (1979a). Tracheal fluid in fetal lambs: spontaneous decrease prior to birth. *J. Appl. Physiol.* **47**, 985–9.

Kitterman, J. A., Liggins, G. C., Clements, J. A. & Tooley, W. H. (1979b). Stimulation of fetal breathing movements in fetal sheep by inhibitors of prostaglandin synthesis. *J. Dev. Physiol.* **1**, 453–66.

Kitterman, J. A., Liggins, G. C., Fewell, J. E. & Tooley, W. H. (1983). Inhibition of breathing movements in fetal sheep by prostaglandins. *J. Appl. Physiol.* **54**, 687–92.

Koos, B. (1982). Central effects on breathing in fetal sheep of sodium meclofenamate. *J. Physiol.* **330**, 50–1P.

Lahiri, S., Nishino, T., Mokasha, A. & Milligan, E. (1980). Interaction of dopamine and haloperidol with $O_2$ and $CO_2$ chemoreception in the carotid body. *J. Appl. Physiol.* **49**, 45–51.

Liggins, G. C., Vilos, G. A., Campos, G. A., Kitterman, J. A. & Lee, C. H. (1981). The effect of bilateral thoracoplasty on lung development in fetal sheep. *J. Dev. Physiol.* **3** 275–82.

McCrimmon, D. R. & Lalley, P. M. (1982). Inhibition of respiratory neural discharges by clonidine and 5-hydroxytryptophan. *J. Pharm. Exp. Ther.* **222**, 771–77.

McGrath, J. C. & Stuart-Smith, K. (1982). Human umbilical artery is contracted by oxygen, KCl or 5-HT but not by α-adrenoreceptor agonists. *Br. J. Pharmacol.* **76**, 258P.

McLeod, W., Brien, J., Loomis, C., Carmichael, L., Probert, C. & Patrick, J. (1983). Effect of maternal ethanol ingestion on fetal breathing movements, gross body movements, and heart rate at 37 to 40 weeks gestational age. *Am. J. Obs. Gynecol.* **145**, 251–7.

Maloney, J. E. (1983). Review of experimental studies on the functional development of the respiratory system in the fetal lamb. *Aust. J. Biol. Sci.* **36**, 1–14.

Mayock, D. E., Standaert, T. A., Guthrie, R. D. & Woodrum, D. E. (1983). Dopamine and carotid body function in the newborn lamb.*J. Appl. Physiol.* **54**, 814–20.

Merlet, C., Hoerter, J., De Villeneuve, C. & Tchobroutsky C. (1970). Mise en evidence de mouvements respiratoires chez le foetus d'agneau *in utero* au cours de dernier mois de la gestation. *C.r. hebd. Seanc. Acad. Sci. Paris* **270**, 2642–4.

Metz, B. (1966). Hypercapnia and acetylcholine release from the cerebral cortex and medulla. *J. Physiol.* **186**, 321–32.

Millhorn, D. E., Eldridge, F. L. & Waldrop, T. G. (1980). Prolonged stimulation of respiration by endogenous central serotonin. *Resp. Physiol.* **42**, 171–88.

Millhorn, D. E., Eldridge, F. L., Waldrop, T. G. & Klinger, L. E. (1983). Centrally and peripherally administered 5-hydroxytryptophan have opposite effects on respiration. *Brain Res.* **264**, 349–54.

Milligan, D. W. A. (1979). Cerebral blood flow and sleep state in the normal newborn infant. *Early Hum. Dev.* **3**, 321–8.

Mitchell, R. A. & Herbert, D. A. (1975). Potencies of doxapram and hypoxia in stimulating carotid body chemoreceptors and ventilation in anaesthetized cats. *Anaesthesiol.* **42**, 559–66.

Mitchell, R. A., Loeschke, H. H., Massion, W. H. & Severinghaus, J. W. (1963). Respiratory responses mediated through superficial chemosensitive areas on the medulla. *J. Appl.Physiol.* **18**, 523–33.

Murata, Y., Martin, C. B., Miyake, K., Socol, M. & Druzin, M. (1981). Effects of catecholamines on fetal breathing activity in rhesus monkeys. *Am. J. Obs. Gynecol.* **139**, 942–7.

Natale, R. J., Patrick, J. & Richardson, B. (1978). Effect of human maternal venous plasma glucose concentrations on fetal breathing movements. *Am. J. Obs. Gynecol.* **132**, 36–41.

Nathanielsz, P. W., Bailey, A., Poore E. R., Thorburn, G. D. & Harding, R. (1980). The relationship between myometrial activity and sleep state and breathing in fetal sheep during the last third of gestation. *Am. J. Obs. Gynecol.* **138**, 653–9.

Nishino, T., Mokashi, A. & Lahiri, S. (1982). Stimulation of carotid chemoreceptors and ventilation by doxapram in the cat. *J. Appl. Physiol.* **52**, 1261–5.

Parmeggiani, P. L. (1979). Integrative aspects of hypothalamic influences on respiratory brain stem mechanisms during wakefulness and sleep. In *Central Nervous Control Mechanisms in Breathing* (eds. C. von Euler & H. Lagercrantz), Oxford: Pergamon Press.

Philipson, E. A. (1978). Respiratory adaptations in sleep. *Ann. Rev. Physiol.* **40**, 133–56.

Piercy, W. N., Day, M. A., Neims, A. H. & Williams, R. L. (1977). Alteration of ovine respiratory-like activity by diazepam, caffeine and doxapram. *Am. J. Obs. Gynecol.* **127**, 43–9.

Poore, E. R.& Walker, D. W. (1980). Chest wall movements during fetal breathing in sheep. *J. Physiol.* **301**, 307–15.

Quilligan, E. J., Clewlow, F., Johnston, B. M. & Walker, D. W. (1981). Effect of 5-hydroxytryptophan on electrocortical activity and breathing movements of fetal sheep. *Am. J. Obs. Gynecol.* **141**, 271–15.

Rosenfeld, M. & Snyder, F. F. (1936). Foetal respiration in the rabbit. *Proc. Soc. Exp. Biol. Med.* **33**, 576.

Scremin, O. U., Sonnenschein, R. R. & Rubinstein, E. H. (1983). Cholinergic cerebral vasodilatation in the rabbit: absence of concomitant metabolic activation. *J. Cerebr. Blood Flow Metab.* **2**, 241–7.

Szeto, H. H. & Umans, J. G. (1985). The effects of a stable adenosine analog on fetal behavioural, respiratory and cardiovascular functions. In *Physiological Development of the Fetus and Newborn* (eds C. T. Jones & P. W. Nathanielsz). London: Academic Press.

van der Wildt, B. (1982). Heart rate, breathing movements and brain activity in fetal lambs. Doctoral thesis, University of Nijmegen.

Walker, D. W., Davies, A. M. & Thorburn, G. D. (1985). Prolonged effect of heat stress on fetal breathing. *Proceedings of XIIth Annual Meeting, Society for the Study of Fetal Physiology*, July 1985, Haifa, Israel.

Wigglesowrth, J. S. & Desai, R. (1979). Effect on lung growth of cervical cord section in the rabbit fetus. *Early Hum. Dev.* **3**, 51–65.

Wilds, P. L. (1978). Observations of intrauterine fetal breathing — a review. *Am. J. Obs. Gynecol.* **131** 315–38.

Yamada, K. A., Norman W. P. Hamosh, P. & Gillis, R. A. (1982). Medullary ventral surface GABA receptors affect respiratory and cardiovascular function. *Brain Res.* **248**, 71–8.

Yamasaki, K. & Lico, M. C. (1981). Electroencephalographic serotonin synchronization: area postrema and solitary tract nucleus. *Am. J. Physiol.* **241**, R158–61.

# 3

# The role of vagal afferents in the peripheral control of respiration in birds

**M. Gleeson***

*Department of Veterinary Physiology, Royal (Dick) School of Veterinary Studies, University of Edinburgh, Edinburgh EH9 1QH, UK*

## 3.1. Introduction

Birds and mammals have developed respiratory systems that are different from each other in both anatomical aspects and to some extent in certain aspects of their peripheral control of rhythmic breathing. In both these vertebrate classes the primary function of the respiratory control system is to maintain adequate levels of lung oxygen and carbon dioxide by matching ventilation to the demand placed on it by tissue metabolism. This paper discusses (a) briefly the structure of the avian respiratory system; (b) methods used in the study of the peripheral control of breathing in birds; and (c) the location, stimulus specificity and physiological function(s) of receptors with vagal axons that influence respiration in birds.

Most of the evidence concerning the peripheral control of breathing in birds has been obtained from experiments performed on domesticated species, particularly the chicken and duck. These are not perhaps the ideal representatives of their class — the chicken being a non-flier and the duck a diving animal — but they have the not inconsiderable advantages of being large, domesticated, convenient and inexpensive experimental animals.

## 3.2. Structural and functional aspects of the avian respiratory system

Detailed descriptions of the avian lung air sac system have been given by King (1966, 1975), King & Molony (1971), Duncker (1971) and McClelland & Molony (1983), and only a brief description will be given here in order to familiarise the non-avian physiologist with the anatomical 'essentials' of the system. The lungs lie in the dorsal thoracic cavity, deeply indented by the medial surfaces of the vertebral parts of the ribs. The avian lungs are

*Present address and address for correspondence: Department of Biological Sciences, Coventry Polytechnic, Priory Street, Coventry CV1 5FB, UK.

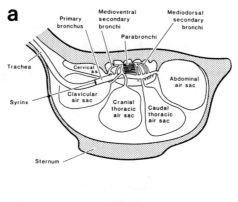

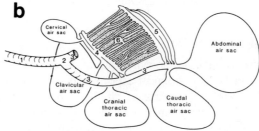

Fig. 3.1.   (a) General arrangement of the lung and air sacs in the bird, left side view, based on the domestic goose. (After Brackenbury, 1974.) All sacs except the clavicular sac are paired. In songbirds the clavicular and cranial thoracic sacs are fused. The syrinx is the vocal organ and lies at the junction between the trachea and the two primary bronchi. (b) Schematic diagram of the parabronchial lung (lateral view of left lung) and air sacs in phylogenetically 'primitive' forms such as emus, penguins and storks. In the more 'advanced' forms such as songbirds and gamebirds there is an additional area of parabronchi, the neopulmo, which connects the abdominal and caudal thoracic sacs directly to the mediodorsal secondary bronchi and the caudal part of the primary bronchus. 1, Trachea; 2, syrinx; 3, primary bronchus; 4, medioventral secondary bronchi; 5, mediodorsal secondary bronchi; 6, parabronchi. The diagram is not drawn to scale. The size of the air sacs has been reduced relative to the size of the lung.

relatively rigid structures, and while they may expand to a small extent due to movements of the ribs, it is predominantly the pressure changes in the extensive voluminous air sacs (Fig. 3.1) that allow gases to enter the respiratory system during inspiration and force gas out of the system during expiration. Thus, active contraction of respiratory muscles occurs during both phases of the respiratory cycle (Kadono *et al.*, 1963; Fedde *et al.*, 1964). The trachea divides into two primary bronchi, one of which passes through each lung in the shape of a drawn-out S and tapers towards its terminal connection with the abdominal air sac (Fig. 3.1). Two series of secondary bronchi arise from the cranial and caudal parts of the primary bronchus respectively, the medioventral secondary bronchi and the mediodorsal secondary bronchi, and these are connected by several hundred, more or less parallel tertiary bronchi (parabronchi) each of which is approximately 1 mm in diameter. The parabronchi are the sites of gas exchange, their walls consisting of two interlocking series of air and blood capillaries. The air capillaries arise from the bases of numerous pockets (atria) within the wall of each parabronchus, the openings to which are surrounded by smooth muscle. Details of the structure and arrangement of the blood and air capillaries are well described by Duncker (1971).

The air sacs arise as evaginations from the embryonic secondary bronchi and retain direct connections with the latter in the adult bird. The air sacs can be divided into two groups. A cranial group, comprising the paired cervicals and cranial thoracics and the unpaired interclavicular sac, connect to the medioventral secondary bronchi, and a caudal group, consisting of the paired caudal thoracics and abdominals, connect to the caudal parts of the primary bronchi (Fig. 3.1).

A simplified schematic representation of the avian respiratory system (Fig. 3.2) illustrates how air circulates in the lower respiratory tract of birds as a result of the pressure gradients developed by the respiratory musculature and the bellows-like action of the air sacs in the two phases of the respiratory cycle. During inspiration the respiratory musculature effects an increase in the volume of the thoracoabdominal cavity (there is no equivalent of the mammalian diaphragm in birds) and all the air sacs expand. The caudal sacs inhale a mixture of dead-space gas and fresh air directly from the primary bronchus which is stored for the remainder of the inspiratory phase; the cranial sacs draw stale air out of the parabronchi replacing it with a stream of fresh air from the primary bronchus, which enters the parabronchi via the mediodorsal secondary bronchi. During the ensuing expiration the relatively fresh air stored in the caudal sacs is injected into the mediodorsal secondary bronchi and aerates the parabronchi for a second time before finally re-entering the primary bronchus via the medioventral secondary bronchi. Here it is joined by stale air simultaneously expelled from the collapsing cranial air sacs. Thus air flows through the parabronchi in the same direction during both phases of the respiratory cycle. The roles of the cranial and caudal air sacs are reflected in their gas composition, gas in the cranial sacs being similar to end-expired gas, that in the caudal sacs being much closer to atmospheric (see reviews by Bouverot & Dejours, 1971, and Brackenbury, 1981). The process of air flow rectification which results in unidirectional ventilation of the parabronchi is mainly dependent on aerodynamic forces acting between the primary bronchus and secondary bronchi, although active constriction of the airways by bronchial smooth muscle cannot be ruled out.

# a. Inspiration

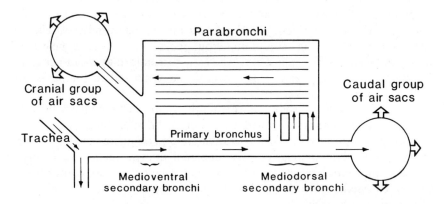

Parabronchi

Cranial group
of air sacs

Caudal group
of air sacs

Trachea

Primary bronchus

Medioventral
secondary bronchi

Mediodorsal
secondary bronchi

# b. Expiration

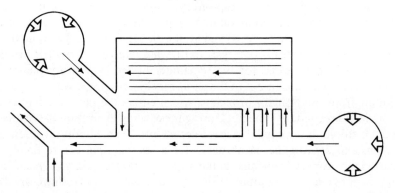

Fig. 3.2.   Diagram of the lung–air sac system to show the airflow pattern during (a) inspiration, and (b) expiration. Air flows through the parabronchi in the same direction during both phases of respiration. Arrows indicate direction of air flow (dotted arrow: flow uncertain).

### 3.3. **Methods used in the study of the peripheral control of avian respiration**

The following presentation is an attempt briefly to mention and comment on the significance of some of the techniques that have been used in investigations on the peripheral control of breathing in birds. The list is by no means exhaustive, but concentrates on the methods that have yielded important information on avian peripheral respiratory control mechanisms. Where applicable, the potential usefulness of some of these techniques in studies on the mechanism of action of peripheral chemoreceptors in general is emphasised.

### 3.3.1. *Light and electron microscopy: anatomical evidence for receptors in the respiratory tract and systemic arteries*

The problems of identifying afferent nerve endings in the avian respiratory tract with the light and electron microscope were analysed by King *et al.* (1974). Much of the evidence from light microscope studies is based on empirical staining techniques with their well known limitations (Groth, 1972). Bower *et al.* (1975) have used radioactive leucine to trace afferent nerve fibres from their cell bodies in the nodose ganglion (of the vagus nerve) into the respiratory tract; observations for the extrapulmonary bronchi reveal both simple and complex endings in the epithelium.

Electron microscopy has revealed axon profiles which satisfy many of the criteria for afferent endings. They have been found in the epithelium of the trachea (Walsh & McClelland, 1978) and in various parts of the lung, including a site close to the parabronchial lumen just below the atrial epithelium (King *et al.*, 1974). Possible afferent nerve endings have also been described in the air sac and bronchoperitoneal membranes (Bennett & Malmfors, 1970; Groth, 1972).

Electron microscopy of the carotid body in the chicken (Hodges *et al.*, 1975; King *et al.*, 1975) and the duck (Osborne & Butler, 1975) indicates that, as in mammals, two main types of cell are present, the type I epithelioid (glomus) cell and the type II (sustentacular) cell. The relationship of these cells to each other and to the nerve supply appears similar to that in the mammal. The topographical anatomy of the carotid body has been established for the chicken by Abdel-Magied & King (1978). In the chicken, receptor tissue similar to that in the carotid body has also been identified in several other arterial sites (Abdel-Magied, 1978a, b).

### 3.3.2. *Artificial unidirectional ventilation*

The parallel arrangement of the bronchi of the avian lung coupled with the extensive air-sac system allows the use of unidirectional, artificial ventilation (Burger & Lorenz, 1960; Fedde & Burger, 1962) in the study of peripheral receptors involved in the control of breathing. The anaesthetised bird can be prepared for this kind of artificial ventilation by cannulating the trachea in the midcervical region and cannulating one or more of the air sacs with wide-bore tubing. A steady stream of humidified gas is then passed into the trachea, through the lungs, into the air sacs and out to the atmosphere through the air-sac cannulae. Alternatively some of the air sacs, usually the

abdominals and thoracics, can be ruptured and the ventilating gas stream
allowed to exit through an incision or a wide-bore cannula in the abdominal
wall.

Respiratory movements occur at a normal rate if the ventilating gas
contains approximately 6% $CO_2$. If the gas flow rate is sufficiently high
(three to four times normal minute volume), a constant air-capillary gas
composition is maintained irrespective of changes in the metabolic $CO_2$
production or $O_2$ consumption of the bird.

The artificial unidirectional ventilation system offers the considerable
advantages of almost total elimination of dead-space gas and allows rapid
and independent control of the pulmonary gas composition while maintaining the gas flow rate constant. Blood gas tensions may be altered rapidly and
precisely by changing the composition of the gas stream, and the outflowing
gas is usually close to equilibrium with arterial blood. The preparation
therefore allows greater control over the stimuli presented to pulmonary and
arterial chemoreceptors than can be achieved by tidal ventilation of the
mammal, either in the steady state or in the unsteady state. Since the steady-
state stimulus–response characteristics of arterial chemoreceptors in the
duck are virtually indistinguishable from those in the mammal (Nye &
Powell, 1984), unidirectionally ventilated birds could provide an inexpensive,
convenient and useful model for the study of the mechanism of excitation of
arterial chemoreceptors in general.

In the unidirectionally ventilated bird any respiratory movement in
response to changes in the ventilating gas composition is a direct reflection of
the activity of the central nervous system and is not influenced by the
ventilatory system *per se* as is the case with the use of reciprocating pumps in
mammals. Also, it is possible to artificially ventilate the bird with a
unidirectional gas stream passed in the reverse direction, i.e. by passing gas
through a manifold into cannulae in the air sacs, through the lungs and out
of the trachea.

Receptors sensitive to $CO_2$ in birds are found both in the lung and in the
extrapulmonary circulation. It is possible to dissociate the $PCO_2$ affecting
intrapulmonary and extrapulmonary $CO_2$-sensitive receptors by ligating the
left pulmonary artery, denervating the right lung (by cutting the right vagus)
and artificially ventilating each lung separately (Osborne *et al.*, 1977a).

### 3.3.3. *The open-loop preparation*

To study respiratory central activity in mammals under open-loop conditions (i.e. in the absence of feedback from the periphery to the respiratory
centre), Cohen (1964) recorded phrenic nerve discharge in vagotomised cats
with spinal section and pneumothorax. To achieve the same effect in birds, it
is only necessary to record respiratory motor nerve activity in the paralysed

bird on unidirectional ventilation. There is no equivalent of the diaphragm and phrenic nerve in birds, but intercostal nerves are accessible with minimal surgery for measurement of purely inspiratory or expiratory motor activity (Jones & Bamford, 1976).

### 3.3.4. *Electrical stimulation of the vagus nerves*

For the vagus and its branches it is inconceivable that electrical stimulation can excite only one modality of fibre, although in some vagal stimulation experiments one pattern of reflex activity may predominate. Stimulation of the central end of the cut vagus in the chicken produces an inspiratory response (McClelland, 1970).

### 3.3.5. *Electrophysiological studies of afferent axons in the vagus nerves*

In birds the majority of afferent nerve fibres from lower respiratory tract and carotid body receptors run in the vagus nerves. Birds in general possess a relatively longer neck than mammals of comparative body size, and this facilitates electrical recording from vagal afferent fibres in the cervical region. The function of vagal fibres studied by electrical recording can be determined only by correlating their behaviour with patterns of reflex activity. It is especially important to obtain single-unit fibre recordings, so that the results are quantitative and so that different stimuli can be shown unequivocally to act on the same unit. In this context, single units may be defined as those units in a filament that can be distinguished from all others at all times and, in particular, in the compound action potential when the vagus is stimulated at several times the threshold (volts) of the most sensitive unit present.

In birds, activity of single vagal afferent fibres has been correlated with respiratory changes (King *et al.*, 1968, 1969; Jones, 1969; Fedde & Peterson, 1970). Two main types of receptor have been revealed by these studies. The $CO_2$-sensitive receptors located in the lower respiratory tract that fire in phase with breathing movements have been investigated in great detail and in several species including the chicken, duck, emu, goose and pigeon. Slowly adapting mechanosensitive receptors with vagal axons and a regular respiratory modulation have also been reported, but have been studied in less detail (Fedde & Peterson, 1970; Leitner & Roumy, 1974; Molony, 1974).

A few electrophysiological studies of afferent axons in the vagus assumed to originate in the carotid and aortic bodies have been carried out in the chicken (Bouverot & Leitner, 1972) and duck (Bamford & Jones, 1976; Nye & Powell, 1984).

The characteristics of these receptors and their possible functional significance in the peripheral control of avian respiration will be discussed in the following section.

### 3.3.6. *Nerve section or block*

Section of a nerve or blockage of its impulse traffic (e.g. by cooling, local anaesthetics, pressure or anodal currents) may indicate the overall tonic action of the cut nerve. If a reflex disappears after section of a nerve (which does not contain the motor path of the reflex), the usual interpretation is that the nerve contains the afferent fibres for the reflex; this conclusion is valid provided that the nerve section has not created new conditions in which the reflex, even with pathways intact, cannot be elicited.

Denervation of the carotid bodies in chickens and ducks (for details of surgical techniques see Bouverot *et al.*, 1974; Tallman & Kunz, 1982) has established their exclusive role in provoking rapid changes in ventilation in response to changes in arterial $PO_2$ (Jones & Purves, 1970; Bouverot *et al.*, 1974). Denervation experiments have also demonstrated that the chemoreflex drive from the carotid bodies contributes about 30% of the resting ventilatory drive in ducks at sea level, and 50–60% in hypoxic conditions corresponding to an altitude of 4000 m (Bouverot & Sébert, 1979).

The main reflex respiratory change after bilateral midcervical vagotomy in birds is slower and deeper breathing (Fedde *et al.*, 1963a; Richards, 1969). Furthermore, bilateral thoracic vagotomy, which leaves the innervation of the carotid bodies, common carotid arteries and aortic bodies intact, produces alterations of respiratory pattern identical to those produced by bilateral cervical vagotomy (Fedde *et al.*, 1963b). Thus, it is likely that receptors responsible for the maintenance of normal breathing are supplied by fibres of those vagal branches which traverse to the pulmonary region.

It has long been known that artificial unidirectional ventilation of the avian respiratory system with $CO_2$-free gas results in a very rapid apnoea. This response has been shown to be a reflex mediated via afferents running in pulmonary branches of the vagus nerves (Peterson & Fedde, 1968), and to a lesser extent in pulmonary branches of thoracic sympathetic nerves (Burger & Estavillo, 1978).

Reflex inhibition of breathing by inflation of the lower respiratory tract of birds was studied by several workers before the importance of hypocapnic stimulation of $CO_2$-sensitive receptors became apparent (Graham, 1940; Richards, 1968). There is only limited evidence for a vagally mediated reflex inhibition of breathing in response to inflation which is not dependent upon increased activity of intrapulmonary $CO_2$-sensitive receptors (Eaton *et al.*, 1971; Leitner, 1972; Molony, 1974; Miller, 1978; Ballam *et al.*, 1984).

### 3.3.7. *Chemicals and drugs that affect receptor activity*

In minimal doses, by appropriate routes of administration, certain chemicals or drugs may influence (inhibit, stimulate, sensitise or desensitise) one particular group of receptors. However, larger doses invariably introduce further actions.

How breathing and respiration-related vagal afferent activity is influenced by various chemicals, including those encountered in physiological conditions (viz. $O_2$, $CO_2$, $H^+$) is covered in the following section.

## 3.4. Receptors involved in the peripheral control of avian respiration

In mammals it is known that suitable electrical stimulation of any visceral and somatic nerve will change breathing, and it is now established that most modalities of sensory and afferent endings can have some respiratory action (Widdicombe, 1964). From the multiplicity of afferent pathways that also exist in birds some can be selected for prime consideration since they change lung ventilation or the breathing pattern in response to normal and frequent physiological events.

Of particular importance in the peripheral control of breathing in birds is the afferent impulse traffic conveyed to the respiratory centres by the vagus nerves which innervate not only the lung–air sac system but also the carotid and aortic bodies. The following account is restricted to the influence of receptors with vagal axons on the control of breathing in birds. It should be borne in mind that reflexes from other (extravagal) physiological chemo-receptors, mechanoreceptors, thermoreceptors and nociceptors also influence breathing in the wide variety of conditions, normal, abnormal and patho-logical, that may be encountered by the animal.

### 3.4.1. *Intrapulmonary carbon dioxide sensitive receptors*

In contrast to the peripheral control of breathing in mammals, one of the most important receptor systems involved in the control of avian breathing is the intrapulmonary $CO_2$-sensitive receptor system. It has been demonstrated to exist in several species of bird (Fedde & Peterson, 1970; Peterson & Fedde, 1971; Fedde *et al.*, 1974a; Osborne & Burger, 1974). These receptors increase their discharge frequency as the $PCO_2$ of intrapulmonary gas is decreased in the unidirectionally, artificially ventilated preparation (Fedde *et al.*, 1974a). The abrupt removal of $CO_2$ from the gas flowing through the lung of a unidirectionally, artificially ventilated bird is shortly followed, in about 0.3 s, by an increased activity of vagal afferents sensitive to $CO_2$ and also provokes an apnoea within about 0.5 s in the chicken (Peterson & Fedde, 1968), duck, pheasant, pigeon and turkey (Peterson & Fedde, 1971). This response has been shown to be a reflex mediated via afferents running in the vagus nerves (Peterson & Fedde, 1968), and to a lesser extent in pulmonary branches of thoracic sympathetic nerves (Burger & Estavillo, 1978). Apnoea is also observed in a chicken with separately ventilated lungs, in which arterial $PCO_2$ is held constant by ventilating one perfused, denervated lung and $CO_2$ is reduced in the other innervated unperfused lung (Osborne *et al.*, 1977a). Section of the pulmonary branches of the vagi abolishes these rapid

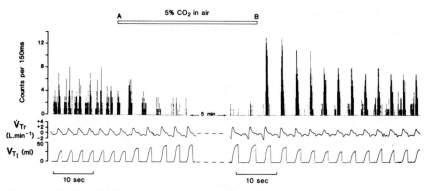

Fig. 3.3.   'On' and 'off' transient responses of breathing and an intrapulmonary $CO_2$ receptor unit (discharge counted by computer in consecutive 150 ms bins) to addition and removal of 5% $CO_2$ in the inspired gas. The 5% $CO_2$ was added to the inspired air at the 'on' (A) and was removed at the 'off' (B). Five minutes separated these events. Note the immediate abolition of inspiratory discharge when $CO_2$ is added to the inspired air, and its immediate return when the $CO_2$ is removed from the inspired air. Note also that in the 'off' transient response inspiratory discharge is related to the depth of breathing. $\dot{V}_{Tr}$, Tracheal air flow rate; $V_{TI}$, inspiratory tidal volume. Data are from a decerebrate chicken (M. Gleeson, unpublished observations).

neurophysiological and ventilatory responses to $CO_2$ removal. A greatly delayed apnoea is still seen after about 5 s but it is almost certainly related to secondary involvement of the central and systemic humoral $CO_2$–$H^+$ chemical drives.

Activity of single vagal afferent fibres has been correlated with respiratory changes (King *et al.*, 1968, 1969; Jones, 1969; Fedde & Peterson, 1970), and $CO_2$-sensitive receptors in the lower respiratory tract revealed in these studies (Fig. 3.3) have been investigated in great detail. They discharge rhythmically during spontaneous breathing and during artificial ventilation with a reciprocating pump. The majority of these receptors have peak discharge frequencies during inspiration, but some discharge also in expiration or solely in expiration (Fedde *et al.*, 1974a; Molony, 1972, 1974).

The average discharge frequency of the intrapulmonary $CO_2$-sensitive receptor (IPC) population has been described in both pump-ventilated ducks (Fedde & Scheid, 1976) and self-ventilating ducks (Berger *et al.*, 1980) and chickens (Gleeson, 1985) (Fig. 3.4). Under both these experimental conditions the average IPC discharge was strongly cyclical: peak discharge frequency occurred about midway through inspiration, and discharge fell in the latter part of inspiration. In self-ventilating animals, during expiration, IPC discharge fell quickly to a steady low level (Berger *et al.*, 1980; Gleeson, 1985) whereas in pump-ventilated ducks IPC discharge exhibited an early peak followed by a gradual decline in discharge throughout the remainder of inspiration (Fedde & Scheid, 1976). The inspiratory peak discharge

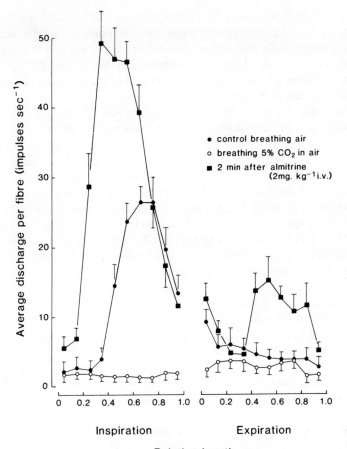

Fig. 3.4. Average discharge and standard errors of a population of intrapulmonary $CO_2$ receptors ($n = 16$) in an entire respiratory cycle during eupnoea, breathing air (●); hyperpnoea, 4 min after the addition of 5% $CO_2$ to the inspired air (○); and hyperpnoea, produced by administration of a respiratory stimulant drug, almitrine (2mg kg$^{-1}$ i.v.), breathing air (■). Note the abolition of the peak inspiratory discharge by $CO_2$, and the increased inspiratory and expiratory discharge following stimulation of breathing by almitrine. For eupnoea (●), $T_I = 1.09 \pm 0.11$ s; $T_E = 1.58 \pm 0.20$ s; $V_{TI} = 22.5 \pm 1.1$ ml. 4 min after the addition of 5% $CO_2$ to the inspired air (○), $T_I = 1.35 \pm 0.21$ s; $T_E = 1.83 \pm 0.25$ s; $V_{TI} = 60.5 \pm 3.8$ ml. 2 min after the injection of almitrine (■), $T_I = 0.96 \pm 0.04$s; $T_E = 1.18 \pm 0.14$ s; $V_{TI} = 39.8 \pm 1.6$ ml. The analysis of discharge was done according to a bin-averaging technique that has been applied to these receptors in earlier studies (Fedde & Scheid, 1976; Berger *et al.*, 1980). Briefly, this technique divides inspiration into 10bins of equal duration and calculates the discharge frequency within each bin. The discharge within a given bin is then averaged for all receptors. Expiration is also divided into 10 equal-length bins and the same analysis is performed. In each state (●, ○, ■) the discharge from four consecutive breaths was analysed and used for the bin averaging. The data are from eight decerebrate chickens. (After Gleeson, 1985.)

frequency can be explained by the arrival, after the dead space is washed out, of fresh air (low $CO_2$) that stimulates the intrapulmonary $CO_2$-sensitive endings. The gradually reduced activity in late inspiration and in expiration most probably is related to a progressive increase in the $PCO_2$ in the microenvironment of the receptor, due to decreasing gas flow rate and to parabronchial gas exchange.

Undoubtedly, the most important characteristic of these $CO_2$-sensitive receptors is their specific sensitivity to both static and dynamic changes in the $PCO_2$ of their microenvironment. Responses to static changes in $PCO_2$ are well described by several authors (Osborne & Burger, 1974; Fedde *et al.*, 1974a; Scheid *et al.*, 1978). Over a physiological range of $F_1CO_2$ from 0·01 to 0·05, activity of these receptors shows an almost linear decrease.

Responses to dynamic changes have also been described by Osborne *et al.* (1977a). These receptors can respond extremely quickly to abrupt changes in $PCO_2$ (Fig. 3.3) and can follow rapid oscillations up to at least 160 cycles $min^{-1}$. Some of these receptors show asymmetry in their dynamic responsiveness, their response to a step increase in $PCO_2$ (inhibition) being much faster than their response to a step decrease (excitation). Although several authors have noted that activity generated by dynamic changes in $PCO_2$ predominates in the normal self-ventilating animal, adequate emphasis has yet to be given to this activity. Other characteristics of these receptors include small myelinated afferent axons, conduction velocity $7·1 \pm 3·1$ m $s^{-1}$, insensitivity to distension of airways and insensitivity to hyperoxia or hypoxia. These receptors are inhibited by volatile anaesthetics such as halothane (Molony, 1974) and can be sensitised by veratridine (Molony, 1972).

There has been much concern over the specificity of these receptors, in particular the possibility of their sensitivity to mechanical changes as well as chemical ($CO_2$) changes in their microenvironment. No substantial evidence has been found for mechanical sensitivity (Fedde *et al.*, 1974a, b; Burger *et al.*, 1974; Barnas *et al.*, 1978). Investigation of their static chemosensitivity suggests that they are sensitive to both the $PCO_2$ and carbonic anhydrase-dependent pH changes associated with the changes in the partial pressure of $CO_2$ (Powell *et al.*, 1978). Thus in the unidirectionally, artificially ventilated duck, administering acetazolamide, a substance known to inhibit carbonic anhydrase and therefore slowing down the rate of $CO_2$ hydration, leads to a higher discharge frequency of the vagal $CO_2$-sensitive afferents at any $F_1CO_2$. There is also some evidence that intracellular pH may be as important as extracellular pH in the transduction processes of such receptors (Scheid *et al.*, 1978). The activity of these receptors does not, however, appear to be affected by the pH of the mixed venous blood. Acid injections into the pulmonary circulation do not reproduce the effects of $CO_2$ (Burger *et al.*, 1974).

Since these receptors are signalling static and dynamic information related to $CO_2$ in their microenvironment, the precise anatomical relationship between the receptors, the luminal $PCO_2$ and the $PCO_2$ of the mixed venous blood of the capillaries is extremely important. Physiological studies designed to localise these receptors have been carried out (Burger *et al.*, 1974; Banzett & Burger, 1977; Osborne *et al.*, 1977b; Nye & Burger, 1978; Powell *et al.*, 1978; Crank *et al.*, 1980; Powell *et al.*, 1980; Boon *et al.*, 1982; Hempelman & Burger, 1984). These studies have located a major population of $CO_2$-sensitive receptors within the parabronchi of the paleopulmo, but only a few receptors were found in other parts of the respiratory tract. Neural recording studies by Scheid *et al.* (1974) and Nye & Burger (1978) localised most of these receptors to the caudal part of the paleopulmonic parabronchi, near the entry site of fresh gas. In contrast, a reflex study by Powell *et al.* (1980) suggested that IPC $CO_2$ sensitivity was uniformly distributed in the lung: flow reversal through the artificially ventilated lungs of chickens had no significant effect on respiratory movements, indicating a symmetrical distribution of intrapulmonary $CO_2$ sensitivity. To reconcile this observation with IPC distribution of Scheid *et al.* (1974) or Nye & Burger (1978) requires a central modification of afferent input, reducing the reflex 'strength' of the numerous caudal IPCs relative to the few cranial IPCs. Recent experiments by Hempelman and Burger (1984) suggest that many IPCs have multiple endings forming chemoreceptive fields that extend, in many cases, 75% of the parabronchial length. Such a distributed receptive ending system has inherent symmetry, and approximately equal reflex effects would be expected on flow reversal without any central modification of the pattern of afferent input. IPC chemoreceptive fields might detect an average lung $PCO_2$. However, in the avian lung, cross-current exchange between the blood and gas phases creates a characteristic profile of $CO_2$ tensions. Hempelman & Burger (1984) frequently observed shifts in apparent IPC position with reversal of ventilatory flow in their artificially ventilated ducks, which is consistent with a 'pacemaker' mechanism of receptor excitation (Scheid *et al.*, 1978).

Attempts to locate the receptive endings more precisely in relation to the peripheral and luminal sides of the mantle or in the luminal epithelium of the parabronchi have not been conclusive. Anatomical studies have not been able to resolve this problem. Boon *et al.* (1982) predict that diffusion resistance in the gas phase (e.g. air capillaries) can cause a radial stratification of $CO_2$ between the parabronchial lumen and blood capillaries. Powell *et al.* (1980) postulate that receptor site $PCO_2$ lies somewhere between the $PCO_2$ values in the parabronchial lumen and the mixed venous blood, the exact $PCO_2$ being dependent on the depth of the receptor in the parabronchial mantle and $CO_2$ flux at the receptor location.

If, as seems most likely (Banzett & Burger, 1977), IPCs sense $CO_2$ which has evolved into the airways, these receptors would monitor the effects of mixed $CO_2$ load combined with effects of pulmonary ventilation. Differing

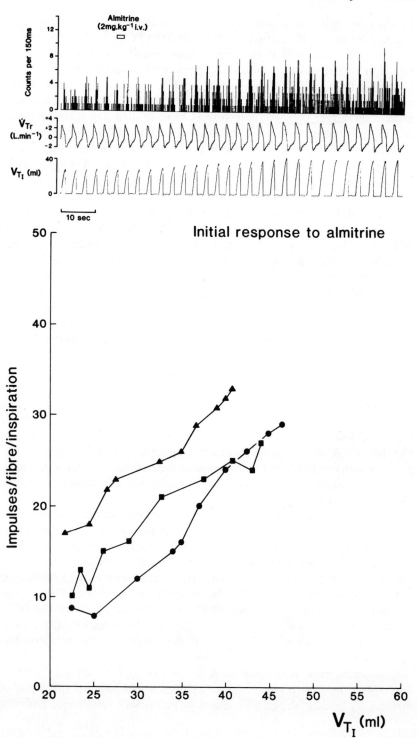

Initial response to almitrine

ratios of ventilation–perfusion would affect different individual IPCs, giving a range of $PCO_2$ chemoreception within the total IPC population from the $PCO_2$ of inhaled gas to the $PCO_2$ of arterial blood, providing the animal with some component of mixed venous chemoreception in addition to arterial blood chemoreception.

Increased activity of $CO_2$-sensitive receptors has been related to inhibition of breathing, and it has been shown, although less clearly, that these receptors are concerned in the control of parabronchial ventilation and perfusion. The details of how such effects are brought about is unclear but several interesting possibilities are under investigation.

It has been shown in the duck (Fedde & Scheid, 1976; Berger *et al.*, 1980), chicken (Gleeson, 1985) and emu (Burger *et al.*, 1976a) that the average discharge of a population of IPCs reaches a peak in inspiration. Thus as air flow through the parabronchial lung washes away $CO_2$ from the receptor site, the discharge of the IPCs increases and inhibits further inspiratory effort. Intrapulmonary $CO_2$-sensitive receptors may all act in a similar manner to inhibit inspiration, the level of inhibition being directly related to the instantaneous activity of the entire population of receptors. In the unidirectionally artificially ventilated bird a good correlation has been shown between the activity of $CO_2$-sensitive receptors and changes in ventilation of the system (Osborne & Mitchell, 1978; Powell *et al.*, 1978; Scheid *et al.*, 1978). In the spontaneously breathing decerebrate chicken there is a good correlation between the activity of $CO_2$-sensitive receptors and changes in inspiratory tidal volume when inspiratory time remains constant (Fig. 3.5). Thus the discharge of these $CO_2$-sensitive receptors appears to be related to the extent of each ventilatory effort (Fig. 3.5).

Increased afferent activity from IPCs appears to inhibit inspiratory and expiratory motor activity (Peterson & Fedde, 1968, 1971; Osborne *et al.*, 1977a). Increased afferent activity from other peripheral chemoreceptors such as those in the carotid body causes stimulation of inspiratory and expiratory flow (Bouverot, 1978). Therefore, the IPC–CNS interaction appears to be unusual for a peripheral chemoreceptor. Besides being stimulated by decreased $F_ICO_2$ in the unidirectionally ventilated preparation, IPCs can also be stimulated by increases in gas flow through the lungs

Fig. 3.5. (a) Initial effects of administration of the respiratory stimulant drug almitrine (2 mg kg$^{-1}$ i.v.) on tracheal air flow rate ($\dot{V}_{Tr}$), inspiratory tidal volume ($V_{TI}$) and the discharge of an intrapulmonary $CO_2$ receptor unit (IPC) (discharge counted by computer in consecutive 150 ms bins). Note the progressive increase in inspiratory discharge as $V_{TI}$ increases following administration of almitrine. Expiratory discharge is also increased. The data are from a decerebrate chicken, breathing air (M. Gleeson, unpublished observations). (b) Relationship between inspiratory IPC discharge (number of impulses per inspiration) and inspiratory tidal volume ($V_{TI}$) for three different IPC units in the first ten breaths after the administration of the respiratory stimulant drug, almitrine (2 mg kg$^{-1}$ i.v.). Data are from three decerebrate chickens, breathing air (M. Gleeson, unpublished observations).

(Banzett & Burger, 1977). Since IPC activity inhibits inspiratory or expiratory flow generated by breathing movements, the IPC may function in a negative-feedback mechanism controlling moment by moment the air flow through the lungs as suggested by Berger (1981). In comparison with the effects on respiratory timing this reflex behaviour is somewhat different from that of a mammalian Hering–Breuer stretch-receptor reflex. In mammals, stimulation of stretch receptors is believed to have little effect on the rate of inspiratory motor output and to cause the rate of expiratory motor output to increase (Farber, 1982).

$CO_2$-sensitive receptors may have different effects on the phases of breathing according to the time within the breathing cycle at which their activity reaches the central respiratory neurones. It has been shown that changing the normal phasic relationship between the activity of the $CO_2$-sensitive receptors and the phases of the cycle, by alteration of the inspired $PCO_2$ profile, will provoke reflex changes in the period of respiratory oscillation as well as changes in ventilation (Miller & Kunz, 1977; Berger *et al.*, 1980). Changing the profile of IPC discharge during inspiration under conditions in which the breathing pattern changes may alter the phase-switching mechanism. The IPC discharge profile could be affected by:

(a) the $PCO_2$ of dead-space gas;
(b) the $PCO_2$ of mixed venous blood, and hence changes in metabolic $CO_2$ production;
(c) changes in inspiratory gas flow rate ($V_T/T_I$).

Different $CO_2$-sensitive receptors may have different actions on breathing according to their location within the system, and be used to control the patterns of air flow within the lower respiratory tract or the ventilation–perfusion ratio of different parts of the lungs. However, little evidence exists to support such proposals.

It is clear that in birds pulmonary $PCO_2$ acts as an important controlling variable for breathing, and that activity of the intrapulmonary $CO_2$-sensitive receptors has a significant, although limited, ability to rapidly modify ventilation and/or perfusion of the exchange tissue. The response of this aspect of the control system may be sufficiently rapid for it to act in a feed-forward fashion to support homeostasis of arterial $PCO_2$, including the smoothing out of breath-by-breath oscillations. This capacity of the system is conceivably responsible for the ventilatory responses to small increases in inspired $PCO_2$ which occur without a detectable change in $P_aCO_2$ (Osborne & Mitchell, 1978) and which are dependent on the vagi being intact (Mitchell & Osborne, 1979). However, recent attempts to demonstrate that this mechanism operates under physiological conditions where venous $PCO_2$ is increased, rather than in the artificial situation where inspired $PCO_2$ is increased, have been unsuccessful (Boon *et al.*, 1980; Tallman & Grodins, 1982a). In experiments in which the circulation time to the carotid bodies and brain was prolonged by vascular loops placed in both brachiocephalic arteries of anaesthetised ducks, changes in mixed venous $CO_2$ load elicited a rapid ventilatory response which was attributed to effects on intrapulmonary chemoreceptors (Fedde *et al.*, 1982). However, the increase in ventilation was not enough to prevent a rise in $P_aCO_2$. Tallman & Grodins (1982a) reported that both low-level $CO_2$ inhalation and loading of $CO_2$ into the mixed venous blood resulted in a hypercapnic hyperpnoea. The slope of the $CO_2$ response curve ($\triangle \dot{V}_E$ versus $\triangle P_aCO_2$) was the same for both forms of loading. Thus, sensitivity of peripheral or central chemoreceptors to changes in $P_aCO_2$ appeared sufficient to explain the ventilatory response to either route of $CO_2$ administration. This finding is consistent with the results from a number of similar studies in mammals (Greco *et al.*, 1978; Lewis, 1975). However, unlike the responses measured in baboons (Lewis, 1975) and dogs (Greco *et al.*, 1978) ducks showed a significant difference in their breathing pattern. At a given level of $P_aCO_2$, $\dot{V}_E$ was not different but breathing was slower and deeper during inhaled loading compared with the breathing patterns measured during venous $CO_2$ loading. The IPCs were most probably responsible for these pattern differences, and in the spontaneously breathing duck IPCs showed a differential sensitivity to inhaled versus infused $CO_2$ loading (Tallman & Grodins, 1982b). $CO_2$ inhalation resulted in a large diminution of IPC discharge, whereas venous $CO_2$ loading did not. If a reduction in IPC discharge were to stimulate ventilation as has been suggested (Scheid *et al.*, 1978), then $CO_2$ inhalation should have given a steeper $CO_2$-response curve than venous-loaded $CO_2$. Since this is not the case (Tallman & Grodins, 1982a; Milsom *et al.*, 1981) it would appear that avian IPCs are not affecting the level of $\dot{V}_E$ under these conditions. These findings are in agreement with the work of Burger *et al.* (1978) who could not demonstrate any ventilatory stimulation by IPCs during increased metabolic rate in chickens.

When the $PCO_2$ of mixed venous blood is increased, it would be expected that expiratory and tonic IPC discharge will be reduced since airway $CO_2$ concentration increases in expiration, while the phasic discharge accompanying each inspiration when fresh air crosses the lung will be increased. Under such conditions increases in ventilation stem primarily from changes in breathing frequency (Milsom *et al.*, 1981). When the bird inhales $CO_2$, tonic discharge will again be reduced by the rise in venous $PCO_2$ but phasic discharge will be greatly reduced, and now increases in ventilation stem primarily from changes in tidal volume. If the animal is bilaterally vagotomised eliminating all tonic and phasic discharge arising from the IPCs and other peripheral respiratory-related receptors, breathing frequency is further reduced (Milsom *et al.*, 1981).

These findings are consistent with predictions from models of the central integration of pulmonary stretch receptor input in mammals (Bradley *et al.*, 1974; Euler, 1983) supporting suggestions (Banzett & Burger, 1977; Burger *et al.*, 1974, 1978; Fedde *et al.*, 1974a; Jones, 1976; Milsom *et al.*, 1981; Molony, 1972, 1974) that avian IPCs are the afferent limb of an inspiratory–inhibitory reflex which uses the rate and extent of $CO_2$ washout during inspiration as the sensory signal rather than the rate and extent of lung expansion. The IPCs, although contributing significantly to the regulation of the breathing pattern, do not appear to contribute to the ventilatory response to blood hypercapnia (Milsom *et al.*, 1981; Tallman & Grodins, 1982a, b).

This conclusion is at variance with some previous reports in the literature (Burger & Estavillo, 1978; Mitchell & Osborne, 1979; Osborne & Mitchell, 1978; Osborne *et al.*, 1977b) which have suggested that avian IPCs play a dominant role in the ventilatory responses to $CO_2$. In anaesthetised unidirectionally ventilated chickens, with opened thoracoabdominal cavities, respiratory sensitivity to $CO_2$ has been reported as being small following bilateral midcervical vagotomy (Burger & Estavillo, 1978). Similarly, Mitchell & Osborne (1979) observed a marked depression in ventilatory responsiveness to inhaled $CO_2$ following bilateral midcervical vagotomy in anaesthetised spontaneously breathing chickens. An important factor that could reconcile these contradictory findings is that the lack of respiration-related afferent traffic may be in itself of importance in changing the responses of the animal to variations in blood gases, though the mechanism by which such a change could occur is not presently understood. The open-loop respiratory chemosensitivity experiments (Section 3.3) of Cohen (1964) showed that pulmonary feedback was necessary for the normal pattern of respiratory chemosensitivity to be shown in the cat, and that when pulmonary afferent traffic was abolished by bilateral vagotomy the normal stimulatory effect of $CO_2$ became an inhibitory effect. A similar situation has been shown to exist in the chicken and duck (Jones & Bamford, 1976). In a lightly anaesthetised unidirectionally ventilated preparation the respiratory responses (as estimated from the motor discharges of an intercostal nerve) to hypercapnia were profoundly altered after removal of respiratory feedback. These were manifest as a respiratory insensitivity to $CO_2$ in the apnoeic chicken and as a $CO_2$-mediated respiratory depression in the duck.

### 3.4.2. *Mechanoreceptors in the respiratory tract*

Slowly adapting mechanosensitive receptors with vagal axons and a regular respiratory modulation have been reported (Fedde & Peterson, 1970; Fedde *et al.*, 1974b; Leitner & Roumy, 1974; Molony, 1974). These receptors are sensitive to inflation of the respiratory system (Molony, 1972, 1974; Fedde *et al.*, 1974b; Leitner & Roumy, 1974) and are insensitive to hypoxia or hypercapnia (Molony, 1974). They fire soon after the beginning of inspiration until the end of inspiration, and exhibit varying degrees of cardiovascular modulation. These receptors appear to be particularly sensitive to a mechanical stimulus that remains relatively constant throughout inspiration

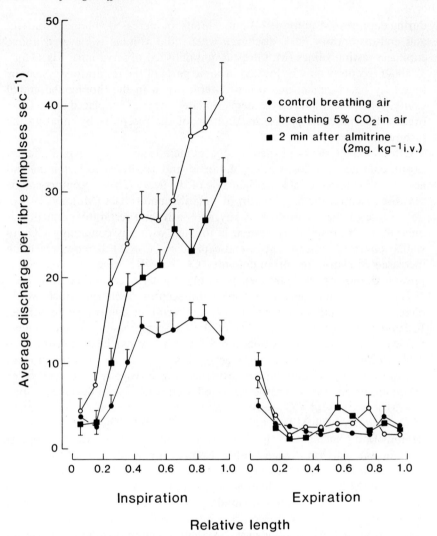

Fig. 3.6. Average discharge and standard errors of a population of presumed respiratory mechanoreceptors ($n = 16$) in an entire respiratory cycle during eupnoea, breathing air (●); hyperpnoea, 4 min after the addition of 5% $CO_2$ to the inspired air (○); and hyperpnoea produced by administration of a respiratory stimulant drug, almitrine (2 mg kg$^{-1}$ i.v.), breathing air (■). For eupnoea (●), $T_I = 1.12 \pm 0.08$ s; $T_E$ = $1.49 \pm 0.15$ s; $V_{TI} = 25.6 \pm 2.9$ ml. 4 min after addition of 5% $CO_2$ to the inspired air (○), $T_I = 1.78 \pm 0.16$ s; $T_E = 2.15 \pm 0.32$ s; $V_{TI} = 56.9 \pm 5.7$ ml. 2 min after the injection of almitrine (■), $T_I = 1.06 \pm 0.16$ s; $T_E = 1.32 \pm 0.19$ s; $V_{TI} = 43.1 \pm 3.7$ ml. The analysis of discharge was done according to the same bin-averaging technique described in the legend of Fig. 3.4. Standard errors are not drawn for most points in expiration to reduce clutter. Where omitted, standard errors were not greater than those plotted for the nearest points. The data are from 11 decerebrate chickens (M. Gleeson, unpublished observations).

during eupnoea (Molony, 1974) but exhibits an increased volume sensitivity and end-inspiratory peak discharge when tidal volume is elevated above eupnoeic resting values (M. Gleeson, unpublished observations: Fig. 3.6).

These receptors may be located in some parts of the respiratory system or they may be in almost any other visceral organ in the thoracoabdominal cavity. When the respiratory system is inflated, stresses are placed on all these organs; this prevents precise localisation of the receptors by inflating the respiratory system.

Other characteristics of these receptors include small myelinated afferent axons, conduction velocity $8.6 \pm 4.4$ ms$^{-1}$ and sensitivity to histamine and acetylcholine injected into the right side of the heart. These receptors can be sensitised (within the first breath) by volatile anaesthetics (Molony, 1974).

The role of these receptors, if any, in controlling respiratory function is unclear. If the respiratory system is inflated with gas containing $CO_2$ in similar concentration to that of end-expired gas (5-8%) thereby preventing increased discharge of intrapulmonary $CO_2$-sensitive receptors, apnoea is prevented and breathing frequency is only slightly decreased (Eaton *et al.*, 1971). That would suggest that mechanoreceptor discharge which would increase in the inflation may not be significant in controlling breathing. Because of the great distensibility of the air sacs, possibly only extremely feeble inspiration-inhibitory inflation reflexes, if any, can be demonstrated in birds within the physiological range of tidal volume and intrapulmonary pressure. There is only limited evidence for a vagally mediated reflex inhibition of breathing in response to inflation which is not dependent upon increased activity of $CO_2$-sensitive receptors (Eaton *et al.*, 1971; Leitner, 1972; Molony, 1974; Miller, 1978; Ballam *et al.*, 1984). The main difficulty in demonstrating such a reflex has been to stimulate or inhibit stretch receptors without, at the same time, either exciting or inhibiting $CO_2$-sensitive receptors or other receptors with actions on breathing. This problem can be overcome (Miller, 1978; Ballam *et al.*, 1981, 1982, 1984) by using unidirectional ventilation to clamp pulmonary $PCO_2$, and thus the activity of pulmonary $CO_2$-sensitive receptors, while changing the volume of the lower respiratory tract. Also, using a servo-system to clamp the pressure in the air sacs (Ballam *et al.*, 1984) allows the animal to inflate or deflate the air sacs with breathing movements without affecting intrapulmonary pressures. Recent evidence from such experiments (Miller, 1978; Ballam *et al.*, 1981, 1982, 1984) indicates that volume feedback may contribute to ventilatory timing in the chicken. Pressure loading experiments demonstrate that inspiratory and expiratory durations are altered by positive and negative loads (Ballam *et al.*, 1981). The effect of pressure loading on the timing of efferent motor output is dependent on an intact vagus, implicating the contribution of vagal mechanoreceptors. The dependence of inspiratory and expiratory durations on air-sac volume (Ballam *et al.*, 1982) is consistent with the time-dependent volume-threshold model currently popular in describing mammalian ventilatory behaviour (Euler, 1973; Bradley *et al.*, 1974). $CO_2$ influences the volume dependence of inspiratory and expiratory durations in the bird (Ballam *et al.*, 1982), indicating that inspiratory and expiratory phase durations are a function of both mechanical and chemical feedback. These findings are consistent with a hypothesis of convergence of the inputs of intrapulmonary $CO_2$-sensitive receptors and mechanoreceptors on the rhythm-generating mechanisms in the brainstem.

### 3.4.3. *Systemic arterial chemoreceptors*

That moderate changes in $P_aCO_2$ and $P_aO_2$ reflexly affect breathing in birds through systemic chemoreceptors was discussed by Jukes (1971). Receptors in the carotid bodies play a definite role in effecting these reflexes and controlling breathing in birds. The carotid bodies in birds are located in the thoracic cavity and receive their arterial supply from small branches of the common carotid arteries, and are innervated mainly by the vagus nerves.

Electrophysiological studies of afferent axons in the vagus assumed to originate in the carotid bodies have been carried out in chickens (Bouverot & Leitner, 1972) and ducks (Bamford & Jones, 1976; Nye & Powell, 1984). In normoxic conditions these receptors fired irregularly in short high-frequency bursts and their discharge frequency increased when arterial $PO_2$ was decreased or arterial $PCO_2$ was increased (Bouverot & Leitner, 1971), and during asphyxia in the duck (Bamford & Jones, 1976). The steady-state stimulus–response characteristics of arterial chemoreceptors to changes in arterial $PO_2$ and $PCO_2$ in the duck were very similar to those found in mammals (Nye & Powell, 1984), which suggests that both avian and mammalian chemoreceptors are excited by the same basic mechanism.

Transient increases of $PO_2$ in the arterial blood cause a decrease in the discharge frequency of arterial chemoreceptors which is accompanied in parallel time course by a decrease in the minute volume of ventilation (Bouverot & Leitner, 1972). Decreases in arterial $PO_2$ which stimulate arterial chemoreceptors elicit hyperventilation in birds, and the minute volume of ventilation is usually augmented mainly by increases in respiratory frequency (Butler, 1970; Bouverot *et al.*, 1974; Butler & Taylor, 1974). Intravenous injection of chemicals that stimulate the carotid body chemoreceptors in mammals, such as sodium cyanide, sodium dihydrogen phosphate, 2,4-dinitrophenol (2,4-DNP) and almitrine, also increase the activity of presumptive arterial chemoreceptor afferent vagal fibres in birds, and with short delay elicit hyperventilation (Bouverot & Leitner, 1972; Nye & Powell, 1984; Gleeson *et al.*, 1985; M. Gleeson, unpublished observations).

Nye & Powell (1984) located the receptive fields of three arterial chemoreceptor preparations by observing their responses to i.v. injections of 2,4-DNP before, during and after occlusion of various arteries. The responses of two preparations were consistent with their location in the ipsilateral carotid body, but the responses of one, containing two active fibres, suggested that its discharge originated in aortic bodies.

In awake ducks, after chronic denervation of the carotid bodies, no ventilatory changes are observed in the course of a transient hyperoxia (Jones & Purves, 1970) or hypoxia (Bouverot *et al.*, 1974). Thus the rapid ventilatory responses to changes in arterial $PO_2$ appear to require intact innervation of the carotid bodies. In birds, as in mammals, the hypoxic stimulus to ventilation appears to act on the central pattern generator exclusively through a peripheral chemoreflex mechanism originating in the carotid bodies.

Systemic arterial chemoreceptors in ducks (Jones & Purves, 1970; Bouverot *et al.*, 1974) and chickens (Bouverot & Leitner, 1972) play an important role in the ventilatory response to transient changes in $P_aCO_2$ and may play a role in the steady-state response to step changes in $P_aCO_2$. In conscious ducks after chronic denervation of the carotid bodies the ventilatory responses to transient hypercapnia are sluggish and reduced compared with the responses in intact animals (Jones & Purves, 1970; Bouverot *et al.*, 1974), similar to the effect of carotid body denervation in mammals (Dejours, 1975). In steady-state conditions in denervated ducks the relationship between ventilation and $P_aCO_2$ at various constant $P_aO_2$ values is shifted to higher $P_aCO_2$ values (viz. a higher $CO_2$ threshold) and its slope is greatly reduced (viz. reduced $CO_2$ sensitivity). In intact hypoxic ducks the ventilation/$P_aCO_2$ line is shifted to lower $P_aCO_2$ values and is steeper than in normoxic animals (Bouverot *et al.*, 1974). Thus, in ducks as in mammals (Dejours, 1962), the hypoxic and $CO_2-H^+$ blood stimuli interact positively through a peripheral chemoreflex mechanism.

Changes in $P_aCO_2$ without concomitant changes in intrapulmonary $PCO_2$ affect breathing; increasing $P_aCO_2$ increases ventilation by increasing tidal volume while there is a concurrent decrease in respiratory frequency (Osborne *et al.*, 1977a). Increases in intrapulmonary (airway) $PCO_2$ without concomitant changes in $P_aCO_2$ also increase the depth of breathing and decrease respiratory frequency (Burger *et al.*, 1978; Osborne & Mitchell, 1978). Interaction between the effects of changing arterial and pulmonary $PCO_2$ has been studied by Osborne & Mitchell (1978). They suggested that these two variables affect ventilation in different ways such as that they act synergistically with respect to changes in tidal volume and antagonistically with respect to changes in respiratory frequency. This interaction was found to be greater under hypocapnic conditions than under hypercapnic conditions.

Changes in $P_aCO_2$, $P_aO_2$ and $pH_a$ at each breath and the timing of the arrival of these oscillations at the systemic arterial chemoreceptors may have significant effects upon breathing in mammals (Cross *et al.*, 1979). Oscillations of arterial blood gases and pH have not been investigated in birds, but changes in $P_aCO_2$, $P_aO_2$ and $pH_a$ at each breath may be expected to be less than in mammals due to the almost continuous ventilation of the lung of birds. Some oscillations may exist since gas flow through the lung during the respiratory cycle is not constant. A consequence of this could be that the sensitivity of the arterial chemoreceptors is greater in order to detect the changes present, although this does not appear to be the case in the duck (Nye & Powell, 1984), the arterial chemoreceptors of which showed steady-state stimulus–response characteristics remarkably similar to those of the cat (Lahiri & Delaney, 1975). Alternatively a signal may be generated by other receptors such as the $CO_2$-sensitive receptors in the lungs.

### 3.4.4. *Other receptors with vagal axons*

There are probably many other types of receptor with vagal axons that influence respiration in birds. Dawes & Mott (1950) showed that intravenous injection of certain amidines (e.g. phenyl diguanide) into cats causes apnoea followed by rapid shallow breathing. The response was named the pulmonary respiratory chemoreflex, and it has been established for the cat that phenyl diguanide works mainly by stimulating alveolar nociceptive (type J) receptors with vagal non-myelinated nerve fibres (Paintal, 1969). A similar vagally mediated respiratory chemoreflex has been demonstrated in the chicken (Molony, 1972) and goose (Callanan *et al.*, 1974). The site and nature of the receptors stimulated by phenyl diguanide in the bird have not been determined, but it is possible that both birds and mammals have similar visceral nociceptive systems in the lungs which give rise to similar vagally mediated reflex responses.

Some electrophysiological recordings of afferent vagal nerve fibre activity in birds are claimed to originate from receptors in the heart (Jones, 1969; Estavillo & Burger, 1973). At normal arterial blood pressure the majority of these receptors discharge with each heart beat, the proportion of receptors with irregular discharge patterns decreasing markedly as the arterial blood pressure is raised (Estavillo & Burger, 1973). Somewhat imprecise attempts at localisation have shown that the main receptor area for this activity is in the ventricle near the base of the aorta in the region of the aortic valve (Jones, 1969; Estavillo & Burger, 1973). This is extremely close to, and may be identical with, the main grouping of systemic arterial baroreceptors at the base of the aorta (Jones, 1969), so it is possible that much of the so-called cardiac afferent vagal activity originates from baroreceptors (West *et al.*, 1981). Increased discharge of vagal ventricular baroreceptors has been shown to decrease respiratory movements in the chicken (Estavillo & Youther, 1978). Transient increases in arterial blood pressure which increase the rate of baroreceptor activity produce a decrease in respiratory movements for the duration of the pressure increase.

Some authors have reported slowly adapting mechanosensitive receptors with vagal axons that increase their activity during expiration (King *et al.*,

1968; Jones, 1979; Molony, 1972). However, as mentioned previously the location of such receptors, firing in phase with respiration, cannot be inferred from recordings of vagal activity since such activity could be produced by pressure receptors in almost any visceral organ or by other receptors stimulated by movements of the body wall as the animal breathes.

## 3.5. Summary

The respiratory system of birds consists of a pair of inexpansible lungs that are ventilated by a series of air sacs. In the intact bird, air flows through the lungs in the same direction in inspiration and expiration, and it is possible, by cannulating the trachea and air sacs, to artificially unidirectionally ventilate the animal.

Because the avian vagus contains afferent fibres from mechanoreceptors and chemoreceptors inside the thoracoabdominal cavity, either or both of these could be implicated in the peripheral control of respiratory pattern. As far as chemoreceptors are concerned, there is now strong evidence that the specifically $CO_2$-sensitive intrapulmonary chemoreceptors can affect the rate and depth of breathing. It has been suggested that these receptors act as the afferent limb of an inspiratory–inhibitory reflex which uses the rate and extent of $CO_2$ washout from the lung as the sensory signal rather than the rate and extent of lung expansion. Mechanoreceptors, possibly located in the air-sac walls or associated membranes, may also have inspiratory–inhibitory reflex effects.

Physiological observations have demonstrated the ventilatory effects of a mammalian-like peripheral systemic arterial chemoreceptor system in birds, innervated mainly by the vagus nerves.

There are probably other types of receptor with vagal axons that influence respiration in birds. A vagally mediated baroreceptor reflex exists, and birds appear to have a mammalian-like visceral nociceptive system in the lungs which gives rise to a vagally mediated reflex response. The receptors responsible for the latter reflex have not yet been identified.

## References

Abdel-Magied, E. M. (1978a). Accessory carotid body tissue of the domestic fowl. *J. Anat.* **126**, 430.

Abdel-Magied, E. M. (1978b). Encapsulated sensory receptors in the wall of the avian common carotid artery. *J. Anat.* **127**, 196–7.

Abdel-Magied, E. M. & King, A. S. (1978). The topographical anatomy and blood supply of the carotid body region of the domestic fowl. *J. Anat.* **126**, 535–46.

Ballam, G. O., Clanton, T. L. & Kunz, A. L. (1982). Ventilatory phase duration in the chicken: role of mechanical and $CO_2$ feedback. *J. Appl. Physiol.* **53**, 1378–85.

Ballam, G. O., Clanton, T. L. & Kunz, A. L. (1984). Ventilatory pressure loading at constant pulmonary $FCO_2$ in *Gallus domesticus*. *Resp. Physiol.* **58**, 197–206.

Ballam, G. O., Kunz, A. L., Clanton, T. L. & Michal, E. K. (1981). A stretch reflex in chickens at constant $F_{LCO2}$. *Fed. Proc.* **40**, 453.

Bamford, O. S. & Jones, D. R. (1976). The effects of asphyxia on afferent activity recorded from the cervical vagus in the duck. *Pflügers Arch.* **366**, 95–9.

Banzett, R. B. & Burger, R. E. (1977). Response of avian intrapulmonary chemoreceptors to venous $CO_2$ and ventilatory gas flow. *Resp. Physiol.* **29**, 63–72.

Barnas, G. M., Mather, F. B. & Fedde, M. R. (1978). Are avian intrapulmonary $CO_2$ receptors chemically modulated mechanoreceptors or chemoreceptors? *Resp. Physiol.* **35**, 237–43.

Bennett, T. & Malmfors, T. (1970). The adrenergic nervous system of the domestic fowl. *Z. Zellforsch. mikrosk. Anat.* **106**, 22.

Berger, P. J. (1981). Changes in ventilatory flow rate in ducks in response to a single inspiration of air containing 5% $CO_2$. *Resp. Physiol.* **43**, 241–8.

Berger, P. J., Tallman, R. D. & Kunz, A. L. (1980). Discharge of intrapulmonary chemoreceptors and its modulation by rapid $FI_{CO_2}$ changes in decerebrate ducks. *Resp. Physiol.* **42**, 123–30.

Boon, J. K., Fedde, M. R. & Scheid, P. (1982). A method for localizing intrapulmonary chemoreceptors in the parabronchial mantle of the duck. *Comp. Biochem. Physiol.* **72A**, 463–8.

Boon, J. K., Kuhlmann, W. O. & Fedde, M. R. (1980). Control of respiration in the chicken: effects of venous $CO_2$ loading. *Resp. Physiol.* **39**, 169–81.

Bouverot, P. (1978). Control of breathing in birds compared with mammals. *Physiol. Rev.* **58**, 604–55.

Bouverot, P. & Dejours, P. (1971). Pathway of respired gas in the air sacs–lung apparatus of fowl and ducks. *Resp. Physiol.* **13**, 330–42.

Bouverot, P. & Leitner, L.-M. (1972). Arterial chemoreceptors in the domestic fowl. *Resp. Physiol.* **15**, 310–20.

Bouverot, P. & Sébert, P. H. (1979). $O_2$-chemoreflex drive of ventilation in awake birds at rest. *Resp. Physiol.* **37**, 201–18.

Bouverot, P., Hill, N. & Jammes, Y. (1974). Ventilatory responses to $CO_2$ in intact and chronically chemodenervated Peking ducks. *Resp. Physiol.* **22**, 137–56.

Bower, A. J., Molony, V. & Brown, C. M. (1975). An autoradiographic technique for demonstration of the vagal afferent innervation of the lower respiratory tract of *Gallus domesticus*. *Experientia* **31**, 620–2.

Brackenbury, J. H. (1974). Pressure relationships of airflow in the avian respiratory system, and their influence on haemodynamics. Ph.D. thesis, University of Cambridge, UK.

Brackenbury, J. H. (1981). Airflow and respired gases within the lung–airsac system of birds. *Comp. Biochem. Physiol.* **68A**, 1–8.

Bradley, G. W., Euler, C. von, Marttila, I. & Roos, B. (1975). A model of the central and reflex inhibition of inspiration in the cat. *Biol. Cybernet.* **19**, 105–16.

Burger, R. E. & Estavillo, J. A. (1978). The alteration of $CO_2$ respiratory sensitivity in chickens by thoracic visceral denervation. *Resp. Physiol.* **32**, 251–63.

Burger, R. E. & Lorenz, F. W. (1960). Artificial respiration in birds by unidirectional air flow. *Poultry Sci.* **39**, 236–7.

Burger, R. E., Barker, M. R. Nye, P. C. G. & Powell, F. L. (1978). Effects of intrapulmonary chemoreceptors in perfused and non-perfused lungs. In *Respiratory Function in Birds, Adult and Embryonic*, pp. 156–63 (ed. J. Piiper). New York: Springer.

Burger, R. E., Coleridge, J. C. G., Coleridge, H. M., Nye, P. C. G., Powell, F. L., Ehlers, C. & Banzett, R. B. (1976a). Chemoreceptors in the paleopulmonic lung of the emu: discharge patterns during cyclic ventilation. *Resp. Physiol.* **28**, 249–59.

Burger, R. E., Nye, P. C. G., Powell, F. L., Ehlers, C., Barker, M. & Fedde, M. R. (1976b). Response to $CO_2$ of intrapulmonary chemoreceptors in the emu. *Resp. Physiol.* **28**, 315–24.

Burger, R. E., Osborne, J. L. & Banzett, R. G. (1974). Intrapulmonary chemoreceptors in *Gallus domesticus*: adequate stimulus and functional localization. *Resp. Physiol.* **22**, 87–98.

Butler, P. J. (1970). The effect of progressive hypoxia on the respiratory and cardiovascular systems of the pigeon and duck. *J. Physiol. Lond.* **211**, 527–38.

Butler, P. J. & Taylor, E. W. (1974). Responses of the respiratory and cardiovascular system of chickens and pigeons to changes in $PaO_2$ and $PaCO_2$. *Resp. Physiol.* **21**, 351–63.

Callanan, D., Dixon, M., Widdicombe, J. C. & Wise, J. C. M. (1974). Responses of geese to inhalation of irritant gases and injections of phenyl diguanide. *Resp. Physiol.* **22**, 157–66.

Cohen, M. I. (1964). Respiratory periodicity in the paralysed, vagotomized cat: hypocapnic polypnea. *Am. J. Physiol.* **206**, 845–54.

Crank, W. D., Kuhlmann, W. D. & Fedde, M. R. (1980). Functional localization of avian intrapulmonary $CO_2$ receptors within the parabronchial mantle. *Resp. Physiol.* **41**, 71–85.

Cross, B. A., Grant, B. J. B., Guz, A., Jones, P. W., Semple, S. J. G. & Stidwell, R. P. (1979). Dependence of phrenic motoneurone output on the oscillatory component of arterial blood gas composition. *J. Physiol. Lond.* **290**, 163–84.

Dawes, G. S. & Mott, J. C. (1950). Circulatory and respiratory reflexes caused by aromatic guanidines. *Brit. J. Pharmacol.* **5**, 65–76.

Dejours, P. (1962). Chemoreflexes in breathing. *Physiol. Rev.* **42**, 335–58.

Dejours, P. (1975). *Principles of Comparative Respiratory Physiology*, p. 253. Amsterdam: North-Holland.

Duncker, H. R. (1971). The lung air sac system of birds. *Ergebs. Anat. Entwicklungsgesch.* **45**, Heft 6.

Eaton, J. A., Fedde, M. R. & Burger, R. E. (1971). Sensitivity to inflation of the respiratory system of the chicken. *Resp. Physiol.* **11**, 167–77.

Estavillo, J. A. & Burger, R. E. (1973). Avian cardiac receptors: activity changes by blood pressure, carbon dioxide and pH. *Am. J. Physiol.* **225**, 1067.

Estavillo, J. A. & Youther, M. L. (1978) Effect of middle cardiac nerve stimulation upon the respiratory response to $PaCO_2$ in the chicken. In *Respiratory Function in Birds, Adult and Embryonic*, pp. 175–81 (ed. J. Piiper). New York: Springer-Verlag.

Euler, C. von (1983). On the central pattern generator for the basic breathing rhythmicity. *J. Appl. Physiol.* **55**, 1647–59.

Farber, P. J. (1982). Pulmonary receptor discharge and expiratory muscle activity. *Resp. Physiol.* **47**, 219–29.

Fedde, M. R. & Burger, R. E. (1962). A gas heating and humidifying accessory for the unidirectional respirator. *Poultry Sci.* **51**, 679.

Fedde, M. R. & Peterson, D. R. (1970) Intrapulmonary receptor responses to changes in airway-gas composition in *Gallus domesticus*. *J. Physiol. Lond.* **209**, 609–25.

Fedde, M. R. & Scheid, P. (1976). Intrapulmonary $CO_2$ receptors in the duck. IV. Discharge pattern of the population during a respiratory cycle. *Resp. Physiol.* **26**, 223–7.

Fedde, M. R. Burger, R. E. & Kitchell, R. L. (1963a). Localization of vagal afferents involved in the maintenance of normal avian respiration. *Poultry Sci.* **42**, 1224–36.

Fedde, M. R., Burger, R. E. & Kitchell, R. L. (1963b). The effect of anesthesia and age on respiration following bilateral, cervical vagotomy in the fowl. *Poultry Sci.* **42**, 1212–23.

Fedde, M. R., Burger, R. E. & Kitchell, R. L. (1964). Electromyographic studies of the effects of bilateral, cervical vagotomy on the action of the respiratory muscles of the domestic cock. *Poultry Sci.* **43**, 1119–25.

Fedde, M. R., Gatz, R. N., Slama, H. & Scheid, P. (1974a). Intrapulmonary $CO_2$ receptors in the duck. I. Stimulus specificity. *Resp. Physiol.* **22**, 99–114.

Fedde, M. R., Gatz, R. M., Slama, H. & Scheid, P. (1974b) Intrapulmonary $CO_2$ receptors in the duck. II. Comparison with mechanoreceptors. *Resp. Physiol.* **22**, 115–21.

Fedde, M. R., Kiley, J. P., Powell, F. L. & Scheid, P. (1982). Intrapulmonary $CO_2$ receptors and control of breathing in ducks: effects of prolonged circulation time to carotid bodies and brain. *Resp. Physiol.* **47**, 121–40.

Gleeson, M. (1985). Changes in intrapulmonary chemoreceptor discharge in response to the adjustment of respiratory pattern during hyperventilation in domestic fowl. *Quart. J. Exp. Physiol.* **70**, 503–13.

Gleeson, M., Haigh, A. L., Molony, V. & Anderson, L. S. (1985). Ventilatory and cardiovascular responses of the unanaesthetized chicken, *Gallus domesticus*, to the respiratory stimulants etamiphylline and almitrine. *Comp. Biochem. Physiol.* **81c**, 367–74.

Graham, J. D. P. (1940). Respiratory reflexes in the fowl. *J. Physiol. Lond.* **97**, 525–32.

Greco, E. C., Jr. Fordyce, W. E., Gonzalez, F., Jr, Reischl, P. and Grodins, F. S. (1978). Respiratory responses to intravenous and intrapulmonary $CO_2$ in awake dogs. *J. Appl. Physiol.* **45**, 109–14.

Groth, H.-P. (1972). Licht und fluoreszenmikroscopische Untersuchungen zur Innervation des Luftsacksystems der Vögel. *Z. Zellforsch. mikrosk. Anat.* **127**, 87–115.

Hempelman, S. C. & Burger, R. E. (1984). Receptive fields of intrapulmonary chemoreceptors in the Pekin duck. *Resp. Physiol.* **57** 317–30.

Hodges, R. D., King, A. S., King, D. Z. & French, E. I. (1975). The general ultra-structure of the carotid body of the domestic fowl. *Cell Tiss. Res.* **162**, 483–97.

Jones, D. R. (1969). Avian afferent vagal activity related to respiratory and cardiac cycles. *Comp. biochem Physiol.* **28**, 961–5.

Jones, D. R. (1976). The control of breathing in birds with particular reference to the initiation and maintenance of diving apnoea. *Fed. Proc.* **35**, 1975–82.

Jones, D. R. & Bamford, O. S. (1976). Open-loop respiratory chemosensitivity in chickens and ducks. *Am. J. Physiol.* **230**, 861–7.

Jones, D. R. & Purves, M. J. (1970). The effect of carotid body denervation upon the respiratory response to hypoxia and hypercapnia in the duck. *J. Physiol. Lond.* **211**, 295–309.

Jukes, M. G. M. (1971). Control of respiration. In *Physiology and Biochemistry of the Domestic Fowl* vol. 1, pp. 171–85. (eds D. J. Bell & B. M. Freeman. New York: Academic Press.

Kadono, J., Okada, T. & Ono, K (1963). Electromyographic studies on the respiratory muscles of the chicken. *Poultry Sci.* **42**, 121–8.

King, A. S. (1966). Afferent pathways in the vagus and their influence on avian breathing: a review. In *Physiology of the Domestic Fowl*, pp. 302–10 (eds C. Horton-Smith & E. C. Amoroso). Edinburgh: Oliver & Boyd.

King, A. S. (1975). Aves, respiratory system. In *The Anatomy of the Domestic Animals*, 5th edn, Chapter 64 (ed. Getty) Philadelphia, PA: Saunders.

King, A. S. & Molony, V. (1971). The anatomy of respiration. In *Physiology and Biochemistry of the Domestic Fowl* pp. 93–169 (eds D. J. Bell & B. M. Freeman). New York: Academic Press.

King, A. S., King, D. Z., Hodges, R. D. & Henry, J. (1975). Synaptic morphology of the carotid body of the domestic fowl. *Cell Tiss. Res.* **162**, 459–73.

King, A. S., McClelland, J., Cock, R. D., King, D. Z. & Walsh, C. (1974). the ultrastructure of afferent nerve endings in the avian lung. *Resp. Physiol.* **22**, 21–40.

King, A. S., McClelland, J., Molony, V. & Mortimer, M. F. (1969). Respiratory afferent activity in the avian vagus: eupnea, inflation and deflation. *J. Physiol. Lond.* **201**, 35–6P.

King, A. S., Molony, V., McClelland, J., Bowsher, D. R. & Mortimer, M. F. (1968). Afferent respiratory pathways in the avian vagus. *Experientia* **24**, 1017–18.

Lahiri, S. & Delaney, R. G. (1975). Stimulus interaction in the response of carotid body chemoreceptor single afferent fibres. *Resp. Physiol.* **24**, 249–66.

Leitner, L.-M. (1972). Pulmonary mechanoreceptor fibres in the vagus of the domestic fowl. *Resp. Physiol.* **16**, 232–44.

Leitner, L.-M. & Roumy, M. (1974). Vagal afferent activities related to the respiratory cycle in the duck: sensitivity to mechanical, chemical and electrical stimuli. *Resp. Physiol.* **22**, 41–56.

Lewis, S. M. (1975). Awake baboon's ventilatory response to venous and inhaled $CO_2$ loading. *J. Appl. Physiol.* **39**, 417–22.

McClelland, J. (1970). The innervation of the air passages of the avian lung and observations on afferent vagal pathways concerned in the regulation of breathing. Ph.D. thesis, University of Liverpool, UK.

McClelland, J. & Molony, V. (1983). Respiration. In *Physiology and Biochemistry of the Domestic Fowl* vol. 4, pp. 63–89 (ed. B. M. Freeman). London: Academic Press.

Miller, D. A. (1978). Effect of stretch on the respiratory pattern of a chicken. In *Respiratory Function in Birds, Adult and Embryonic*, pp. 188–95. (ed. J. Piiper). New York: Springer Verlag.

Miller, D. A. & Kunz, A. L. (1977). Evidence that a cyclic rise in avian pulmonary $CO_2$ triggers the next inspiration. *Resp. Physiol.* **31**, 193–202.

Milsom, W. K., Jones, D. R. & Gabbott, G. R. J. (1981). On chemoreceptor control of ventilatory responses to $CO_2$ in unanaesthetized ducks. *J. Appl. Physiol.* **50**, 1121–8.

Mitchell, G. S. & Osborne, J. L. (1979). Ventilatory responses to carbon dioxide inhalation after vagotomy in chickens. *Resp. Physiol.* **37**, 81–8.

Molony, V. (1972). A study of vagal afferent activity in phase with breathing and its role in the control of breathing in *Gallus domesticus*. Ph.D. thesis, University of Liverpool, UK.

Molony, V. (1974). Classification of vagal afferents firing in phase with breathing in *Gallus domesticus*. *Resp. Physiol.* **22**, 57–76.

Nye, P. C. G. & Burger, R. E. (1978). Chicken intrapulmonary chemoreceptors: discharge at static levels of intrapulmonary carbon dioxide and their location. *Resp. Physiol.* **33**, 299–322.

Nye, P. C. G. & Powell, F. L. (1984). Steady-state discharge and bursting of arterial chemoreceptors in the duck. *Resp. Physiol.* **56**, 369–84.

Osborne, J. L. & Burger, R. E. (1974). Intrapulmonary chemoreceptors in *Gallus domesticus*. *Resp. Physiol.* **22**, 75–85.

Osborne, J. L. & Mitchell, G. S. (1978). Intrapulmonary and systemic $CO_2$ chemoreceptor interaction in the control of avian respiration. *Resp. Physiol.* **33**, 349–57.

Osborne, J. L., Burger, R. E. & Stoll, P. J. (1977a). Dynamic responses of $CO_2$-sensitive avian intrapulmonary chemoreceptors. *Am. J. Physiol.* **233**, R15–22.

Osborne, J. L. Mitchell, G. S. & Powell, F. L. (1977b). Ventilatory responses to $CO_2$ in the chicken: intrapulmonary and systemic chemoreceptors. *Resp. Physiol.* **30**, 369–82.

Osborne, M. P. & Butler, P. J. (1975). New theory for receptor mechanism of carotid body chemoreceptors. *Nature, London* **254**, 701–3.

Paintal, A. S. (1969). Mechanism of stimulation of type J pulmonary receptors. *J. Physiol. London* **203**, 511–32.

Peterson, D. F. & Fedde, M. R. (1968). Receptors sensitive to carbon dioxide in lungs of chicken. *Science* **162**, 1499–1501.

Peterson, D. F. & Fedde, M. R. (1971). Avian intrapulmonary $CO_2$-sensitive receptors: a comparative study. *Comp. Biochem. Physiol.* **40A**, 425–30.

Powell, F. L., Barker, M. R. & Burger, R. E. (1980). Ventilatory response to the $PCO_2$ profile in chicken lungs. *Resp. Physiol.* **35**, 361–72.

Powell, F. L., Fedde, M. R., Gratz, R. K. & Scheid, P. (1978). Ventilatory response to $CO_2$ in birds. I. Measurements in the unanaesthetised duck. *Resp. Physiol.* **35**, 349–59.

Richards, S. A. (1968). Vagal control of thermal panting in mammals and birds. *J. Physiol. London* **199**, 89–101.

Richards, S. A. (1969). Vagal function during respiration and the effects of vagotomy in the domestic fowl (*Gallus domesticus*). *Comp. Biochem. Physiol.* **29**, 955–64.

Scheid, P., Slama, H., Gratz, R. K. & Fedde, M. R. (1974). Intrapulmonary chemoreceptors in the duck: III. Functional localization. *Resp. Physiol.* **22**, 123–36.

Scheid, P., Gratz, R. K., Powell, F. L. & Fedde, M. R. (1978). Ventilatory response to $CO_2$ in birds. II. Contribution by intrapulmonary $CO_2$ receptors. *Resp. Physiol.* **35**, 361–72.

Tallman, R. D. & Grodins, F. S. (1982a). Intrapulmonary $CO_2$ receptors and ventilatory response to lung $CO_2$ loading. *J. Appl. Physiol.* **52**, 1272–7.

Tallman, R. D. & Grodins, F. S. (1982b). Intrapulmonary $CO_2$ receptor discharge at different levels of venous $PCO_2$. *J. Appl. Physiol.* **53**, 1386–91.

Tallman, R. D. & Kunz, A. L. (1982). Changes in breathing pattern mediated by intrapulmonary $CO_2$ receptors in chickens. *J. Appl. Physiol.* **52**, 162–7.

Walsh, C. & McClelland, J. (1978). The development of the epithelium and its innervation in the avian extra-pulmonary respiratory tract. *J. Anat.* **125**, 171–82.

West, N. H., Lowell Langille, B. & Jones, D. R. (1981). Cardiovascular system. In *Form and Function in Birds*, vol. 2, pp. 235–339 (eds A. S. King & J. McClelland). London: Academic Press.

Widdicombe, J. G. (1964). Respiratory reflexes. In *Handbook of Physiology. Respiration*, vol. I, Chapter 24. (eds W. O. Fenn & H. Rahn). Washington, DC: American Physiological Society.

# 4

# Neural control of gill ventilation in decapod Crustacea

**B. M. H. Bush**[1]**, A. J. Simmers**[2] **and V. M. Pasztor**[3]

[1]*Department of Physiology, University of Bristol, Bristol BS1 5LS, UK;* [2]*C. N. R. S. Laboratoire de Neurobiologie et Physiologie Comparées, Arcachon, France;* [3]*Department of Biology, McGill University, Montreal, Canada*

## 4.1. Introduction

Respiratory gas exchange in crabs, lobsters and other large decapod Crustacea takes place over the gills, which lie beneath the carapace and are attached at the bases of the walking legs and chelipeds. Ventilation of the gills results from a water current which enters the gill chamber at the limb bases and leaves through two exhalent apertures located rostrally beneath the eyecups. Occasionally the direction of water flow reverses. These 'reversals' may serve to clean the gills, or promote ventilation in hypoxic conditions.

The water currents are produced by the rhythmic beating of the bilateral pair of scaphognathites, or 'gill bailers', the horizontally flattened, longi-tudinally elongated, exopodite 'blades' of the second maxillae. The longi-tudinal undulations of the scaphognathites propel the surrounding water anteriorly on both the upstroke (levation) and downstroke (depression). These movements are produced by two antagonistic sets of muscles, five levators and five depressor muscles. Each muscle is innervated by two or three excitatory motoneurones, making up a total population of a dozen or so motoneurones for each direction of movement. Periodic bursts of impulses occurring in antiphase in the levator and depressor motoneurones elicit alternating contractions of their respective muscle groups. The resulting movements are monitored and probably regulated by various mechanorecep-tors of the second maxillae, notably a stretch receptor within the scaph-ognathite, the 'oval organ'.

This chapter is concerned with central and peripheral components of the neural control of the ventilatory rhythm, and the mechanisms of switching between forward and reversed beating. A brief description of the typical motor output patterns, as recorded electrophysiologically with extracellular electrodes on the motor nerves, will precede an analysis from intracellular microelectrode recordings of the physiological characteristics of the different types of motoneurones and interneurones implicated in ventilatory motor pattern generation. The roles of descending 'command' interneurones in the circumoesophageal connectives from the brain (cerebral ganglion) to the suboesophageal ganglion containing the central pattern generator (CPG) for ventilation will be outlined. The principal mechanoreceptor input from the scaphognathite will be described, but chemosensory control, e.g. by oxygen or $CO_2$ receptors, will not be considered since little is known about its neural mechanisms. The possible involvement of certain neurohormones at various sites in the ventilatory system will also be briefly discussed.

Most of the experiments on the neural basis of ventilatory motor pattern generation were carried out on the common shore crab, *Carcinus maenas*, whereas those on the oval organ were done mainly on the lobster, *Homarus gammarus*. However, comparative studies on other species suggest that the main conclusions apply to all Decapoda Reptantia. Our major findings in the crab are reviewed in Simmers (1981) and Simmers & Bush (1985); more detailed accounts can be found in Simmers & Bush (1980, 1983*a*, b). Other reviews covering selected aspects of respiratory (and circulatory) control in Crustacea appear under 'Core readings'.

## 4.2. Ventilatory motor output pattern

The motoneurones innervating the muscles of each scaphognathite lie within the ipsilateral suboesophageal ganglion, anteriorly in the fused thoracic ganglionic mass (Fig. 4.1b). This is shown by cobalt backfilling of the cut central ends of the two main motor nerves to the scaphognathite, the 'levator nerve' (LN) and the 'depressor nerve' (DN), innervating the levator and depressor muscles, respectively. The procedure reveals a well defined neuropilar plexus of cell bodies and dendritic processes, with no gross anatomical separation of levator and depressor motoneurones (Fig. 4.1c).

Extracellular recordings made *in situ* from the exposed but otherwise intact levator and depressor nerves reveal alternating bursts of impulses of several units in each nerve (Fig. 4.1d). These bursts correspond closely to the alternating levation and depression movements of the ipsilateral scaphognathite. The different individual motoneurones fire with characteristic phase relations in each burst. Overall burst frequency is generally about 0·5–2 per second, this being within the normal range of forward beat frequencies of the gill bailers in the intact animal. The burst frequencies on the two sides of the animal commonly differ somewhat, showing at most only loose bilateral coupling (Wilkens & Young, 1975; Best, 1982: see also Figs 4.4e, 4.7b). Occasionally the burst frequency spontaneously increases, and the spike patterns within the bursts change, to those characteristic of reversed beating. These two principal burst patterns are represented diagrammatically in Fig. 4.1a.

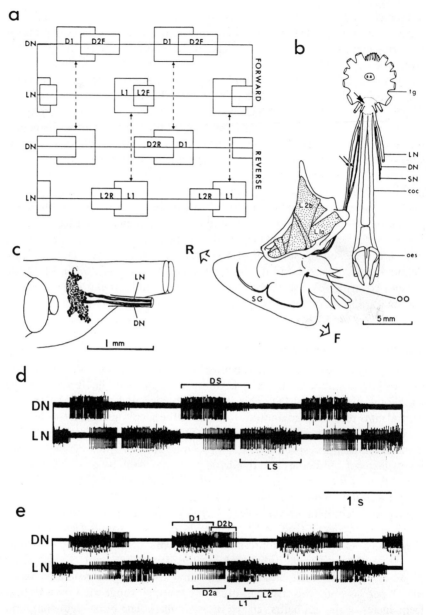

Fig. 4.1.   Anatomy and discharge patterns of ventilatory motoneurones in the crab, *Carcinus maenas*. (a) Diagram of the relative timing of the bursts of impulses in the main functional subgroups of depressor (D) and levator (L) motoneurones during forward and reverse ventilation (see text for further explanation). (b) Gross anatomy of the ventilatory nervous system, showing: the position of the ventilatory neuropile (large arrow) anteriorly in the thoracic ganglion (tg) complex; the *levator nerve* (LN) and the *depressor nerve* (DN) carrying motor axons to the *scaphognathite* (SG) — two

Virtually identical patterns of rhythmic motor output can be recorded from the cut central ends of the levator and depressor nerves in the completely isolated thoracic central nervous system of the crab (Fig. 4.1e). This implies the existence of a 'central pattern generator' (CPG) for ventilatory activity, located within the thoracic ganglia. Since all the segmental ganglia in crabs are fused into one ganglionic mass, it is difficult experimentally to isolate individual ganglia. However, evidence from intra-cellular recordings (see below) strongly implicates the ipsilateral suboeso-phageal ganglion as the locus of the CPG for the motor output to each scaphognathite, specifically the region demarcated by cobalt backfilling of the ventilatory nerves, referred to above (see Fig. 4.1c). For convenience this region will be termed the 'ventilatory rhythm centre' (VRC). It should be emphasised, however, that other parts of the crab's nervous system can also influence ventilation.

### 4.2.1. *Intracellular recordings from motoneurones*

The neurones most commonly encountered by microelectrodes impaling cells within the VRC are ventilatory motoneurones. They are identified as levator or depressor motoneurones by (a) the 1:1 correlation of their spikes with those of a 'unit' in the corresponding peripheral nerve; (b) the excitatory or inhibitory effects on the peripherally recorded unit, of positive or negative current, respectively, injected into the cell through the recording micro-electrode (using a bridge circuit) (Figs 4.2, 4.5 and 4.6). In the resting, non-rhythmic condition, ventilatory motoneurones usually show a resting membrane potential between $-50$ and $-60$ mV. During the expression of rhythmic motor output they exhibit large, 15–25 mV oscillations in mem-brane potential at the frequency of the prevailing rhythm. Levator and depressor motoneurones depolarise and produce spikes in phase with the

levator muscles are labelled; the sensory nerve (SN), with the three large afferents from the *oval organ* (OO); and the circumoesophageal connectives (coc) which run round the oesophagus (oes) to the brain. (c) Central projections and cell bodies of the levator and depressor motoneurones (right side view) as shown by cobalt backfilling. (d) Typical burst patterns recorded *in situ* from the depressor (DN) and levator (LN) nerves (at the points indicated by small arrows in b) during rhythmic ventilatory movements of the ipsilateral scaphognathite, showing the depressor (DS) and levator (LS) sessions of three complete beat cycles. (e) Similar burst patterns recorded from the central cut ends of the motor nerves in a completely *isolated central nervous system* preparation, with the two main component parts (1 and 2) of each burst indicated; the depressor unit D2a runs in the 'levator nerve' at the usual recording point (small arrows in b) and therefore appears in the LN trace. The relative spike sizes of the different motor axons varies between preparations, but the overall pattern of discharge closely resembles that seen in 'semi-intact' preparations (i.e. with all nerves intact). (From Simmers & Bush, 1983a, b.)

extracellularly recorded impulse bursts in LN (e.g. Fig. 4.2a, c) and DN (Fig. 4.2d), respectively.

The amplitude of the membrane potential oscillations is commonly increased during injection of depolarising (i.e. positive) current, while small hyperpolarising currents lead to reduced amplitude (Fig. 4.2b). With increasing negative currents the oscillations wane and disappear (Figs 4.2c, g), but then reappear at still greater current levels; now, however, they are reversed in phase, with the depolarising portions being in phase with the *antagonistic* motor impulse bursts (Fig. 4.2e). That is, the membrane has been driven through a 'reversal potential' for the slow waves (Figs 4.2c, g) which lies somewhat more negative than the resting potential.

This constitutes strong evidence for a chemical inhibitory synaptic input which periodically hyperpolarises the motoneurones at the frequency of the ventilatory rhythm. Two further experimental observations lend support to this hypothesis: (1) Spikes recorded intracellularly in a motoneurone on antidromic stimulation of the appropriate motor nerve during the hyperpolarising phase of the membrane potential oscillation were up to 75% smaller than those evoked during resting conditions; and (2) strong depolarising currents (up to 20 nA) injected into a motoneurone could not evoke orthodromic spikes when injected during the hyperpolarising phase, although less than 2 nA was often effective at other times (DiCaprio & Fourtner, 1984). These observations are most readily explained by a large increase in motoneurone membrane conductance during the hyperpolarising phase, such as could occur as a result of strong (inhibitory) chemical synaptic input. Periodic excitatory inputs in antiphase with the inhibition cannot as yet be ruled out but, if present, they must be considerably less potent to account for the observed changes produced by injected currents. Nevertheless some form of excitation seems likely in order to raise the membrane potential to the threshold for spike initiation, relative to the normal subthreshold resting potential seen in the quiescent, inactive condition. This may include purely tonic, non-rhythmic synaptic excitation superimposed upon the periodic inhibition, but postinhibitory rebound excitation of the motoneurones themselves probably also contributes to burst generation (see Section 4.5).

The question then arises as to whether the periodic inhibition is due to bursts of impulses in inhibitory pre-motor neurones, or to some form of slow, graded, non-spiking inhibitory input, as is known for other invertebrate motor systems (see e.g. Burrows & Siegler, 1978; Graubard, 1978; Raper, 1979). The absence of any discrete, unitary postsynaptic potentials, either excitatory or inhibitory, superimposed upon the slow oscillations (Figs 4.2b–e) favours the latter explanation. The 'spikes' riding on top of the depolarising phases are clearly not postsynaptic potentials but rather electrotonic reflections of all-or-none impulses in the motoneurone, since they are abruptly abolished, not increased (or decreased), by injection of

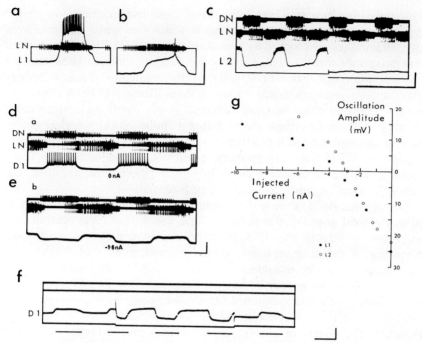

Fig. 4.2. Ventilatory motoneurone characteristics during spontaneous rhythmic activity, as revealed by intracellular recordings in the ventilatory neuropile, with simultaneous extracellular recordings from the motor nerves (DN and LN). (a) Single cycle of membrane potential oscillation in an L1 levator motoneurone, with spikes superimposed on the depolarising wave; (b) same cell during steady hyperpolarising current injection through the recording microelectrode so as to just block most impulses: note the absence of discrete postsynaptic potentials (and also the loss of the larger unit's spikes in the LN trace). (c) Cyclical activity in an L2 motoneurone (identified as such since its discharge is phase-locked to the later part of the extracellularly recorded levator bursts) is abolished by hyperpolarising current ($-3$ nA: bottom trace) which brings it to the 'reversal potential' for the slow waves. (d) Long plateau-like waves underlie spikes in a depressor motoneurone, active during the D1 phase of the rhythm; (e) these waves are phase-inverted by adequate hyperpolarising current ($-1.6$ nA here), which also suppresses the D1 spike (and the corresponding unit in the DN trace). (f) After addition of tetrodotoxin (TTX, 1 µM) to the bathing solution (same preparation as d, e) all impulses are now eliminated, yet the slow waves (sustained in this case by 100 nM dopamine — see text) can continue, and are still inverted in polarity by hyperpolarising current ($-2$ nA; bridge circuit not balanced; bars beneath record indicate expected times of depolarising phases in the absence of current). (g) Variation of slow wave amplitude with strength of negative current injected into the two levator (L1 and L2) motoneurones represented in a and c; with currents greater than $-3$ nA in each case the polarity (or phase) of the waves reverses. Calibrations: 20 mV (intracellular traces only); 1 s. (From Simmers & Bush, 1983a.)

hyperpolarising current (Fig. 4.2b). More definitive evidence for graded synaptic input comes from experiments in which slow waves continue even after all impulses are blocked by tetrodotoxin (Fig. 4.2f). Sometimes in such experiments the slow oscillations cease, but they can generally be reactivated by the addition of dopamine (100 µM), a neuromodulator with a facilitatory effect upon several crustacean motor systems (Raper, 1979; Anderson & Barker, 1981). Injection of steady currents in this condition causes similar changes to those described above before impulse block: the slow waves increase in amplitude with positive current, and reverse in sign (and hence phase: Fig. 4.2f) with hyperpolarising current, at the same membrane potential as that recorded previously in the presence of impulses (i.e. somewhat more negative than the resting potential).

The fact that the slow-wave oscillations in the motoneurones can occur at all in the total absence of impulses — and hence of discrete postsynaptic potentials — implies that they must be due to endogenous membrane properties of the motoneurones themselves, and/or to graded release of transmitter on to the motoneurones. The possibility that some form of unstable membrane properties in the motoneurones, in addition to the postinhibitory rebound mentioned above, may contribute to the potential oscillations in the motoneurones cannot be excluded (see Section 4.5). However, the effects of current injection into motoneurones upon the amplitude and sign of the slow waves are consistent with the hypothesis that periodic, graded, chemical inhibitory synaptic input to the motoneurones provides a major source of oscillatory drive. What is its origin?

### 4.3. 'Oscillator' interneurones underlying ventilatory rhythm

One of two functional types of interneurone found in the suboesophageal ganglion shows physiological characteristics well suited to providing the required periodic oscillatory drive to the motoneurones (Mendelson, 1971; Simmers & Bush, 1980). Both types lack axons and appear to be restricted to their own hemiganglion, so that they can be classified as *'local'* interneurones (Pearson, 1979; Siegler, 1984). They are moreover *non-spiking* neurones, since action potentials have never been recorded in these neurones, either on penetration by a microelectrode, or during expression of the ventilatory motor rhythm, or in response to depolarising currents up to 20 nA or more (in contrast to any of the nearby motoneurones, which discharge impulses in all these circumstances and with positive injected currents as small as 1–2 nA).

In the absence of rhythmic motor discharge in the peripherally recorded ventilatory motor nerves, both these types of local interneurone show stable, often quite low membrane potentials. During rhythmic motor output, however, the membrane potential of the first type oscillates with large slow waves, somewhat resembling those seen in some motoneurones but smaller in

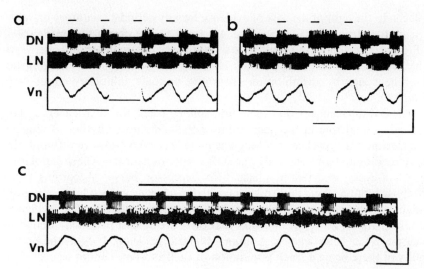

Fig. 4.3. Two non-spiking oscillator interneurones, showing membrane potential fluctuations (Vn) whose depolarising waves occur in phase with either levator (a and b) or (c) depressor motor bursts, recorded in the two extracellular traces. Depolarising (a) or hyperpolarising (b) current pulses injected into either cell (but not illustrated for the cell represented by c) reset the complete rhythm: short bars above the DN traces indicate when the D1 bursts would have occurred without the current pulses. (c) When the motor pattern for 'reversed ventilation' is spontaneously expressed (bar above record), the interneurone's membrane potential continues to oscillate, still with the same phase relationship to the extracellularly recorded rhythm. Calibrations: 10 mV, 1 s. (From Simmers & Bush, 1980, 1983b.)

amplitude, typically 8–12 mV at the site of impalement, and without any superimposed impulses (Fig. 4.3). As in the motoneurones, the oscillations are strictly phase-locked to the peripherally recorded motor rhythm, varying in frequency in precise, constant relationship to the motor bursts. A brief current pulse injected into this type of interneurone resets the whole rhythm, depending upon the polarity of the injected pulse and its timing in the cycle (Figs 4.3a, b; see also Simmers & Bush, 1980). This 'resetting' capacity is generally taken as a necessary criterion for the neurones in question being regarded as integral elements in any rhythm-generating network (see, for example, Calabrese & Peterson, 1983; Heitler, 1983).

Two sub-types of these *'oscillator' interneurones* can be distinguished. In one the depolarising phase of each oscillation coincides with the levator burst in each cycle (Figs 4.3a, b); in the other it is synchronous with the depressor burst (Fig. 4.3c). Depolarising each of these interneurones at any point in its activity cycle, or during quiescent, non-rhythmic periods, results in activation of those motoneurones which normally discharge during the interneurone's depolarising phase and simultaneous inhibition of the antagonistic motoneurones; hyperpolarising it tends to produce the reverse effects. In the light of the lack of evidence for any periodic excitatory drive to the motoneurones (but see Sections 4.2 and 4.5), the simplest interpretation of these effects involves reciprocal inhibitory interconnections between the two oscillator sub-types, thus allowing the activation of antagonistic motoneurones by disinhibition from the periodic inhibitory input (see Fig. 4.9).

These results suggest that these non-spiking oscillator interneurones play a fundamental role in the generation of the ventilatory rhythm. A similar conclusion was reached by Mendelson (1971) who, however, found (in hermit crabs and lobsters) only one such oscillator neurone, whose depolarising half-cycle occurred in phase with depressor bursts. Accordingly he proposed that a single non-spiking oscillator neurone in each hemi-ganglion might be the source of the complete ventilatory rhythm. The evidence outlined above, however, indicates that there are at least two such 'oscillator neurones' per hemi-segmental suboesophageal ganglion. Indeed, the possibility of there being a small population of each sub-type cannot be excluded on present evidence.

### 4.4. Frequency-modulating interneurones

As noted above, the repetition frequency of the impulse bursts recorded in the ventilatory motor nerves, and of the synchronous oscillations in the foregoing oscillator interneurones, varies over a limited range. Typical cycle periods in our partly or fully isolated nervous system preparations are $0·5-2$ s, but in intact animals a wider range is seen. *In vivo*, this variation in ventilatory rhythm frequency probably depends upon a variety of influences, including chemoreceptor and other sensory inputs, presumably serving to adapt the animal's respiratory performance to varying environmental factors and metabolic requirements (see McMahon & Wilkens, 1982; Taylor, 1982, for recent reviews covering these aspects).

Many if not all these influences on the frequency of the ventilatory rhythm may be integrated in and mediated by a second type of non-spiking, local interneurone encountered in the suboesophageal ganglion, an example of which is illustrated in Fig. 4.4c. In contrast to the foregoing oscillator interneurones, these latter interneurones exhibit only very small (0.5–2 mV) oscillations in membrane potential during expression of the ventilatory rhythm (Figs 4.4a, b, e). Brief current pulses have little or no overt effect, but maintained currents have a marked influence upon the overall rhythm frequency (or cycle period). They have accordingly been termed '*frequency-modulating interneurones*', and three sub-types of these neurones have been described, designated FM1, FM2 and FM3 (DiCaprio & Fourtner, 1983, 1987). The first type, FM1, physiologically identical to an interneurone described by Mendelson (1971) and by Simmers & Bush (1980), is excitatory in its effects, whereas FM2 and FM3 are both inhibitory.

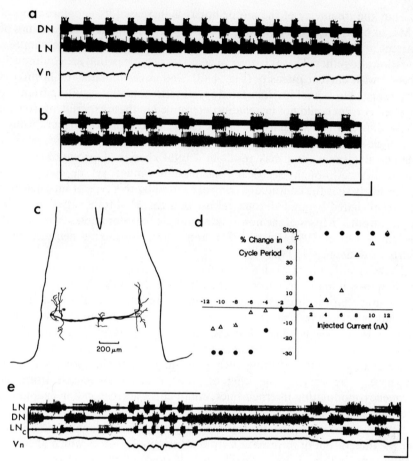

Fig. 4.4. Two non-spiking frequency-modulating interneurones (Vn), with either excitatory (a, b) or inhibitory (c–e) effects on the overall rhythm. (a) Depolarising, or (b) hyperpolarising, currents (bottom traces) injected into FM1 increase or decrease, respectively, the extracellularly recorded burst frequency. (c) Morphology of FM2 as revealed by Lucifer Yellow injection. (d) Variation in ventilatory cycle period with steady hyperpolarising (negative) and depolarising currents injected into FM2: note that cycle frequency *decreases* with increasing positive current, the rhythmic bursting eventually stopping with the higher currents; ● = ipsilateral, △ = contralateral to the impaled interneurone. (e) Modulation of membrane potential (Vn) of FM2 during a spontaneous 'reversal' (bar above record), followed by a brief arrhythmic period. Note the prolonged hyperpolarisation during the reversal period, and the transient small hyperpolarisations coincident with both ipsilateral (LN) and contralateral (LN$_c$) levator bursts. Calibrations: 10 mV, 1 s. (a, b from Simmers & Bush, 1980; c–e from R. A. DiCaprio & C. R. Fourtner, unpublished.)

Thus the frequency of the motor bursts is increased by depolarisation of FM1, or by hyperpolarisation of FM2 or FM3, while the reverse polarities of current in each case lower burst frequency or, if sufficiently intense, suppress bursting altogether. These changes in ventilatory cycle period are continously graded with current intensity (Fig. 4.4d), and cover most of the normal *in vivo* range. The actual interneuronal membrane potential resulting from the injected current could not be reliably determined in these experiments (owing to the difficulty of balancing the bridge circuit used to inject current through the single microelectrode), but it presumably varies directly with current over the effective range, and may result in a total change of potential of some 10–20 mV. Although electrical transmission cannot yet be rule out, it seems likely that the continuous control exerted by this type of interneurone is also mediated by graded, tonic release of a chemical transmitter, as in the tonic output synapses of the non-spiking muscle receptor afferents in the crab (Blight & Llinas, 1980; Bush, 1981), and other non-spiking neurones (e.g. Burrows & Siegler, 1978).

There is little direct evidence on the connectivity of these two types of local, non-spiking interneurones. The available data are consistent with the hypothesis that the latter, frequency-modulating interneurones feed directly or indirectly to the former, oscillator neurones to modulate their cycle period. If, as seems likely, the cyclical fluctuations in potential of the oscillator neurones depend upon some form of voltage-dependent conductance changes, simply shifting their prevailing membrane potential up or down, e.g. by varying the level of tonic transmitter release from the frequency-modulating interneurones, could effect corresponding changes in the oscillator frequency.

The frequency-modulating neurones might themselves constitute a locus for the integration of information from a variety of sources which affect the ventilatory rhythm. These probably include descending, higher order 'command' influences, various sensory inputs, neuromodulators, and recurrent feedback from motoneurones and other elements in the ventilatory system, and perhaps also other neural systems. These will be considered in the following sections.

### 4.5. Motoneurone involvement in ventilatory pattern generation

Evidence that some if not all ventilatory motoneurones themselves may contribute to the ventilatory motor pattern comes mainly from experiments in which current is injected into individual motoneurones. Four out of five possible types of influence have been observed, two being dependent upon intrinsic membrane properties of the motoneurones and three upon collateral or recurrent synaptic connections (Simmers & Bush, 1983a; DiCaprio & Fourtner, 1984).

### 4.5.1. *Intrinsic properties*

The first of these, postinhibitory rebound excitation, has been seen in many motoneurones following hyperpolarising pulses (Section 4.2). Though transient, this effect varies in intensity with the strength and duration of the negative current (see Simmers & Bush, 1983a, Fig. 5e–g), and probably reflects a graded reduction in the degree of spike inactivation at the prevailing membrane potential. Presumably it could contribute to normal spike generation following each hyperpolarising trough during the cyclical membrane potential oscillations underlying rhythmic bursting in the motoneurones.

A second endogenous property which might play a part in the ventilatory motor pattern is that in which certain voltage-dependent conductances (probably involving calcium and possibly potassium) result in a bistable condition in which adequate depolarising inputs initiate 'driver' or 'plateau potentials' (Benson & Cooke, 1984). Although tests have so far not yielded any definitive evidence for such a property, the shape of the oscillations recorded in some ventilatory motoneurones (e.g. Figs 4.2d, 4.5b) is quite reminiscent of membrane potential changes meeting the criteria for plateau potentials in other systems (see e.g. Sillar & Elson, 1986).

### 4.5.2. *Synaptic influences*

Some 10% of ventilatory motoneurones tested were found to have inhibitory effects upon one or more antagonistic motoneurones. Depolarising current injected into a depressor motoneurone, for example, not only elicits impulses in the impaled neurone itself but may also suppress ongoing tonic activity in levator motoneurones; this inhibition may be followed by transient rebound excitation of the levator cell. Such collateral inhibitory connections, however restricted in extent, would clearly help to reinforce the alternation of bursting in antagonistic motoneurones. Excitatory coupling between synergistic motoneurones has not been seen, but cannot be ruled out.

Secondly, brief current pulses of either polarity injected during the depolarising phase of a motoneurone's membrane potential oscillations can reset the rhythm (Figs 4.5b, c; DiCaprio & Fourtner, 1984). In eight different motoneurones so tested, a 100–250 ms, 2–5 nA hyperpolarising pulse delayed the onset of the next motor burst; another motoneurone produced only phase advance, and one caused either advance or delay of the next burst, depending on the precise timing of the current pulse within the cycle period (Fig. 4.5d).

Thirdly, small steady currents ($< 10$ nA) injected into many motoneurones can alter the overall frequency of the ventilatory rhythm, in a similar, graded manner to the FM1 interneurones described above (Fig. 4.5a). Thus the rhythm period decreases in proportion to the strength of depolarising

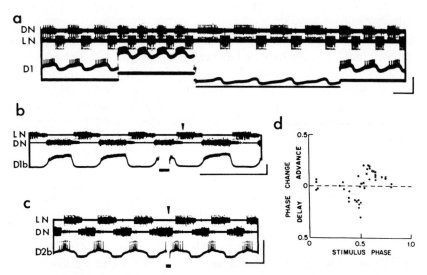

Fig. 4.5.  Motoneuronal influences on frequency and timing of motor discharge in the ventilatory rhythm. (a) Depolarising current (upward deflection of bottom trace = 4.5 nA) injected into a (D1) motoneurone not only excites the neurone itself but increases the frequency of bursts in the whole pattern, while hyperpolarising it blocks its spikes — note dropout of this unit in the DN trace — and reduces burst frequency (stronger negative current stops bursting altogether). (b, c) Brief (hyperpolarising) current pulses injected into two depressor motoneurones during the depolarising phases of their own rhythms induce phase advance (b) or delay (c) in the overall burst pattern. (d) This rhythm 'resetting' effect depends on the timing of the stimulating pulse (dots, for records as in c, from same D2b motoneurone), and occurs even when impulses are blocked by sustained hyperpolarisation (crosses); zero 'stimulus phase' = start of depressor burst; stimulus pulses: −3 nA, 250 ms. Calibrations: 20 mV, 1 s. (a, From Simmers & Bush, 1983a; b–d, from DiCaprio & Fourtner, 1984.)

current, while hyperpolarising the motoneurone slows (Fig. 4.5a) and, if strong enough, may in some cases stop the alternating motor bursts altogether.

These last two observations indicate that the motoneurones have access to the pre-motor circuit that controls them, probably via either the oscillator interneurones or, for the last effect, the frequency-modulating neurones. The capacity of some if not all motoneurones to reset the rhythm, in particular, implies that they should be regarded as intrinsic elements of the ventilatory pattern generator. Moreover, since both the graded modulation of cycle period (Fig. 4.5a) and the resetting effect persist even when all impulses are blocked by steady hyperpolarising current, they too may depend, at least in part, upon subthreshold release of transmitter from tonic, graded chemical synapses. In these respects, the ventilatory rhythm generating system recalls other motor pattern generating systems in crustaceans, notably those of the stomatogastric ganglion (see Selverston *et al.*, 1983), and the abdominal ganglia controlling swimmeret beating in the crayfish (Heitler, 1983).

### 4.6. Reversal of ventilation: neural mechanisms

As already noted, spontaneous switches to the 'reversed' motor output pattern recorded from the ventilatory nerves occur from time to time, whether the nervous system be intact within the thorax or completely isolated. Small changes in the burst intensity, duration or frequency are not uncommon, but the most striking modification to the motor pattern involves a sudden increase in burst frequency, usually to around twice the prevailing frequency, together with a consistent change in the sequence and identity of certain motor units in the nerve record (Figs 4.4e, 4.6a, b, d). In essence, one or two of the smaller-spike units (D2, L2) which normally fire towards the end of each burst in both the levator and depressor records are replaced by other small units firing early in each burst (see Fig. 4.1a). What is the neuronal basis of this change?

Intracellular recordings from individual levator or depressor moto-neurones during such 'reversals' reveal one of three distinct effects, each characteristic of a particular category of motoneurones:

(1) The membrane potential of the motoneurone continues oscillating throughout the period of the reversal, with almost constant oscillation amplitude but at the new, higher frequency of the overall rhythm recorded in the peripheral nerves (Fig. 4.6a). Superimposed upon the depolarising peaks of the oscillations, as before, are bursts of attenuated spikes.

(2) Other motoneurones resemble those of the first type in the normal forward pattern, but become hyperpolarised during the reversal period (Fig. 4.6b). Small-amplitude oscillations, at the same frequency as the reverse rhythm, may be present during the reversals, but spikes are here totally lacking (Fig. 4.6c).

(3) A third group of ventilatory motoneurones show large oscillations only during, and at the frequency of, the reverse rhythm (Fig. 4.6d). The attenuated spikes riding upon the depolarised peaks once again show the expected 1:1 correlation with a unit recorded extracellularly — in this example one which fires at the beginning of each levator burst (Fig. 4.6e).

Following the terminology of Young (1975) and Simmers & Bush (1983b), six functional subgroups of motoneurones can now be distinguished:

(a) '*bimodal*' depressor (D1) and levator (L1) units, active during both forward and reverse ventilation;

(b) *forward*-only units (D2F and L2F), which fire late in each forward rhythm burst; and

*Control of ventilation*

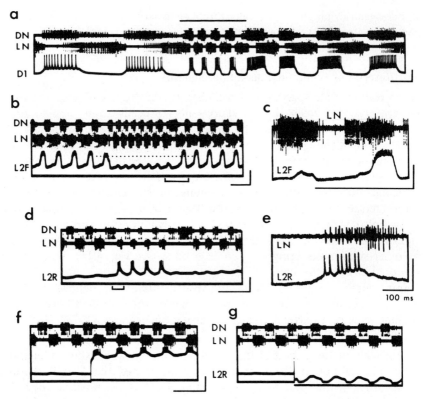

Fig. 4.6. Motoneurone types seen during spontaneous rhythm reversals (indicated by bars above the records). Note the changes in structure as well as frequency of the DN and LN bursts during the periods of 'reversed' rhythm. (a) 'Bimodal' motoneurone which continues to fire bursts of impulses throughout both the forward and the reversed rhythms. (b, c) Motoneurone which discharges spikes only during the forward rhythm, although its membrane potential continues to oscillate during reversals, albeit with much reduced amplitude (dotted line represents resting membrane potential during pauses in rhythmic activity); the small spikes (electrotonic reflections of impulses) on the depolarising waves are clearer in the faster recording (c) of the section of b indicated. (d, e) Slow and fast timebase recordings from a 'reversal' motoneurone, whose membrane oscillations are suppressed during the forward rhythm; note in e the 1:1 correspondence between intracellular (L2R) spikes and a unit in the extracellular trace (LN). (f) Depolarising this motoneurone during the normal (forward) rhythm elicits spikes superimposed upon the now larger, suprathreshold oscillations, while (g) hyperpolarising current causes phase reversal of the slow waves, indicating that during the forward rhythm it was effectively clamped at or near the reversal potential for a periodic inhibitory synaptic input. Calibrations: 20 mV, 1 s (100 ms in e). (From Simmers & Bush, 1983b.)

(c) *reversal* units (D2R and L2R), firing early in the corresponding reverse rhythm burst.

The sequence of activity in these different subgroups is thus D1, D2F, L1, L2F, D1 ... for forward beating; and D2R, D1, L2R, L1, D2R ... in reversed beating (Fig. 4.1a). That is, the phase relationships of the four main muscle groups, D1, D2, L1 and L2, change in a manner so as to reverse the direction of thrust of the power strokes — both depressor and levator muscles contributing, in either direction, to the propulsion of the water.

Throughout the reverse pattern the membrane potential of the forward-only (D2F and L2F) motoneurones hyperpolarises to a level comparable with that during the troughs between the oscillatory waves in forward beating; whereas the D2R and L2R motoneurones remain at a similarly hyperpolarised level during forward ventilation and, when the rhythm reverses, they oscillate between this level and their depolarising peaks. This suggests that the forward motoneurones are tonically inhibited during reversals, whereas the reversal motoneurones are inhibited throughout the normal forward pattern. In support of this hypothesis, when increasing amounts of steady hyperpolarising current are injected into the forward-only motoneurones, the small oscillations often evident during reversal periods at first diminish and disappear, and then reappear with inverted polarity — i.e. with their phase reversed with respect to the peripherally recorded burst pattern. A similar result follows the same protocol for the reversal motoneurones during the forward rhythm (Fig. 4.6g). Incrementing depolarising currents, on the other hand, result in progressively increasing oscillation amplitudes during the motoneurones' non-active periods. With sufficiently large positive currents, spikes appear on the peaks of the now 10–15 mV slow waves (Fig. 4.6f), and corresponding unitary impulses are recruited in the extracellular recording, with the phase relationship appropriate to its usual active period. The bimodal motoneurones are not inhibited during either forward or reverse beating.

The neural switching between ventilatory modes therefore occurs by synaptic inhibition of the inappropriate motoneurones, that is, a 'gating' mechanism acting at the level of the motoneurones themselves. Such tonic inhibition may derive from as yet unidentified inhibitory interneurones in the VRC, with appropriate synaptic connections to the motoneurones. Interneurones having an analogous mode-switching effect have been reported in the crayfish abdominal nervous system, where they can induce reversal in the direction of metachronal coordination of beating swimmerets in adjacent abdominal segments (Heitler, 1985). What is the source of the reversed rhythm?

One possibility could be that, in addition to the motoneurones being appropriately gated, reverse-mode oscillator interneurones, similar to those for forward beating but with a higher intrinsic oscillation frequency, come into play while the normal forward ones are shut off. However, no such neurones have yet been encountered, though in view of the infrequent occurrence of reversals the probability of finding them would be rather low.

The alternative, a combined forward- *and* reverse-mode oscillator, whose frequency increases abruptly at the onset of reverse ventilation, is supported by the available evidence. Thus, the non-spiking oscillator interneurones described previously continue to exhibit their large oscillations in membrane potential during the reversed ventilatory pattern, with the same overall phase relationship to the extracellularly recorded depressor and levator bursts but now at the higher frequency characteristic of the reversed rhythm (Fig. 4.3c). This has been seen for both sub-types of oscillator neurone, depolarising in phase with either levators or depressors, respectively. Further, the forward-only and reverse-mode motoneurones continue to show membrane potential oscillations (albeit very small ones) at the prevailing burst frequency throughout their 'inactive' mode. If different oscillators were responsible for the two modes, it would seem unlikely that both types would connect with both forward- and reverse-mode motoneurones.

### 4.7. Descending 'command' inputs to the VRC

A variety of types of influence upon the ventilatory rhythm can be elicited by repetitive pulse stimulation of either circumoesophageal connective (COC) linking the cerebral ganglion ('brain') with the suboesophageal ganglion (Fig. 4.1b). These include initiation, acceleration, inhibition or suppression of the overall rhythm, and 'switching' between forward and reverse motor patterns, depending upon which fibres, or fibre bundles, are stimulated (Best, 1982).

Sometimes two or more distinct effects could be evoked by a single bundle. In one instance (Fig. 4.7a), slowly increasing intensity of stimulation at 60 Hz first initiated the normal forward ventilatory pattern in the quiescent preparation, or accelerated it if already active, then produced further acceleration; and finally, at a still higher intensity, the bursting rhythm was suddenly suppressed. Subsequently reducing the stimulus intensity resulted in the reverse sequence of changes, each at a similar threshold. The smplest interpretation of this observation is that this bundle contained two or three fibres having discrete 'command' influences upon the ventilatory rhythm generating network in the suboesophageal ganglion. Other filaments isolated from one COC often produced only one effect upon the ventilatory rhythm, normally at a single, clearly defined threshold intensity (e.g. Figs 4.7b, e). Presumably such single-threshold filaments contained one descending 'command fibre' affecting the ventilatory system; some may have comprised a single axon only, though histological support for this is lacking.

Many of the effects observed in these experiments were graded in intensity with frequency of stimulation, within a limited range. Only occasionally did variation in stimulus strength produce a graded response, suggesting recruitment of several fibres wth a similar function. The most common form of response gradation was in the frequency of the motor bursts (or inter-burst period) recorded in the ventilatory nerves. Thus COC fibres which initiated and/or accelerated the rhythm commonly produced an increase in burst frequency with each increase in stimulation frequency (Fig. 4.7c), while most inhibitory COC fibres caused progressive slowing of the rhythm with increasing stimulus frequency (Fig. 4.7d) before eventually rhythmic bursting stopped altogether. A few COC units, however, either initiated or suppressed the ventilatory rhythm, with no effect on its frequency. Others evoked a sudden change to the reverse mode (e.g. Fig. 4.7f), and yet others had a graded action on the frequency of the reverse rhythm but no effect on the forward rhythm.

There is as yet no direct evidence (e.g. from intracellular recordings in the VRC) on the manner by which the foregoing 'descending' COC units exert their effects upon the ventilatory pattern generating system. Graded accelerating or decelerating effects on the whole rhythm could be achieved via depolarising or hyperpolarising synaptic inputs to the frequency modulating interneurones (see Section 4.4), while initiation or suppression of rhythmic bursting might be induced by inputs to the oscillator neurones (Section 4.3). COC-mediated rhythm reversal might be mediated by the postulated 'reverse-mode' interneurones in the VRC (Section 4.6), with inhibitory synapses upon the purely forward-mode motoneurones, and possibly also — though evidence for this is lacking — excitatory connections with the reversal motoneurones; conversely, one or more similar 'forward-mode' inter-neurones with opposite connections might sustain the forward rhythm. Although the descending reversal units (or any of the other COC units) could conceivably act directly on the motoneurones, such a mechanism alone would not explain the spontaneous reversals (or other changes in the rhythm) seen occasionally in the completely isolated thoracic CNS preparation.

Simultaneous recordings from the ventilatory nerves on both sides of the suboesophageal ganglia reveal that a minority of these COC units have bilateral effects. Several have similar but weaker or less consistent influences on the contralateral motor output in addition to their ipsilateral action (e.g. Fig. 4.7b). None has purely contralateral actions. *In vivo*, any one COC unit, or various combinations of them acting in concert, may exert overall control of the pattern-generating system in the suboesophageal ganglia. The sources of input to these COC units themselves are as yet unknown, but it seems likely that various sensory receptors in the head region, including the antennules and antennae, will be implicated (see below).

## 4.8. Sensory feedback from the scaphognathite

Rhythmical output from the ventilatory central pattern generator is subject to modulation from a wide variety of sensory stimuli impinging upon most

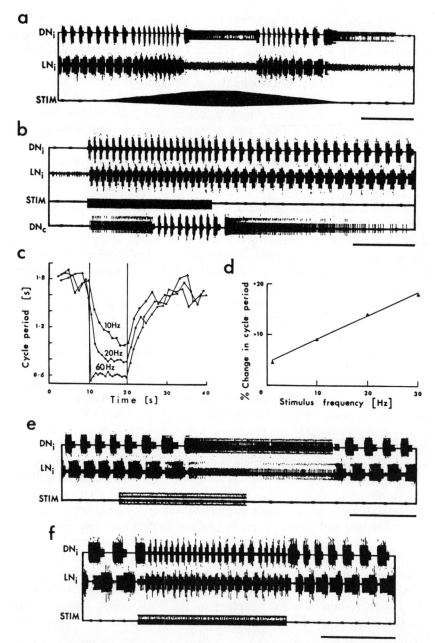

Fig. 4.7.  Descending 'command fibre' influences on the ventilatory rhythm, elicited by repetitive pulse (10–60 Hz) stimulation (STIM) of different nerve fibre bundles isolated from the circumoesophageal connectives ('coc' in Fig. 4.1b). Extracellular recordings only, from ipsilateral depressor (DN$_i$) and levator (LN$_i$) and contralateral depressor (DN$_c$) nerves. (a) Increasing stimulus intensity (maximum 2 V) recruits first

regions of the body (see reviews by McMahon & Wilkens, 1982; Taylor, 1982). Responses commonly involve transient decreases in beat frequency, temporary apnoea and, in crabs, reversed scaphognathite beating. This suggests that short-term sensory influences on the CPG originating from other segmental ganglia are mostly inhibitory. Stimulation of one branchial chamber frequently evokes an ipsilateral response, supporting the inference (see above) that left and right pattern generators can be modulated independently. Long-term shifts in pump performance can also occur; for example, scaphognathite frequency and stroke volume increase under chronic hypoxic conditions, a tonic excitatory effect which may stem at least in part from oxygen receptors in the gills. However, the sensory and neural bases of these various extrinsic sensory influences on ventilation are as yet largely unknown.

The only known source of proprioceptive feedback within the ventilatory system is a single stretch receptor (in contrast to the wealth of proprioceptive information from the legs: see Bush & Laverack, 1982). This is the 'oval organ', a unique mechanoreceptor found within the second maxilla of all decapod Crustacea studied (Pasztor, 1969, 1979; see Fig. 4.1b). A conical array of some 200–300 connective tissue strands spans the region of maximum flexion and extension near the base of the scaphognathite blade. These strands support the rich dendritic arborisations and bulbous peripheral terminals of three large afferent fibres, whose cell bodies lie within the suboesophageal ganglion. Their branching central terminals share the same restricted lateral neuropile as the scaphognathite motoneurones, and the apparent close interlacing of sensory and motor branches suggests the possibility of synaptic interactions.

In isolated preparations of the oval organ and suboesophageal ganglion of *Homarus*, the three sensory afferents are readily distinguishable from one another and from other nerve fibres in the desheathed nerve truck (SN) by their large diameters (20–45 µm). They have been labelled X, Y and Z in descending order of size. Afferent responses to stretch stimuli, recorded

a COC 'unit' (i.e. producing one functional effect) which accelerates the rhythm, then at a higher threshold an inhibitory unit (these two effects could also be evoked separately by appropriate steady voltages); following stimulation the inhibition appears to outlast excitation. (b) Constant-intensity stimulation of another COC bundle initiates rhythmic bursts (or accelerates the ongoing rhythm) ipsilaterally; the contralateral response is weaker and delayed in onset. (c) Effect on the ventilatory cycle period of three different frequencies of stimulation, for 10 s (between vertical bars), of an excitatory unit. (d, e) Other COC bundles slow the rhythm, in proportion to stimulus frequency, up to a maximum of 20% increase in cycle period (*d*) before it stops altogether, usually in the D1 phase (e). (f) 'Switching' to the motor pattern of the reversed rhythm results from stimulation of a third class of COC bundle. These responses may be purely ipsilateral, or weak contralateral effects may also occur. Calibration bars: 5 s. (From Best, 1982.)

intracellularly 2–8 mm from the confluence of the sensory dendrites, have two components: bursts of impulses superimposed upon slow graded potentials (Fig. 4.8a; Pasztor & Bush, 1982, 1983a). The spikes can be blocked with tetrodotoxin, leaving the graded potentials to be examined separately. They are clearly electrotonic derivatives of depolarising receptor potentials, and follow the parameters of the stretch stimulus faithfully, but with little or no dynamic response and at most a small hyperpolarising undershoot after relaxation. The very large length constant of the afferent fibres — probably well over the measured 1 cm and thus greater than the distance from oval organ to ganglion, due to an unusually high specific membrane resistance ($> 100$ k$\Omega$ cm$^2$) — indicates that the graded potentials can spread electrotonically into central presynaptic terminals with sufficient magnitude to modulate transmitter release (cf. the coxal muscle receptor afferents: see Bush, 1981). This inference is supported by recent intracellular recordings from the afferents, at their entry into the neuropile, of good-sized graded potentials in response to stretch of the oval organ (V. M. Pasztor & B. M. H. Bush, unpublished observations). Reafference from proprioceptor to central pattern generator is thus evidently mediated by both impulses and graded potentials.

In the branchial pump both elevation and depression of the scaphognathite are effective power strokes, so that continuous monitoring of the whole beat cycle would presumably be advantageous. Discrete bursts of impulses at peak stretches of a proprioceptor with few afferent units could not adequately encode all the movement parameters likely to be important as feedback for the scaphognathite motor programme. On the other hand the analogue signal provides a continuous source of information, depolarising and hyperpolarising in phase with the alternating movements of the scaphognathite. The non-impulsive nature of several key elements in the ventilatory CPG, moreover (see Sections 4.3 and 4.4), makes them well adapted to respond to small fluctuations of transmitter released by graded input signals (cf. Burrows & Siegler, 1978; Blight & Llinas, 1980).

The three afferent fibres differ in their receptor potential waveforms, spiking capacity and extent of adaptation (Fig. 4.8a; Bush & Pasztor, 1983b). Fibre X has the largest graded potentials (up to 35 mV) and smallest number of spikes (usually one to six), and shows almost no receptor potential or spike frequency adaptation (within its burst). Fibre Z has the highest threshold, but also attains the highest firing frequencies (100 Hz) and adapts rapidly. Fibre Y is intermediate in all these properties. It has been suggested that X may act as a beat frequency marker during rhythmical scaphognathite beating. Both X and Y respond as position detectors (X in its analogue signal amplitude and Y mainly by impulse frequency coding), while Z is primarily a movement detector with some degree of velocity sensitivity.

During rhythmical beating of the scaphognathite, the oval organ must undergo cyclical variations in length, probably of a more or less sinusoidal

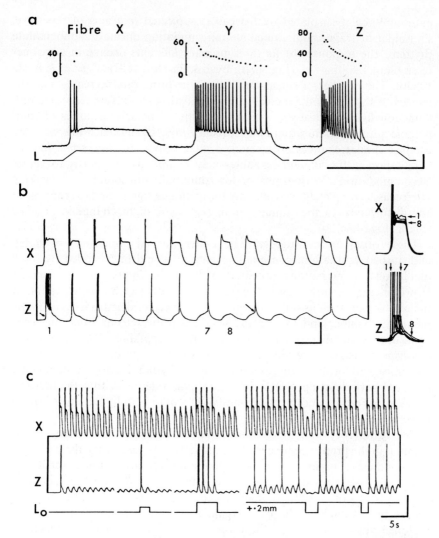

Fig. 4.8. Properties of the lobster 'oval organ', a ventilatory stretch receptor, as revealed by intracellular recordings in the 12–15 mm long afferent fibres taken *c.* 6 mm from their sensory terminals. (a) Distinctive responses of the three afferents, X, Y and Z, to single 0.8 mm-amplitude trapezoidal stretches of the isolated oval organ; note the large receptor potentials in X and Y, and rapid spike accommodation in X and Z. (b) 'Habituation' of the spike responses in fibres X and Z to similar, repetitive pulls, with relatively small decline in the receptor potentials; note the increasing spike latency in Z (but not X) — see superimposed recordings of the same first eight responses (numbered at right). (c) 'Dishabituation' (left half), and loss of spike responses (right half), resulting from small (100 or 200 μm) changes in basal length, $L_o$: increase upwards, upon which the 0.4 mm trapezoidal pulls at 1 Hz are superimposed; note accompanying changes in receptor potentials. Calibrations: 20 mV, 1 s (5 s in c). (From Pasztor & Bush, 1983a, b.)

nature. When the isolated oval organ is subjected to trains of repetitive, sinusoidal or trapezoidal stretch stimuli simulating normal scaphognathite rhythms, the responses of its three primary afferents decline in a manner resembling 'habituation' (Fig. 4.8b); Bush & Pasztor, 1983a; Pasztor & Bush, 1983b). The number of spikes diminishes, the firing rate decreases, and the latency to the first spike increases. The graded potentials undergo less of a reduction than impulse generation. Repetitive depolarising pulses of comparable amplitude, duration and frequency injected into each afferent fibre produce similar changes in the evoked spike responses, suggesting that the habituation in the afferent responses may be due at least partly to neural 'accommodation'. With trains of low-amplitude sinusoidal pulls, spiking often ceases completely, leaving only the analogue signal. Spikes reappear at any disturbance to the stimulus train such as a slight change in baseline length (Fig. 4.8c).

These observations suggest that, under normal conditions of quiet, undisturbed ventilation, continuous feedback would be provided by small oscillations in membrane potential without the intervention of spikes. However, any perturbation in the regular cycle of stretch and relaxation of the oval organ, such as might be caused by a piece of detritus lodging in the pumping chamber and forcing the scaphognathite into an abnormal configuration, would disrupt habituation and restore spiking. Hyperventilation, involving a faster, more powerful stroke, would continue to evoke spiking responses, with prolific firing at any change in rhythm. During the commonly observed periods of apnoea, habituation would decay so that the first few cycles after recommencement of ventilation would be fully monitored by all three sensory units.

The complexity and systematic variation with the parameters of the stimulus in the proprioceptive feedback signals mediated by the three afferent fibres of the oval organ emphasise its potentially important role in regulating ventilation. Weak resistance reflexes can sometimes be demonstrated in semi-isolated oval organ–suboesophageal ganglion preparations. The reflex response to a stretch of the oval organ, a short burst from a few levator motoneurones, is not robust, however, and habituates rapidly to repetitive pulls. Nevertheless this does provide evidence of an excitatory pathway between oval organ afferents and some ventilatory motoneurones, though how significant such reflex actions may be *in vivo* is uncertain.

A more likely role for the reafference from the oval organ might involve a direct influence upon the ventilatory CPG. There are now several examples of phasic input from proprioceptors having immediate, cycle-by-cycle effects on central pattern generators, including insect respiration (Farley & Case, 1968), mammalian respiration (von Euler, 1981), vertebrate locomotion (Grillner, 1985), insect flight (Pearson *et al.*, 1983) and, most recently, crayfish locomotor rhythms (Sillar *et al.*, 1986). Phasic information is clearly available from the oval organ, but modulation of the ventilatory CPG by the oval organ remains to be unequivocally demonstrated.

### 4.9. Neurohormonal modulation in the ventilatory system

There have been many reports of monoamine and neuropeptide activation of motor pattern generators in both vertebrates and invertebrates. In crustacean studies attention has focused on four substances, the monoamines dopamine, octopamine and serotonin, and the pentapeptide proctolin (reviewed by Kravitz *et al.*, 1985). Noradrenaline has not been found in Crustacea. Berlind (1977) recorded changes in scaphognathite beating, notably an increase in occurrence of reversals, when serotonin and peptide extracts of pericardial organ, a major neurohaemal structure, were injected into crabs and crayfish. Recent work in our laboratories and elsewhere indicates that neurohormonal modulation has significant influences on all aspects of ventilatory activity.

Proctolin and octopamine were found to have excitatory effects upon scaphognathite beating in crayfish (Pasztor *et al.*, 1985), whereas serotonin transiently reduced beat frequency. When injected into intact, normoxic animals, proctolin in particular consistently caused prolonged, dose-dependent increases in both beat frequency and amplitude. The increase in beat amplitude is due not only to excitation of the ventilatory rhythm centre, but also to a phasic peripheral action of the neurohormones on the scaphognathite muscles themselves (Pasztor *et al.*, 1985; Mercier & Wilkens, 1985). Octopamine and serotonin also had excitatory actions tending to enhance the vigour of beating. In isolated suboesophageal ganglion preparations, proctolin initiated rhythmical motor bursting in quiescent ganglia, and brought about motoneurone recruitment and elevated firing rates in ganglia with ongoing rhythmicity.

In lobsters, octopamine and serotonin both circulate in the haemolymph at concentrations of $1-5 \times 10^{-8}$ M, which is suprathreshold for many of the physiological effects demonstrated *in vitro*. Proctolin has so far not been detected in the circulation, but the half-life of exogenous proctolin injected into the haemolymph is short (6–10 min), suggesting that it is metabolised or sequestered much more rapidly than are the other neurohormones (Schwarz *et al.*, 1984). These authors speculate that proctolin may act only on target tissues close to release sites. Indeed octopamine, serotonin and proctolin, in addition to being released from neurohaemal organs and acting as circulating hormones, are also released at certain peripheral and central synaptic sites, where they may act as neuromodulators or even neurotransmitters (Kravitz *et al.*, 1985).

Immunocytochemical techniques have made possible the mapping of neurone somata, fibre tracts and central neuropile regions shown thus to contain these neurohormones (e.g. Schwarz *et al.*, 1984). Some of the neurones so mapped have axons extending long distances in the connectives linking central ganglia, suggesting the involvement of 'command' inputs of the kind mentioned above. Several hundred neurone somata in the lobster suboesophageal ganglion show proctolin-like immunoreactivity (IR) (Siwicki & Bishop, 1986), and one large cluster is positioned in the same location as cells which take up cobalt when the scaphognathite nerves are backfilled. Proctolin-like IR has since been found in all branches of the scaphognathite innervation (V.M. Pasztor & K.K. Siwicki, unpublished observations). A large proportion of both levator and depressor motor axons stained well, and it is probable that proctolin is co-localised with the neuromuscular transmitter glutamate in a subset of ventilatory motoneurones.

A surprising observation was that the large mechanosensory afferents of the oval organ also showed proctolin-like IR, and that the complete peripheral arborisation was permeated with punctate staining. This correlated with previous ultrastructural studies showing the bulbous sensory terminals to contain abundant dense cored vesicles (75–90 nm diameter), which also appeared to be streaming distally along dendrite branches or lodged in numerous storage varicosities (Pasztor, 1979). The oval organ receives no efferent innervation, nor do these peripheral sensory dendrites make any synaptic connections.

Since the possibility thus exists for localised release of proctolin in the scaphognathite, from sensory as well as motor endings, it was of interest to ascertain whether proctolin had any effects upon the sensory signals from the oval organ. Intracellular recordings from the three afferents showed that their responses to pull stimuli were enhanced by proctolin, and depressed by octopamine and serotonin, at threshold concentrations of around $10^{-10}$ M (Pasztor & Bush, 1987). Receptor potential amplitudes and rise-times were modulated, with consequent changes in the spike patterns of the afferent signals. It has been shown (Bush & Pasztor, 1983b) that the properties of fibre X are markedly different from those of fibres Y and Z. Under most conditions fibre X showed insignificant modulation by proctolin, octopamine or serotonin, suggesting that *in vivo* its feedback signal remains constant, in contrast to varying signal strengths from the other two oval-organ afferent fibres, according to prevailing neurohormone concentrations.

## 4.10. Summary and conclusion

Recent studies outlined in this chapter now permit a fairly comprehensive account of the neuronal basis of gill ventilation in decapod Crustacea. Although many gaps in the picture still remain, the following summary of the major features of the system is consistent with the evidence to date. The scheme envisaged is represented diagrammatically in Fig. 4.9, and can be regarded as a working hypothesis, each component of which will require testing with more rigorous methods or different analytical approaches, including the use of dual microelectrode penetration of different neural elements to assess the various synaptic interactions proposed.

The rhythmical up-and-down movements of each of the two scaphognathites which propel water through the bilateral branchial chambers for respiratory gill ventilation in crabs and lobsters result from the co-ordinated contractions of five levator muscles alternating with five depressors. These muscle actions are effected by alternating bursts of impulses in levator and depressor motoneurones, two or three per muscle. Usually only a dozen or so of the 25–30 motoneurones in all are active during normal quiet ventilation. Each motoneurone penetrated with a microelectrode shows regular, 10–30 mV amplitude oscillations in membrane potential during expression of the appropriate motor rhythm. These result primarily from cyclical, smoothly graded, chemical synaptic inhibition, with no evidence of discrete, brief, postsynaptic potentials from presynaptic impulses. Tonic excitatory input, as well as postinhibitory rebound excitation, may also contribute, to bring the motoneurones above threshold for impulse generation.

Reversal of the direction of water flow, which occasionally occurs spontaneously, both *in vivo* and as 'fictive reversal' in the isolated nervous system, depends on a switch in part of the population of motoneurones active. Certain 'forward-mode' motoneurones cease firing, and a new group of 'reverse-mode' motoneurones are recruited, while a large core of 'bimodal' motoneurones continue firing in bursts throughout both forward and reverse beating. During reversals the membrane potentials of the forward-mode motoneurones are 'clamped' at a relatively hyperpolarised level, while the oscillatory activity of the reversal motoneurones is similarly suppressed throughout the normal forward rhythm. This tonic, presumably chemical inhibition in both cases, may originate from as yet unidentified interneurones controlling reverse and forward mode ventilation, respectively.

These rhythmic, alternating bursts of impulses in antagonistic sets of scaphognathite motoneurones have been shown to be controlled by a network of neurones, or 'central pattern generator' (CPG), located in the suboesophageal ganglion. The primary oscillatory drive appears to derive from the intrinsic membrane properties of at least two interneurones within each hemi-ganglion. The membrane potentials of these *oscillator neurones* fluctuate at the prevailing frequency of the scaphognathite beat: one depolarises in phase with levation of the ipsilateral scaphognathite, the other with the depression phase of the beat cycle. Neither sub-type of oscillator neurone ever showed any sign of all-or-none impulses, so they are presumed to be non-spiking, local interneurones. In view of the strong evidence for periodic, graded inhibition, we postulate that these oscillator neurones make purely inhibitory synapses with the motoneurones, namely with those oscillating in *anti-phase* with the interneuronal oscillations. The two antagonistic oscillator sub-types may also make reciprocal inhibitory con-

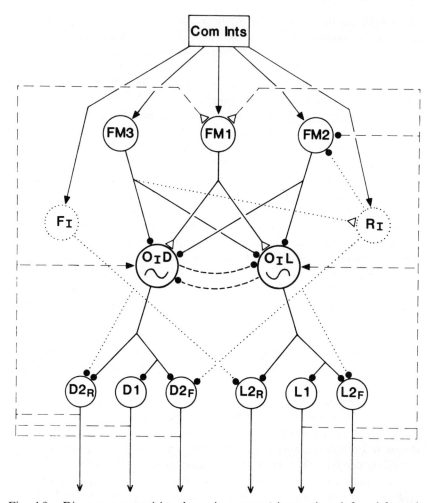

Fig. 4.9.   Diagram summarising the main neuronal interactions inferred from the studies reviewed in this chapter. Com Ints, 'command interneurones' whose axons run in the circumoesophageal connective between cerebral and suboesophageal ganglia. Large open circles represent the three classes of neurones recorded with microelectrodes in the ventilatory neuropile of the suboesophageal ganglion: FM1–3, frequency-modulating interneurones; $O_ID$, $O_IL$, oscillator interneurones inhibiting depressor or levator motoneurones, respectively; D1, L1, bimodal depressor/levator motoneurones; $D2_F$, $L2_F$, depressor/levator motoneurones active only during forward rhythm; $D2_R$, $L2_R$, depressor/levator reversal-mode motoneurones. Dotted circles represent hypothetical interneurones and their connections (dotted lines) postulated to provide tonic inhibition of the inactive motoneurones during forward ($F_I$) and reverse ($R_I$) rhythms. Solid lines represent the simplest connections consistent with the experimental observations; broken lines indicate inferred feedback pathways from motoneurones. Open triangles excitatory, and closed circles inhibitory, synaptic inputs: the latter and at least some of the former comprise graded chemical synapses; arrowheads indicate probable synaptic

nections with each other, thereby reinforcing levator–depressor alternation.

The same oscillator neurones are involved in the control of both forward and reversed ventilation, since both sub-types of these interneurones are active throughout both forms of the ventilatory rhythm. In each sub-type the only change in activity is a sudden increase in frequency of the oscillations, simultaneously with the peripherally recorded switch to the reversed motor pattern. During quiescent periods, when rhythmic motor ouput from the suboesophageal ganglion is absent, the membrane potential of these oscillator neurones is stable, with no sign of oscillatory behaviour.

Overall rhythm frequency is subject to control by at least three different *'frequency-modulating'* interneurones. These are evidently also local non-spiking interneurones, again lacking both impulses and any long fibre projections beyond the confines of the suboesophageal ganglia. Current-induced depolarisation of one of these, FM1, initiates or accelerates the rhythm, while depolarising either of the other two, FM2 and FM3, slows or stops the rhythm altogether; hyperpolarising current has the opposite effect in each case. The smooth gradation, in *both* directions, of these effects on the overall rhythm frequency, as well as the absence of impulses, suggests graded, tonic, chemical synaptic interactions with the oscillator neurones, possibly by affecting the rate of 'pacemaker' depolarisation. Each of these frequency-modulating interneurones also exhibits small ($<$ mV) oscillations in membrane potential, in synchrony with the overt motor rhythm but with different phase relationships with each other; this suggests that they receive recurrent feedback from the oscillator neurones or motoneurones which they control.

The motoneurones themselves also contribute to the generation of the ventilatory motor pattern, in at least four different ways.

(1) Some 30% or more can affect the overall rhythm frequency, in a graded manner similar to that described above for FM1. This effect is most easily explained by tonic, graded excitatory connections from these motoneurones to FM1, and perhaps also inhibitory inputs to FM2/3.

(2) Many ventilatory motoneurones are capable, when injected with brief current pulses, of resetting the complete rhythm. This might be explicable by recurrent synaptic connections from the motoneurones to the oscillator neurones. These observations alone imply that the motoneurones must also be considered as elements in the ventilatory CPG.

(3) Inhibitory interactions have been seen between some antagonistic

inputs but of indeterminate sign or type. Descending 'command fibre' influences are shown on the frequency-modulating and mode-gating interneurones, but they may also act on other ventilatory neurones. Only one side of the neural system controlling ventilation is represented; some bilateral coupling between the two hemi-ganglia must also be present. Additional connections (e.g. between synergistic and antagonistic motoneurones) are omitted for clarity. See text for further details.

motoneurones, implying collateral synaptic influences which could reinforce depressor–levator alternation.
(4) Postinhibitory rebound, an intrinsic property of some motoneurones
    indicated by a transient excitation following hyperpolarising currents,
    would support this reciprocity, and would help also to ensure
    motoneurone re-activation after each inhibitory half-cycle during the
    rhythm.
(5) 'Plateau' or 'driver' potentials, if present, could further reinforce and
    stabilise motor burst production; however, there is as yet no direct
    evidence for them in the ventilatory system.

Descending 'command fibres' in the circumoesophageal connectives
(COCs) from the brain to the thoracic ganglia exert overall control on the
expression of the ventilatory rhythm. Repetitive activity in some of these
neurones initiates or accelerates the rhythm, others inhibit or suppress it, and
yet others can switch the rhythm into the reverse mode. The excitatory and
inhibitory effects are graded with frequency of COC fibre stimulation,
and may be mediated by synaptic inputs to the frequency-modulating interneurones in the suboesophageal ganglion. *In vivo* the overall effect presumably depends upon the precise combination of these COC fibres activated, as
well as their relative firing frequencies. They probably receive a variety of
sensory inputs in the brain (cerebral ganglion), including information about
oxygen tensions in the surrounding water, and perhaps also of the blood.

Sensory feedback from the scaphognathite itself to the ventilatory CPG is
provided by the 'oval organ', a stretch receptor situated at a major region of
articulation at the base of the oscillating appendage. Three large-diameter
afferent fibres, X, Y and Z, with centrally located cell bodies, convey both
impulses and the underlying graded (analogue) potentials to the ganglion,
reflecting the main stimulus parameters in different ways in each fibre. With
repetitive, oscillatory length changes simulating the normal rhythmical
movements of the scaphognathites, the sensory responses 'habituate', the
spikes on each stretch decreasing in frequency and sometimes ceasing
altogether, and the graded potentials declining in amplitude somewhat. It
seems probable that, as in other rhythmic motor systems, this proprioceptive
input will serve to modulate the central motor output pattern so as to adapt it
to prevailing conditions within the branchial chamber.

Proctolin immunoreactivity has been found at various sites in the ventilatory control system, notably in the ventilatory region of the suboesophageal ganglionic neuropile, in some ventilatory motor axons and
neuromuscular junctions, and in the afferent fibres of the oval organ and
their peripheral arborisations. The latter correlates with the ultrastructural
observation of dense-cored vesicles in the afferent terminals, suggesting that
the neuropeptide might be released by stretch of these terminals. In accord
with these observations, proctolin potentiates afferent responses to oval
organ stretch, and increases both the strength and frequency of

scaphognathite beating. Other neurohormones, octopamine and serotonin, though less potent, tend to have inhibitory effects on several aspects of ventilatory performance. *In vivo*, these and perhaps several other neuromodulators probably play a significant role in the overall control of ventilation, by their actions at a variety of sites, both locally at specific synapses, neuromuscular junctions and afferent endings, and more generally as circulating neurohormones.

This brief survey has focused primarily upon the central nervous components of the ventilatory motor pattern generating system. The model presented here, like those for many other invertebrate motor-control systems, is attractive in its simplicity and economy of network design, as well as in the *relative* completeness of the description now possible for this system. Moreover the whole system is in general terms not unlike many other motor systems with alternating, multiphase bursting activity in motor units of antagonistic sets of muscles, and two or more alternative modes (forward and reverse in this case). However, we must caution against assuming either that the present account represents a complete picture of the true physiological condition of the system; or that any inferences about the neural mechanisms of this system can be extrapolated to other motor systems subserving similar functions.

A pertinent lesson can in fact be drawn from previous studies of this system: a model is only as valid as the last experiment. Thus, for example, the elegant simplicity of Mendelson's (1971) hypothesis, of a single non-spiking oscillator neurone controlling the whole ventilatory motor output pattern, proved to be only partially correct (see Section 4.3); yet more than one review dealing with the neural basis of respiration in mammals cited this as an example of what might be learned from invertebrates. Again, our work (Simmers & Bush, 1983a) suggested that the ventilatory motoneurones, apart from inhibitory interactions between antagonists, had only tonic and rebound excitatory effects on ventilation; however, the ability to reset the rhythm by injection of brief pulses into individual motoneurones (DiCaprio & Fourtner, 1984) indicates that they should be regarded as integral elements of the ventilatory 'CPG'.

Perhaps one concluding message might be that, even in such a 'simple system' as that for ventilatory control in this lower animal, the *variety* of contributory mechanisms is impressive, and likely to increase as new discoveries emerge. Whether this makes it more, or less, 'relevant' to the unquestionably more complex yet functionally analogous motor systems of mammals and other vertebrates is arguable. Suffice it to conclude that at least it should not now seem so simple a system as not even to warrant ventilating in the present context of 'higher order' systems.

## Acknowledgements

We thank Dr Ralph DiCaprio for permission to quote unpublished results, Dr Robert Elson for helpful criticism of the manuscript, Sue Maskell for secretarial assistance and Jane Robbins for photographic help. Work in the authors' laboratories was supported by research grants from the SERC (UK) to B.M.H.B. and the NSERC (Canada) to V.M.P.

## Core readings

Bush, B. M. H. & Laverack, M. S. (1982). Mechanoreception. In *The Biology of Crustacea* (ed. D. E. Bliss), *Vol. 3, Neurobiology: Structure and Function*, pp. 399–468 (eds H. L. Atwood & D. C. Sandeman). New York: Academic Press.

Heitler, W. J. (1983). The control of rhythmic limb movements in Crustacea. In *Neural Origin of Rhythmic Movements*, Symposia of the Society for Experimental Biology, vol. 37, pp. 351–82 (eds A. Roberts & B. L. Roberts). Cambridge: Cambridge University Press.

McMahon, B. R. & Wilkens, J. L. (1982). Ventilation, perfusion and oxygen uptake. In *The Biology of Crustacea*, (ed. D. E. Bliss), *Vol. 5, Internal Anatomy and Physiological Regulation* pp. 289–371 (ed. L. H. Mantel). New York: Academic Press.

Pasztor, V. M. & Bush, B. M. H. (1982). Impulse-coded and analog signaling in single mechanoreceptor neurons. *Science* **215**, 1635–7.

Simmers, A. J. (1981). Non-spiking interactions in crustacean rhythmic motor systems. In *Neurones without Impulses*. Society for Experimental Biology Seminar Series, vol. 6, pp. 177–98 (eds A. Roberts & B. M. H. Bush). Cambridge: Cambridge University Press.

Simmers, A. J. & Bush, B. M. H. (1980). Non-spiking neurones controlling ventilation in crabs. *Brain Res.* **197**, 247–52.

Simmer, A. J. & Bush, B. M. H. (1985). Neurogenesis of respiration in Crustacea. In *Neurogenesis of Central Respiratory Rhythm* pp. 41–4 (eds A. L. Bianchi & M. Denavit-Saubié). Lancaster and Boston: MTP Press Ltd.

Taylor, E. W. (1982). Control and co-ordination of ventilation and circulation in crustaceans: responses to hypoxia and exercise. *J. Exp. Biol.* **100**, 289–319.

## Supplementary readings

Anderson, W. W. & Barker, D. L. (1981). Synaptic mechanisms that generate network oscillations in the absence of discrete postsynaptic potentials. *J. Exp. Zool.* **216**, 187–91.

Benson, J. A. & Cooke, I. M. (1984). Driver potentials and the organization of rhythmic bursting in crustacean ganglia. *Trends Neurosci.* **7**, 85–91.

Berlind, A. (1977). Neurohumoral and reflex control of scaphognathite beating in the crab *Carcinus maenas*. *J. Comp. Physiol.* **116**, 77–90.

Best, S. R. (1982). Central and peripheral control of ventilation in the shore crab, *Carcinus maenas*. Ph. D. Thesis, University of Bristol, UK.

Blight, A. R. & Llinas, R. (1980). The non-impulsive stretch–receptor complex of the crab: a study of depolarization–release coupling at a tonic sensorimotor synapse. *Phil. Trans. Roy. Soc. B* **290**, 219–76.

Burrows, M. & Siegler, M. V. S. (1978). Graded synaptic transmission between local interneurones and motor neurones in the metathoracic ganglion of the locust. *J. Physiol.* **285**, 231–55.

Bush, B. M. H. (1981). Non-impulsive stretch receptors in crustaceans. In *Neurones without Impulses* Society for Experimental Biology Seminar Series, vol. 6, pp. 147–76 (eds A. Roberts & B. M. H. Bush). Cambridge: Cambridge University Press.

Bush, B. M. H. & Pasztor, V. M. (1983a). Adaptation and sensory habituation in primary mechanoreceptive afferents of the lobster oval organ. *J. Physiol. Lond.* **343**, 26–7P.

Bush, B. M. H. & Pasztor, V. M. (1983b). Graded potentials and spiking in single units of the oval organ, a mechanoreceptor in the lobster ventilatory system. II. Individuality of the three afferent fibres. *J. Exp. Biol.* **107**, 451–64.

Calabrese, R. L. & Peterson, E. (1983). Neural control of heartbeat in the leech, *Hirudo medicinalis*. In *Neural Origin of Rhythmic Movements*, Symposia of the Society for Experimental Biology, vol. 37, pp. 195–221 (eds A. Roberts & B. L. Roberts). Cambridge: Cambridge University Press.

DiCaprio, R. A. & Fourtner, C. R. (1983). Frequency modulating interneurons in the ventilatory system of the crab, *Carcinus maenas. Soc. Neurosci. Abstr.* **9**, 541.

DiCaprio, R. A. & Fourtner, C. R. (1984). Neural control of ventilation in the shore crab, *Carcinus maenas*. I. Scaphognathite motor neurons and their effect on the ventilatory rhythm. *J. Comp. Physiol.* **155**, 397–405.

DiCaprio, R. A. & Fourtner, C. R. (1987). Neural control of ventilation in the shore crab, *Carcinus maenas*. II. Frequency modulating interneurons. *J. Comp. Physiol.* In press.

Euler, C. von (1981). The contribution of sensory inputs to the pattern generation of breathing. *Can. J. Physiol. Pharmacol.* **59**, 700–6.

Farley, R. D. & Case, J. F. (1968). Sensory modulation of ventilative pacemaker output in the cockroach, *Periplaneta americana. J. Insect Physiol.* **14**, 591–601.

Graubard, K. (1978). Synaptic transmission without action potentials: input–output properties of a non-spiking presynaptic neuron. *J. Neurophysiol.* **41**, 1014–25.

Grillner, S. (1985). Neural control of vertebrate locomotion — central mechanisms and reflex interaction with special reference to the cat. In *Feedback and Motor Control in Invertebrates and Vertebrates*, pp. 35–56 (eds W. J. P. Barnes & M. H. Gladden). London: Croom Helm.

Heitler, W. J. (1985). Motor programme switching in the crayfish swimmeret system. *J. Exp. Biol.* **114**, 521–49.

Kravitz, E. A., Beltz, B., Glusman, S., Goy, M., Harris-Warrick, R., Johnston, M., Livingstone, M., Schwarz, T. & Siwicki, K. K. (1985). The well-modulated lobster: the roles of serotonin, octopamine, and proctolin in the lobster nervous system. In *Model Neural Networks and Behavior*, pp. 339–60 (ed. A. I. Selverston). New York: Plenum Press.

Mendelson, M. (1971). Oscillator neurons in crustacean ganglia. *Science* **171**, 1170–3.

Mercier, A. J. & Wilkens, J. L. (1985). Modulatory effects of proctolin on a crab ventilatory muscle. *J. Neurobiol.* **16**, 401–8.

Pasztor, V. M. (1969). The neurophysiology of respiration in decapod Crustacea. II. The sensory system. *Can. J. Zool.* **47**, 435–41.

Pasztor, V. M. (1979). The ultrastructure of the oval organ, a mechanoreceptor in the second maxilla or decapod Crustacea. *Zoomorphologie* **193**, 171–91.

Pasztor, V. M. & Bush, B. M. H. (1983a). Graded potentials and spiking in single units of the oval organ, a mechanoreceptor in the lobster ventilatory system. I. Characteristics of dual afferent signalling. *J. Exp. Biol.* **107**, 431–49.

Pasztor, V. M. & Bush, B. M. H. (1983b). Graded potentials and spiking in single units of the oval organ, a mechanoreceptor in the lobster ventilatory system. III. Sensory habituation to repetitive stimulation. *J. Exp. Biol.* **107**, 465–72.

Pasztor, V. M. & Bush, B. M. H. (1987). Peripheral modulation of mechanosensitivity in primary afferent neurons. *Nature* **326**, 793–5.

Pasztor, V. M., Katz, R., Weizner, S. & Bush, B. M. H. (1985). Physiological actions of proctolin in the ventilatory system of crayfish and lobster. *Soc. Neurosci. Abstr.* **11**, 711.

Pearson, K. G. (1979). Local neurons and local interactions in the nervous systems of invertebrates. In *The Neurosciences: Fourth Study Program*, pp. 145–57 (eds F. O. Schmitt & F. G. Worden). Cambridge, Mass.: MIT Press.

Pearson, K. G., Reye, D. N. & Robertson, R. M. (1983). Phase dependent influences of wing stretch receptors on flight rhythm in the locust. *J. Neurophysiol.* **49**, 1168–81.

Raper, J. A. (1979). Non-impulse mediated synaptic transmission during the generation of a cyclic motor program. *Science* **205**, 304–6.

Schwarz, T. L., Lee, G. M. H., Siwicki, K. K., Standaert, D. G. & Kravitz, E. A. (1984). Proctolin in the lobster: the distribution, release, and chemical characterization of a likely neurohormone. *J. Neuroscience* **4**, 1300–11.

Selverston, A. I., Miller, J. P. & Wadepuhl, M. (1983). Cooperative mechanisms for the production of rhythmic movements. In *Neural Origin of Rhythmic Movements*, Symposia of the Society for Experimental Biology, vol. 37, pp. 55–87 (eds A. Roberts & B. L. Roberts). Cambridge: Cambridge University Press.

Siegler, M. V. S.(1984). Local interneurones and local interactions in arthropods. *J. Exp. Biol.* **112**, 253–81.

Sillar, K. T. & Elson, R. C. (1986). Slow active potentials in walking-leg motor neurones triggered by non-spiking proprioceptive afferents in the crayfish. *J. Exp. Biol.* **126**, 445–52.

Sillar, K. T., Skorupski, P., Elson, R. C. & Bush, B. M. H. (1986). Two identified afferent neurones entrain a central rhythm generator. *Nature* **323**, 440–3.

Simmers, A. J. & Bush, B. M. H. (1983a). Central nervous mechanisms controlling rhythmic burst generation in the ventilatory motoneurones of *Carcinus maenas*. *J. Comp. Physiol.* **150**, 1–21.

Simmers, A. J. & Bush, B. M. H. (1983b). Motor programme switching in the ventilatory system of *Carcinus maenas*: the neuronal basis of bimodal scaphognathite beating. *J. Exp. Biol.* **104**, 163–81.

Siwicki, K. K. & Bishop, C. A. (1986). Mapping of proctolin-like immunoreactivity in the nervous systems of lobster and crayfish. *J. Comp. Neurol.* **243**, 435–53.

Wilkens, J. L. & Young, R. E. (1975). Patterns and bilateral coordination of scaphognathite rhythms in the lobster *Homarus americanus*. *J. Exp. Biol.* **63**, 219–35.

Young, R. E. (1975). Neuromuscular control of ventilation in the crab *Carcinus maenas*. *J. Comp. Physiol.* **101**, 1–37.

# Part II

# Control of perfusion: the cardiovascular system

# 5

# Cardiovascular control systems in fish

**S. Nilsson and M. Axelsson**

*Comparative Neuroscience Unit, Department of Zoophysiology, University of Göteborg, Sweden*

## 5.1. Introduction

The physiology of the circulatory systems of fish, particularly teleosts and elasmobranchs, has, over the years, been one of the most active and exciting areas in comparative physiology. Comparatively little attention has, however, been devoted to those systems that mediate the control of the circulation in fish, i.e. cardiovascular control via the autonomic nervous system and the related humoral systems (cardio- and vasoactive hormones).

As late as 1970, Campbell could find no record of experiments dealing with the autonomic nervous control of vascular beds in fish, and the knowledge of cardiovascular control mechanisms *in vivo* was fragmentary. There are now several reports on the autonomic innervation and effects of putative regulatory substances on the heart and vasculature of various fish groups, but many problems remain before a comprehensive picture of circulatory control mechanisms in fish can emerge.

The aim of this chapter is to summarise briefly some information about the circulatory control systems in fish, with some comments on the possible actions of these systems during exercise and 'stress'. Particular emphasis will be placed on the adrenergic control systems (adrenergic neurones and circulating catecholamines) that are best known, but it should be acknowledged immediately that several non-adrenergic control mechanisms exist.

## 5.2. Adrenergic control systems

In all vertebrates there are two major groups of peripheral adrenergic cells: the adrenergic neurones and the chromaffin cells (Fig. 5.1; Nilsson, 1983, 1984b). These two cell types share many features, e.g. embryological origin, innervation by preganglionic autonomic neurones and the ability to synthesise, store and release catecholamines. Functionally, the chromaffin cells are thus closely related to the autonomic nervous system, although their content

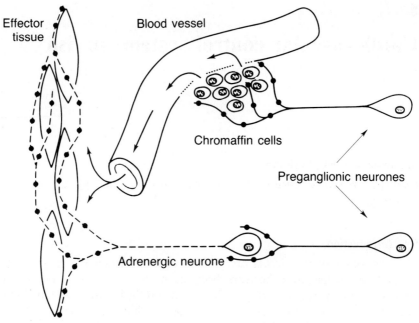

Fig. 5.1. The two main types of adrenergic cells in the vertebrates: the chromaffin cell and the adrenergic neurone. The two types of cell have many features in common, e.g. embryological origin; innervation by preganglionic nerve fibres from the spinal autonomic ('sympathetic') system; and capability of catecholamine synthesis, storage and release. The main difference is the way in which the catecholamines reach the effector tissue: catecholamines released from the chromaffin cells are transported by the blood to the effector tissue ('humoral catecholamines'), while the adrenergic neurones release the catecholamine neurotransmitter directly on to the effector cells. Reprinted with permission from Nilsson, S. Adrenergic control systems in fish. *Marine Biology Letters* **5**. Copyright 1984, Elsevier Biomedical Press B. V., Amsterdam.

is released into the blood (humoral or circulating catecholamines) whereas the adrenergic neurones release catecholamines (in many fish both adrenaline and noradrenaline) directly at the surface of the effector cells (adrenergic neurotransmitters) (Fig. 5.1).

### 5.2.1. *Adrenergic neurones*

According to the terminology introduced by Langley (1921), the autonomic nervous system is composed of three anatomically separated parts: the sympathetic, the parasympathetic and the enteric portions. The arrangement of the autonomic nervous system in non-mammalian vertebrates does not allow a clear distinction of sympathetic and parasympathetic pathways, and a modified terminology has therefore been proposed (Nilsson, 1983). In this terminology the term *cranial autonomic* is used to describe the autonomic pathways leaving the central nervous system via the cranial nerves, and *spinal autonomic* denotes the pathways leaving in the spinal segments. The term *enteric nervous system* is used as originally proposed by Langley (1921).

The spinal autonomic ('sympathetic') nervous pathways consist of two neurones: one preganglionic neurone, which runs from the spinal cord to the paravertebral ganglia (and in the higher vertebrates sometimes also to prevertebral ganglia), and a postganglionic neurone with its cell body within the paravertebral ganglion. In vertebrates other than cyclostomes and elasmobranchs, the paravertebral ganglia are connected longitudinally to form the sympathetic chains.

The adrenergic neurones are, without exception, postganglionic neurones of spinal autonomic ('sympathetic') pathways. In fish the adrenergic nerve fibres may reach their effector tissues/organs either in direct nerves from the paravertebral ganglia (splanchnic nerves), or they may re-enter and run in the spinal or cranial nerves. In the effector tissue the adrenergic axon divides into an extensive terminal plexus (see, for examples, Nilsson, 1983).

### 5.2.2. *Chromaffin cells*

The piscine equivalent of the mammalian adrenal medulla is the chromaffin tissue which is found associated with parts of the vascular system. In fish, chromaffin cells (defined here simply as cells storing large amounts of catecholamines) are found in the walls of blood vessels, notably the large veins (Fig. 5.2) (cyclostomes, dipnoans and actinopterygians), associated with paravertebral ganglia within the posterior cardinal sinuses (elasmobranchs) or within the heart itself (cyclostomes, dipnoans) (Fig. 5.3; Nilsson, 1984b). With the possible exception of the cardiac chromaffin cells in cyclostomes, these cells are innervated by preganglionic (cholinergic) autonomic neurones (see also section 3.1).

It is clear that some forms of 'disturbance' of a fish will result in the release of catecholamines from the chromaffin stores, and release of catecholamines during stimulation of preganglionic nervous pathways has been directly demonstrated in some species (Nilsson *et al.*, 1976; Abrahamsson, 1979).

### 5.3. **Circulatory control at rest**

The boundary between a 'resting' and a 'lightly stressed' fish is not sharp. Some of the earlier measurements of circulatory parameters in 'resting' fish *in vivo* may have to be disregarded, since the conditions of the experiment, particularly the use of anaesthesia during, or shortly before, the experiment, will leave the fish in an abnormal state.

This section will outline the arrangnement of the adrenergic systems involved in cardiovascular control, and give examples of the possible role of these systems *in vivo* at rest.

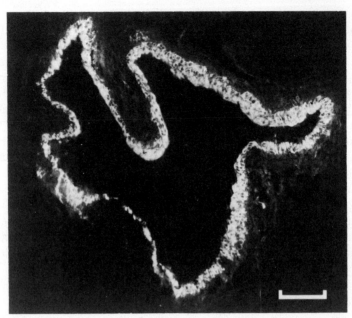

Fig. 5.2. Intensely fluorescent cells lining the walls of the most anterior part of the left cardinal vein of the African lungfish, *Protopterus aethiopicus*. Falck–Hillarp fluorescence histochemistry of catecholamines. Photomontage. Calibration bar = 200 μm. Reprinted with permission from Abrahamsson, T., Holmgren, S., Nilsson, S. & Pettersson, K., On the chromaffin system of the African lungfish, *Protopterus aethiopicus. Acta Physiologica Scandinavica* **107**. Copyright 1979, Scandinavian Physiological Society.

### 5.3.1. *Control of the heart at rest*

There are several modern reviews dealing with the anatomy and physiology of the fish heart, and some of these also give in-depth descriptions of the cardioregulatory control systems (Jones & Randall, 1978; Johansen & Burggren, 1980; Laurent *et al.*, 1983; Nilsson, 1983; Farrell, 1984; Santer, 1985).

The heart of all fish, with the exception of the myxinoids (hagfish), receives a cranial autonomic innervation via the cardiac branch of the vagus (X) nerve (Fig. 5.3). In the lampetroid cyclostomes this innervation is excitatory, acting via nicotinic cholinoceptors of the heart (Augustinsson *et al.*, 1956), whereas in all other vertebrates studied the vagal innervation is instead inhibitory acting via muscarinic cholinoceptors (elasmobranchs: Butler & Taylor, 1971; Taylor *et al.*, 1977; teleosts: e.g. Gannon & Burnstock, 1969; Holmgren, 1977; Cameron, 1979; see also Nilsson, 1983; Laurent *et al.*, 1983).

The hearts of cyclostomes, and also that of the dipnoan *Protopterus aethiopicus*, contain large quantities of adrenaline and noradrenaline stored

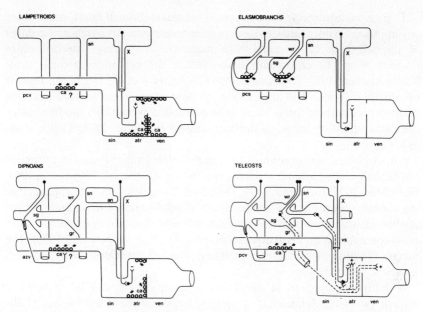

Fig. 5.3. Simplified diagrammatic representation of the pattern of cardiac control in lampetroids, elasmobranchs, dipnoans and teleosts via autonomic nerves and catecholamines released from endogenous (lampetroids and dipnoans) and exogenous chromaffin tissue (ca). In the dipnoans, the sympathetic chains are very thin with hardly visible paravertebral (sympathetic chain) ganglia (sg). The white (wr) and grey (gr) *rami communicantes* in dipnoans and teleosts may be anatomically fused to a single nerve containing both the preganglionic and the postganglionic recurrent neurones. The mode of control of the chromaffin tissue in the posterior cardinal vein of lampetroids is unclear, and although there is a distinct nerve to the azygos vein (azv) in dipnoans, there has been no direct demonstration of an innervation of the chromaffin tissue. an, Anastomosis between the vagus and the 1st spinal nerve; atr, atrium; azv, azygos vein; ca, chromaffin tissue; gr, grey ramus communicans; pcs, posterior cardinal sinus; pcv, posterior cardinal vein; sg paravertebral (sympathetic chain) ganglion; sin, sinus venosus; sn, spinal nerve; ven, ventricle; vs, 'vago-sympathetic trunk'; wr, white ramus communicans; X, vagus nerve (ramus cardiacus). + and − refer to the effects on the pacemaker (positive and negative chronotropic effect) and the cardiac muscle of the atrium and ventricle (positive and negative inotropic effect). Solid lines, cholinergic neurones; broken lines, adrenergic neurones. Reprinted with permission from Laurent, P., Holmgren, S. & Nilsson, S., Review article: nervous and humoral control of the fish heart: structure and function *Comparative Biochemistry and Physiology* **76A**. Copyright 1983, Pergamon Press.

in chromaffin-type cells (Dahl *et al.*, 1971; Abrahamsson *et al.*, 1979; Scheuermann, 1979). The hearts are remarkably insensitive to extrinsic catecholamines, but depletion of the chromaffin stores by injection of reserpine slows or stops the heart of *Myxine* (Bloom *et al.*, 1961). This suggests some function of the endogenous catecholamines in the maintenance of normal cardiac functions in the hagfish.

There is no adrenergic innervation of the elasmobranch heart, nor is there any appreciable intracardiac stores of catecholamines. An adrenergic control of the selachian heart could take place via circulating catecholamines released from the chromaffin tissue within the posterior cardinal sinus (Gannon *et al.*, 1972; Abrahamsson, 1979; Laurent *et al.*, 1983), but there is no direct evidence for this mode of control *in vivo*. Instead, cardiac performance in these fish is likely to be controlled mainly by a modulation of the vagal inhibitory tonus on the heart (Butler & Taylor, 1971; Taylor *et al.*, 1977).

An adrenergic innervation of the heart similar to that found in tetrapods has been described in several teleost species (e.g. Gannon & Burnstock, 1969; Holmgren, 1977; Cameron, 1979; Donald & Campbell, 1982). It appears that the cardiac control at low temperatures depends mainly on changes in the cholinergic vagal tonus (cf. elasmobranchs), while the adrenergic innervation plays some role at higher temperatures (Priede, 1974; Wood *et al.*, 1979). The precise function of the adrenergic innervation of the teleost heart remains, however, to be clarified.

Although many gaps in our knowledge remain, it may be possible to discern a step-wise refinement of the adrenergic control of the fish heart. The most 'primitive' case, with endogenous catecholamine stores of obscure function, is replaced in the elasmobranchs (and possibly also teleosts) by a potential control via circulation catecholamines. In the actinopterygian fish, an adrenergic innervation of the heart allows a rapid and restricted cardiac control, a situation that persists in the higher vertebrates (Fig. 5.3).

### 5.3.2. *Control of the branchial vasculature at rest*

The anatomy and physiology of fish gills has recently been thoroughly reviewed (Hoar & Randall, 1984), and the control systems involved in branchial vasomotor control are dealt with by Laurent (1984), Nilsson (1984a) and Randall & Daxboeck (1984).

An innervation of the branchial vasculature is evident in teleosts only, and changes in the branchial vascular resistance during branchial nerve stimulation in elasmobranchs appear to be due solely to contraction of non-vascular elements (Metcalfe & Butler, 1984). In the elasmobranchs there is, however, the possibility of branchial vasomotor control via circulating catecholamines (and possibly also other humoral agents). Thus Davies & Rankin (1973) reported that blood plasma from 'stressed' dogfish (*Scyliorhinus*) contained enough catecholamine-like material to produce a reduction in the overall vascular resistance of perfused gills. In both elasmobranchs and teleosts, a direct vasoconstrictor effect of hypoxia on the branchial vasculature has been described (Satchell, 1962; Pettersson & Johansen, 1982).

Adrenergic nerve fribres reach the afferent and efferent lamellar arterioles in *Salmo trutta* and *S. gairdneri*, and there is also a rich innervation of

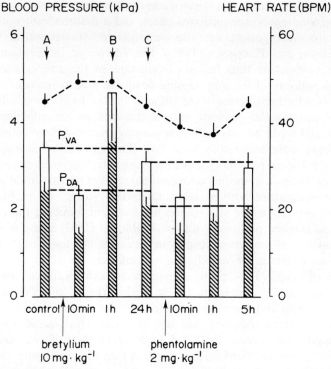

Fig. 5.4. Effects of bretylium (10 mg kg$^{-1}$) and phentolamine (2 mg kg$^{-1}$) injected into conscious cod, *Gadus morhua*, at points indicated in the figure. Blood plasma samples taken at points A, B and C showed no significant variation in catecholamine content between samples. The broken line shows mean values for heart rate. Dorsal aortic blood pressure ($P_{DA}$), but not ventral aortic blood pressure ($P_{VA}$) or heart rate (HR), was significantly lower (P < 0.01) 24 h after bretylium treatment compared with control values. There was no significant reduction in any of the parameters ($P_{DA}$, $P_{VA}$ or HR) 5 h after phentolamine injection compared with the 'bretylium + 24 h' values. The results are interpreted in favour of a solely nervous adrenergic tonus affecting dorsal aortic blood pressure in resting, conscious cod. The figure shows mean values ± SEM from six cod. Blood pressures are expressed in kPa and heart rate in beats per minute (BPM). Reprinted from Smith, D. G., Nilsson, S., Wahlqvist, I. & Eriksson B–M., Nervous control of the blood pressure in the Atlantic cod, *Gadus morhua. Journal of Experimental Biology* **118**. Copyright 1985, Company of Biologists Ltd.

nutritive blood vessels in the gill filaments in these species. In addition, adrenergic fibres occur in the afferent and efferent branchial arteries and at the base of the efferent filamental artery in *S. trutta* (Donald, 1984). In the cod, *Gadus morhua*, changes in the branchial vascular resistance can be elicited by stimulation of the sympathetic chains, and this effect is mediated by adrenergic fibres which innervate branchial blood vessels. The major effect of such nerve stimulation is a constriction of the nutritive vasculature of the gill via an α-adrenoceptor-mediated effect, and a β-adrenoceptor-mediated vasodilatatory component was also demonstrated (Pettersson & Nilsson, 1979; Nilsson and Pettersson, 1981). The adrenergic innervation of the branchial vasculature thus favours blood flow in the arterio-arterial (respiratory) pathway of the gills, closing down the arterio-venous (nutritive) pathway (for further discussion see Nilsson, 1984a). In addition, adrenergic fibres to non-vascular smooth muscle elements in the gills have been observed, and could influence gill functions by changing the position of the gill filaments in the respiratory water flow (Laurent, 1984; Nilsson, 1985).

There is a distinct possibility that circulating catecholamines released from the chromaffin tissue in the posterior cardinal veins of teleosts could affect the branchial vasculature both at rest and during 'stress'. By perfusing the posterior cardinal vein of cod (*Gadus morhua*) and pumping the perfusate through an isolated perfused gill arch, Wahlqvist (1981) was able to show that stimulation of the nervous supply to the chromaffin tissue of the cardinal vein causes a release of catecholamines sufficient to affect the vascular resistance of the gill. In addition, a comparison between the concentration–response curves for adrenaline on isolated perfused gills (Wood, 1974; Wahlqvist, 1980) and the range of catecholamine concentrations in blood plasma of the same species during rest or 'stress' (Nakano & Tomlinson, 1967; Wahlqvist & Nilsson, 1980; P. J. Butler, J. D. Metcalfe, M. Axelsson & S. Nilsson, in preparation) further suggests that the circulating catecholamines affect the branchial vascular resistance *in vivo* (see also Nilsson, 1984a).

In addition to the adrenergic control of the gill vasculature in teleosts, there exists a cholinergic vasomotor control of vagal fibres which presumably innervate the bases of the efferent filamental arteries (Dunel & Laurent, 1977; Smith, 1977). The role of this innervation *in vivo* is unknown.

### 5.3.3. *Control of the systemic vasculature at rest*

The innervation and control of the systemic vasculature in fish has been reviewed by, for example, Johansen (1971, 1982) and Nilsson (1983, 1984b).

Very little is known about the systemic vascular control in elasmobranchs, although a sparse innervation of arteries in *Squalus* has been described (Nilsson *et al.*, 1975; Holmgren & Nilsson, 1983a). A control of the systemic vessels via circulating catecholamines has been suggested (Short *et al.*, 1977; Butler *et al.*, 1978), but further work in this area would be most welcome.

In teleosts there is a well developed adrenergic innervation of the systemic vasculature, and there is good evidence for both an α-adrenoceptor-mediated constrictor mechanism and a β-adrenoceptor-mediated dilatation of the systemic vasculature (see Nilsson, 1983, 1984b; Nilsson & Holmgren, 1985). Even at rest there is an adrenergic tonus affecting the blood pressure of some species (*Salmo gairdneri, Gadus morhua*), and the cause of this tonus (nervous and/or humoral) has been the cause of some discussion (Wahlqvist & Nilsson, 1977; Smith, 1978). In a recent study of the Atlantic cod, *Gadus morhua*, Smith and co-workers (1985) utilised the adrenergic neurone blocking agent bretylium to differentiate between the nervous and humoral adrenergic tonus affecting blood pressure in the resting animal (> 24 h post-anaesthesia/surgery). After establishing the selectivity of the bretylium effect, it was concluded that the adrenergic tonus in resting cod is due solely to adrenergic nerves (Smith *et al.*, 1985).

## 5.4. Circulatory control during exercise

Exercise in fish may be divided into three types: burst, prolonged and sustained swimming (Beamish, 1978; Hoar & Randall, 1978). Burst swimming is chiefly anaerobic and of short duration, whereas the prolonged and sustained types of swimming are aerobic and of longer duration. The control of the cardiovascular system during long-term swimming exercise will be briefly discussed in this section.

Ever since the construction of the first water channels (Fry & Hart, 1948; see also Beamish, 1978), recordings of various circulatory parameters associated with exercise have been made, e.g. heart rate, arterial and venous blood pressure at different sites, cardiac output, cardiac stroke volume, resistance of the major vascular beds, oxygen comsumption, blood parameters such as haematocrit and concentrations of catecholamines. Comparison of data from different investigations is made difficult by differences in the experimental protocol (e.g. temperature, swimming speed, salinity, oxygen and carbon dioxide tension of the respiratory water, diurnal variations, construction of the water channel (with more or less 'stressful' disturbance from vibrations, etc.)), and, of course, the choice of species (Fry & Hart, 1948; Dahlberg *et al.*, 1968; Kutty, 1968; Rao, 1968; Priede, 1974; Beamish 1978; Jones & Randall, 1978; Wood *et al.*, 1979; Bushnell *et al.*, 1984). An attempt to summarise some of the cardiovascular parameters recorded during exercise is offered in Table 5.1.

### 5.4.1. Control of the heart during exercise

The heart rate is comparatively easy to record from swimming fish in the laboratory using ECG leads, or signals from blood-pressure or blood-flow recordings. As mentioned above, experimental conditions may influence the results reported in the literature. Thus Priede (1974) demonstrated that a temperature increase from 5 to 15°C caused an elevation of the heart rate both at rest (from 32·5 to 56 beats min$^{-1}$) and during exercise (from 45·5 to 93 beats min$^{-1}$).

A transient bradycardia at the onset of swimming has been observed in the cod, *Gadus morhua* (Wardle & Kanwisher, 1974; Axelsson & Nilsson, 1986),

Table 5.1. Effects of exercise on some cardiovascular parameters in fish. The figures indicate values during exercise divided by values at rest. Swimming velocities are expressed as body lengths per second (Bl/s), centimetres per second (cm/s) or in terms of critical swimming speed ($U_{crit}$) (see, for example, Beamish 1978).

| Species | Swimming velocity | Temp. (°C) | HR | VAP | DAP | $\dot{Q}$ | SV | $VR_g$ | $VR_s$ | $P_aO_2$ | $P_vO_2$ | Reference |
|---|---|---|---|---|---|---|---|---|---|---|---|---|
| Scyliorhinus stellaris | 0.27 Bl/s | 17–19 | 1.07 | 1.0 | 1.0 | 1.69 | 1.60 | 1.69 | 0.57 | — | — | Piiper et al., 1977 |
| Squalus suckleyi | low | — | 1.25 | — | — | — | — | — | — | — | — | Johansen et al., 1966 |
| Salmo trutta | 2.2 Bl/s | 8 | 1.6–1.7 | — | — | — | — | — | — | — | — | Sutterlin, 1969 |
| Salmo gairdneri | 55 cm/s | 10–12 | 1.15 | 1.40 | ~1.20 | — | — | — | — | — | — | Stevens & Randall, 1967a |
| Salmo gairdneri | 52 cm/s | 4–8 | — | — | — | 4.5 | 5.0 | — | — | 1.0 | 0.85 | Stevens & Randall, 1967b |
| Salmo gairdneri | 2 Bl/s | 9 | 1.13 | — | 1.15 | — | — | — | — | — | — | Smith, 1978 |
| Salmo gairdneri | 1.4 Bl/s | 6.5/15 | 1.7/2.0 | — | — | — | — | — | — | — | — | Priede, 1974 |
| Salmo gairdneri | $U_{crit}$ | 9–10.5 | 1.36 | 1.59 | 1.19 | 2.99 | 2.24 | 1.05 | 0.40 | 0.92 | 0.48 | Kiceniuk & Jones, 1977 |
| Salmo gairdneri | 80% $U_{crit}$ | — | — | — | — | — | — | — | — | 0.98 | 0.41 | Randall & Daxboeck, 1982 |
| Onchorhyncus nerka | $U_{crit}$ | 13–16 | 1.69 | — | 1.25 | — | — | 1.59 | — | — | — | Smith et al., 1967 |
| Anguilla australis | 25 cm/s | 17 | 0.90 | 1.17 | 0.97 | 0.77 | 1.0 | — | 1.08 | — | — | Davie & Foster, 1980 |
| Ictalurus nebulosus | 1 Bl/s | 18–20 | 1.2–1.6 | — | — | — | — | — | — | — | — | Sutterlin, 1969 |
| Carassius auratus | 1.5 Bl/s | 20–25 | 1.6 | — | — | — | — | — | — | — | — | Cameron, 1979 |
| Ophiodon elongatus | low | 9–11 | 1.4 | — | — | ~1.3 | ~1.3 | — | — | — | — | Farrell, 1982 |
| Gadus morhua | 2/3 Bl/s | 10–11 | 1.20 | 1.30 | 1.28 | 1.46 | 1.20 | 1.02 | 0.93 | 1.08 | 0.87 | Axelsson & Nilsson, 1986 |
| Gadus morhua | 1.2 Bl/s | 9 | 1.56 | — | — | — | — | — | — | — | — | Wardle & Kanwisher, 1974 |
| Lepomis gibbosus | 1 Bl/s | 18–22 | 2.28 | — | — | — | — | — | — | — | — | Sutterlin, 1969 |
| Scombrus japonicus | 4–5 Bl/s | 16–20 | 1.54 | — | — | — | — | — | — | — | — | Roberts, 1974 |

*Abbreviations*: HR, heart rate; VAP, ventral aortic blood pressure; DAP, dorsal aortic blood pressure; $\dot{Q}$, cardiac output; SV, cardiac stroke volume; $VR_g$, branchial vascular resistance; $VR_s$, systemic vascular resistance; $P_aO_2$, arterial oxygen tension; $P_vO_2$, venous oxygen tension.

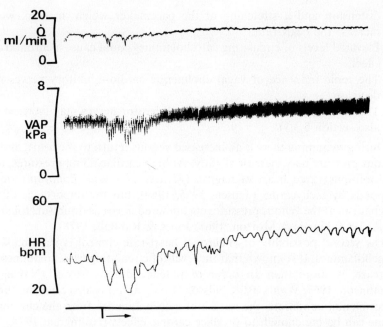

Fig. 5.5.   Recordings of ventral aortic blood flow ($Q$), ventral aortic blood pressure (VAP) and heart rate (beats min$^{-1}$) before and during moderate swimming (2 or 3 body lengths$^{-1}$) in the cod, *Gadus morhua*. Note transient bradycardia at the start of swimming (arrow) and the increase in all three parameters during the swimming.

lingcod, *Ophiodon elongatus* (Stevens *et al.*, 1972; Farrell, 1982), rainbow trout, *Salmo gairdneri* (Priede, 1974) and spiny dogfish, *Squalus acanthias* (Opdyke *et al.*, 1982). This bradycardia is a reflex involving vagal cardio-inhibitory cholinergic fibres, and it is abolished by vagotomy or injection of atropine (Stevens *et al.*, 1972; Priede, 1974; Axelsson & Nilsson, 1986).

Tachycardia during exercise has been described in many different species: *Salmo gairdneri, S. trutta, Caranx crysos, Pomatonius saltatrix, Stenotonius crysops, Oncorphyncus nerka, Lepomis gibbosus, Ictalurus nebulosus, Gadus morhua* (Fig. 5.5), *Scomber scombrus, S. Japonicus, Carassius auratus* and *Scyliorhinus stellaris* (Smith *et al.*, 1967; Stevens & Randall, 1967a; Sutterlin, 1969; Priede, 1974; Roberts, 1974; Wardle & Kanwisher 1974; Kiceniuk & Jones, 1977; Piiper *et al.*, 1977; Cameron, 1979; Axelsson & Nilsson, 1986. In some cases (e.g. *Gadus morhua*), the tachycardia declines with time, leaving only a moderate elevation of heart rate after the first 5–20 min of exercise (Axelsson & Nilsson, 1986).

The increase in heart rate during exercise could be due to at least four different mechanisms, two aneuronal and two neuronal:

(1) Increased venous return due to muscular activity could cause cardiac

distension and a stretching of the pacemaker which, in turn, would increase the heart rate.

(2) Elevated levels of circulating catecholamines could cause a chronotropic effect.

(3) The tonic influence of vagal cholinergic cardio-inhibitory nerves may decrease.

(4) The influence of adrenergic cardio-accelerator nerves may increase (see also section 5.3.1).

During swimming there is an increased venous return to the heart, and the venous pressure may increase slightly. At high cardiac filling pressures, even the non-innervated heart of hagfish (*Myxine glutinosa, Eptatretus stouti*) responds by tachycardia (Jensen, 1965, 1969), but the importance of this mechanism at the venous pressures encountered *in vivo* is doubtful (Johansen *et al.*, 1964; Harris & Morton, 1968; Jones & Randall, 1978).

The second possibility of aneuronal heart-rate control is via circulating catecholamines. It is known that the levels of circulating catecholamines can increase by more than an order of potency during 'stress' (Nakano & Tomlinson, 1967; Wahlqvist & Nilsson, 1980), and it is also clear that under experimental conditions the release of catecholamines from the chromaffin tissue can be big enough to produce cardiac effects (Holmgren, 1977). The few observations of catecholamine levels in teleost blood plasma during exercise do not, however, suggest any dramatic increase associated with moderate swimming (Butler *et al.*, 1986, Axelsson & Nilsson, 1986; see also Opdyke *et al.*, 1982), and it is clear that this possible mode of cardiac control needs further elucidation (see also section 5.3.1).

The mechanisms of nervous cardiac control during exercise are not clear. In some species the exercise tachycardia may be due to a withdrawal of a cholinergic vagal inhibitory tonus on the heart, while in other species (where the heart rate does not increase after atropine or vagotomy) other mechanisms may prevail to explain the tachycardia observed during exercise (Stevens & Randall, 1967; Priede, 1974; Cameron, 1979; Randall, 1982; Axelsson & Nilsson, 1986).

### 5.4.2. *Control of the branchial vasculature during exercise*

Direct measurement of the branchial vascular resistance or the pattern of blood flow within the gills *in vivo* is technically difficult, and the vascular events of the gills are intimately linked to flow and pressure changes caused by altered cardiac performance and systemic vascular resistance.

In rainbow trout there is a *c.* 12–15 times increase in the oxygen uptake during exercise, with more than 90% of the oxygen taken up by the working muscle (Randall & Daxboeck, 1982). It has been estimated that in resting rainbow trout no more than about 60% of the gill lamellae are perfused, but during exercise oxygen transfer at the gills increases substantially indicating vascular changes in the gills such as increased lamellar recruitment (Booth, 1978; Randall, 1982; Randall & Daxboeck, 1982, 1984).

The role of the adrenergic (or other) control systems in the vascular changes of the gills associated with exercise is not at all clear. Due to the compliance of the gill vasculature, an increase in the ventral aortic blood pressure *per se* will reduce the branchial vascular resistance (Farrell *et al.*, 1979, 1980) and it is not yet clear to what extent circulating catecholamines or the innervation of gill blood vessels modify this direct response.

### 5.4.3. *Control of the systemic vasculature during exercise*

Recordings of prebranchial (ventral aortic) and postbranchial (dorsal aortic) blood pressure using chronically implanted catheters have been made in a number of fish species. In cyclostomes, elasmobranchs and some teleosts, there is little or no increase in arterial blood pressure during exercise, but in most teleost species there is a marked increase in both mean arterial (particularly ventral aortic) blood pressure and pulse pressure (Johansen *et al.*, 1966; Piiper *et al.*, 1977; Jones & Randall, 1978; Davie & Foster, 1980). The changes in blood pressure often follow the pattern of the changes in heart rate, and an initial increase with a peak 5–15 min after the start of exercise slowly declines to a steady level above the resting blood pressure (Kiceniuk & Jones, 1977; Jones & Randall, 1978; Randall, 1982; Randall & Daxboeck, 1982; Axelsson & Nilsson, 1986).

The initial increase in blood pressure is independent of the swimming speed at the start of exercise, and it is possible that a general disturbance is responsible for this transient increase. This underlines the importance of differentiating between initial and long-term effects of exercise (Stevens & Randall, 1967a; Kiceniuk & Jones, 1977).

The increase in blood pressure during exercise is the result of an elevated cardiac output (three to six times the resting values; Kiceniuk & Jones, 1977; Randall, 1982). At the same time the systemic vascular resistance falls in association with an increase in the systemic blood flow, particularly to the muscles (Stevens, 1968; Satchell, 1971; Wood, 1975; Jones & Randall, 1978; Randall & Daxboeck, 1982). Both α- (constrictor) and β- (dilatator) adrenoceptors have been demonstrated in the systemic circulation of fish, but the role of the adrenergic control in the changes of systemic vascular resistance associated with swimming are not yet clear (Wood, 1974; Davie, 1981; Jones & Randall, 1978; Nilsson & Holmgren, 1985).

### 5.5. **Circulatory control during 'stress'**

'Stress' is not a unitary conception, and a stress response in the animal may be caused by a wide range of environmental stimuli: severe hypoxia, physical disturbance or damage, changes in temperature, environmental pollutants and illness to name a few. The stress response of the animal may involve cardiovascular changes which are elicited by triggering of the control systems, notably a dramatically increased 'sympathico-adrenal' tonus (see Cannon, 1929; Pickering, 1981; Mazeaud & Mazeaud, 1981).

Physical disturbance of a fish leads to increased levels of circulating catecholamines (see Nilsson, 1983), and in some cases this increase may be big enough to affect cardiac performance and vascular resistance. Experiments with 'stressed' fish *in vivo* are, however, often difficult to interpret, since the stress response of the animal may involve many different links in the control systems depending on the type and degree of 'stress'. Thus transient bradycardia or cardiac arrest is caused by a variety of stimuli (Leivestad *et al.*, 1957; Stevens *et al.*, 1972; Priede, 1974; Wahlqvist & Nilsson, 1980; Smith *et al.*, 1985), and other cardiovascular reflexes may be triggered by, for example, changes in blood pressure or oxygen levels.

### 5.6. Cardiovascular control by non-adrenergic nerves

The control of the fish heart by cholinergic vagal fibres is well established (section 5.3.1), and a cholinergic systemic vasomotor innervation in fish was postulated by Kirby & Burnstock (1969). Later experimentation has not, however, supported the idea of cholinergic vasomotor fibres in fish (see Nilsson, 1983), except in the innervation of the efferent filamental artery of fish gills (see Nilsson, 1984a).

In addition to the adrenergic and cholinergic nerves, there is now increasing evidence for several types of non-adrenergic, non-cholinergic (NANC) neurones in the autonomic nervous system. There is histochemical evidence for the existence of a peptidergic cardiac innervation in mammals, and in the toad, *Bufo marinus*, there is excellent histochemical and physiological evidence for a functional inhibitory control of the heart by neurones releasing both acetylcholine and somatostatin (Campbell *et al.*, 1982). So far, no descriptions of a NANC innervation of the fish heart have been published, but the possibility of a functional NANC innervation of the fish heart deserves elucidation.

Histochemical studies of the fish gut revealed the presence of a number of NANC neurotransmitters in fibres innervating blood vessels. Thus the peptides bombesin, neurotensin and vasoactive intestinal polypeptide (VIP) have been demonstrated in blood vessels from *Squalus acanthias* (Holmgren & Nilsson, 1983a), and VIP is also present in blood vessels in the gut of *Lepisosteus platyrhincus* (Holmgren & Nilsson, 1983b) and in the swimbladder vasculature and coeliac artery of the cod, *Gadus morhua* (Lundin & Holmgren, 1985).

Although the function of the NANC innervation of the vasculature is not known, it is clear that this type of vasomotor innervation must be taken into account when the overall nervous control of the fish vasculature is considered.

## 5.7. Final comments

Future research on the cardiovascular control systems in fish will have to deal with two areas in particular. First, the NANC systems must be taken into account when discussing the arrangement of the cardiovascular control in general. Secondly, the individual building block studies of different vascular beds or isolated heart preparations *in vitro* must be used in the analysis of integrated control *in vivo*. A continuous refinement of techniques will also be necessary to analyse the various links and reflexes of the cardiovascular control systems and to distinguish between 'stress' and specific stimuli applied (exercise, hypoxia, etc.).

## Acknowledgements

We thank Drs PJ Butler and Susanne Holmgren for critical reading of the manuscript. Our own research concerning cardiovascular control in fish is currently supported by the Swedish Natural Science Research Council.

## References

Abrahamsson, T. (1979). Phenylethanolamine-N-methyl transferase (PNMT) activity and catecholamine storage and release from the chromaffin tissue of the spiny dogfish, *Squalus acanthias. Comp. Biochem. Physiol.* **64C**, 169–72.

Abrahamsson, T., Holmgren, S., Nilsson, S. & Pettersson, K. (1979). On the chromaffin system of the African lungfish, *Protopterus aethiopicus. Acta Physiol. Scand.* **107**, 135–9.

Augustinsson, K. B., Fänge, R., Johnels, A. & Östlund, E. (1956). Histological, physiological and biochemical studies on the heart of two cyclostomes, hagfish (*Myxine*) and lamprey (*Lampetra*). *J. Physiol. (London)* **131**, 257–76.

Axelsson, M. & Nilsson, S. (1986). Blood pressure control during exercise in the Atlantic cod, *Gadus morhua, J. Exp. Biol.* **126**, 225–36.

Beamish, F. W. H. (1978). Swimming capacity. In *Fish Physiology* vol. 7 (eds W. S. Hoar & D. J. Randall). London and New York: Academic Press.

Bloom, G., Östlund, E., Euler, U. S. von, Lishajko, F., Ritzen, M. & Adams-Ray, J. (1961). Studies on catecholamine-containing granules of specific cells in cyclostome hearts. *Acta Physiol. Scand.* **53** Suppl. **185**, 1–34.

Booth, J. H. (1978). The distribution of blood in the gills of fish: application of a new technique to rainbow trout (*Salmo gairdneri*). *J. Exp. Biol.* **73**, 119–29.

Bushnell, P. G., Steffensen, J. F. & Johansen, K. (1984). Oxygen consumption and swimming performance in hypoxia-acclimated rainbow trout (*Salmo gairdneri*). *J. Exp. Biol.* **113**, 225–35.

Butler, P. J., Metcalfe, J. D. & Ginley, S. A. (1986). Plasma catecholamines in the lesser spotted dogfish and rainbow trout at rest and during different levels of exercise. *J. Exp. Biol.* **123**, 409–21.

Butler, P. J. & Taylor, E.W. (1971). Response of the dogfish (*Scyliorhinus canicula L.*)

to slowly induced and rapidly induced hypoxia. *Comp. Biochem. Physiol.* **39A**, 307–23.

Butler, P. J., Taylor, E. W. Capra, M. F. & Davison, W. (1978). The effect of hypoxia on the levels of circulating catecholamines in the dogfish *Scyliorhinus canicula.* *J. Comp. Physiol.* **127**, 325–30.

Cameron, J. S. (1979). Autonomic nervous tone and regulation of heart rate in the goldfish, *Carassius auratus. Comp. Biochem. Physiol.* **63C**, 341–9.

Campbell, G. (1970). Autonomic nervous systems. In *Fish Physiology*, vol. 4, pp. 109–32 (eds W. S. Hoar & D. J. Randall). London and New York: Academic Press.

Campbell, G., Gibbins, I. L. Morris, J. L., Furness, J. B., Costa, M., Oliver, A. M., Beardsley, A. M. & Murphy, R. (1982). Somatostatin is contained in and released from cholinergic nerves in the heart of the toad *Bufo marinus. Neuroscience* **7**, 2013–23.

Cannon, W. B. (1929). Organization for physiological homeostasis. *Physiol. Rev.* **9**, 399–431.

Dahl, E., Ehinger, B., Falck, B., Mecklenburg, C., Myhrberg, H. & Rosengren, E. (1971). On the monoamine-storing cells in the heart of *Lampetra fluviatilis* and *L. planeri* (Cyclostomata). *Gen. Comp. Endocrinol.* **17**, 241–6.

Dahlberg, M. L., Shumway, D. L. & Doudoroff, P. (1968). Influence of dissolved oxygen and carbon dioxide on swimming performance of largemouth bass and coho salmon. *J. Fish. Res. Bd Can.* **25**, 49–70.

Davie, P. S. (1981). Vascular responses of an eel tail preparation: alpha constriction and beta dilation. *J. Exp. Biol.* **90**, 65–84.

Davie, P. S. & Foster, M. E. (1980) Cardiovascular responses to swimming in eels. *Comp. Biochem. Physiol.* **67**, 367–73

Davies, D. T. & Rankin, J. C. (1973). Adrenergic receptors and vascular responses to catecholamines of perfused dogfish gills. *Comp. Gen. Pharmacol.* **4**, 139–47.

Donald, J. (1984). Adrenergic innervation of the gills of brown and rainbow trout, *Salmo trutta* and *S. gairdneri. J. Morphol.* **182**, 307–16.

Donald, J. & Campbell, G. (1982). A comparative study of the adrenergic innervation of the teleost heart. *J. Comp. Physiol.* **147**, 85–91.

Dunel, S. & Laurent, P. (1977). La vascularization branchial chez l'Anguille: actione de l'acetylcholine et de l'adrénaline sur la répartition d'une résine polymérisable dans les différents compartiments vasculaires. *C. R. Acad. Sci. Ser. D* **284**, 2011–14.

Farrell, A. P. (1982). Cardiovascular changes in the unanaesthetized lingcod (*Ophiodon elongatus*) during short-term progressive hypoxia and spontaneous activity. *Can. J. Zool.* **60**, 933–43.

Farrell, A. P. (1984). A review of cardiac performance in the teleost heart: intrinsic and humoral regulation. *Can. J. Zool.* **62**, 523–36.

Farrell, A. P., Daxboeck, C. & Randall, D. J. (1979). The effect of input pressure and flow on the pattern and resistance to flow in the isolated perfused gill of a teleost fish. *J. Comp. Physiol.* **133**, 233–40.

Farrell, A. P., Sobin, S. S., Randall, D. J. & Crosby, S. (1980). Intralamellar blood flow patterns in fish gills. *Am. J. Physiol.* **239**, R428–36.

Fry, F. E. J. & Hart, J. S. (1948). Cruising speed of goldfish in relation to water temperature. *J. Fish. Res. Bd Can.* **7**, 169–75.

Gannon, B. J. & Burnstock, G. (1969). Excitatory adrenergic innervation of the fish heart. *Comp. Biochem. Physiol.* **29**, 765–73.

Gannon, B. J. Campbell, G. D. & Satchell, G. H. (1972). Monoamine storage in relation to cardiac regulation in the Port Jackson shark, *Heterodontus portusjacksoni. Z. Zellforsch.* **131**, 437–50.

Harris, W. S. & Morton, M. J. (1968). A cardiac intrinsic mechanism that relates heart rate to filling pressure. *Circulation* **38** Suppl. 6, 95.

Hoar, W. S. & Randall, D. J. (eds) (1978). *Fish Physiology, vol. 7. Locomotion.* New York: Academic Press.

Hoar, W. S. & Randall, D. J. (eds) (1984) *Fish Physiology, vols 10A and 10B Gills.* Orlando, Fla: Academic Press.

Holmgren, S. (1977) Regulation of the heart of a teleost, *Gadus morhua*, by autonomic nerves and circulating catecholamines. *Acta Physiol. Scand.* **99**, 62–74.

Holmgren, S. & Nilsson, S. (1983a). Bombesin-, gastrin/CCK-, 5-hydroxytryptamine-, neurotensin-, somatostatin-, and VIP-like immunoreactivity and catecholamine fluorescence in the gut of the elasmobranch, *Squalus acanthias. Cell Tissue Res.* **234**, 595–618.

Holmgren, S. & Nilsson, S. (1983b). VIP-, bombesin- and neurotensin-like immunoreactivity in neurons of the gut of the holostean fish, *Lepisosteus platyrhincus. Acta Zool. (Stockholm)*, **64**, 25–32.

Jensen, D. (1965) The aneural heart of the hagfish. *Ann. NY Acad. Sci.* **127**, 443–58.

Jensen, D. (1969). Intrinsic cardiac rate regulation in the sea lamprey (*Petromyzon marinus*) and rainbow trout (*Salmo gairdneri*). *Comp. Biochem. Physiol.* **30**, 685–90.

Johansen, K. (1971). Comparative physiology: gas exchange and circulation in fishes. *Ann. Rev. Physiol.* **33**, 569–612.

Johansen, K. (1982). Blood circulation and the rise of air-breathing (passes and bypasses). In *A Companion to Animal Physiology*, pp. 91–105 (eds C. R. Taylor, K. Johansen & L. Bolis). Cambridge: Cambridge University Press.

Johansen, K. & Burggren, W. (1980). Cardiovascular function in the lower vertebrates. In *Hearts and heart-like organs*, vol. 1, pp. 61–117 (ed. G. H. Bourne). London and New York: Academic Press.

Johansen, K., Krog, J. & Reite, O. B. (1964). Autonomic nervous influence on the heart of the hypothermic hibernator. *Finn. Acad. Sci. A* **IV**, 245–55.

Johansen, K., Franklin, D. L. & Van Citters, R. L. (1966). Aortic blood flow in free-swimming elasmobranchs. *Comp. Biochem. Physiol.* **19**, 151–60.

Jones, D. R. & Randall, D. J. (1978). The respiration and circulatory systems during exercise. In *Fish Physiology, vol. 7. Locomotion* (eds W. S. Hoas & D. J. Randall), pp. 425–501. New York: Academic Press.

Kiceniuk, J. W. & Jones, D. R. (1977) The oxygen transport system in trout (*Salmo gairdneri*) during sustained exercise. *J. Exp. Biol.* **69**, 247–60.

Kirby, S. & Burnstock, G. (1969) Comparative pharmacological studies of isolated spiral strips of large arteries from lower vertebrates. *Comp. Biochem. Physiol.* **28**, 307–20.

Kutty, M. N. (1968). Influence of ambient oxygen on the swimming performance of goldfish and rainbow trout. *Can. J. Zool.* **46**, 647–53.

Langley, J. N. (1921). *The Autonomic Nervous System*, Part I. Cambridge: Heffer.

Laurent, P. (1984) Gill internal morphology. In *Fish Physiology*, vol. XA pp. 73–183 (eds W. S. Hoas & D. J. Randall). Orlando, Fla: Academic Press.

Laurent, P., Holmgren, S. & Nilsson, S. (1983). Nervous and humoral control of the fish heart: structure and function. *Comp. Biochem. Physiol.* **76A**, 525–42.

Leivestad, H., Andersen, H. & Scholander, P. F. (1957). Physiological responses to air exposure in codfish. *Science* **126**, 505

Lundin, K. & Holmgren, S. (1984). Vasoactive intestinal polypeptide-like immunoreactivity and effects of VIP in the swimbladder of the cod, *Gadus morhua. J. Comp. Physiol.* 154, 627–33.

Mazeaud, M. M. & Mazeaud, F. (1981). Adrenergic responses to stress in fish. In *Stress and Fish*, pp. 49–75 (ed. A. D. Pickering). New York: Academic Press.

Metcalfe, J. D. & Butler, P. J. (1984). On the nervous regulation of gill blood flow in the dogfish (*Scyliorhinus caniculia*). *J. Exp. Biol.* **113**, 253–67.

Nakano, T. & Tomlinson, N. (1967). Catecholamine and carbohydrate concentration in rainbow trout (*Salmo gairdneri*) in relation to physical disturbance. *J. Fish. Res. Bd Can.* **24**, 1701–15.

Nilsson, S. (1983). *Autonomic Nerve Function in the Vertebrates.* Berlin, Heidelberg, New York: Springer-Verlag.

Nilsson, S. (1984a). Innervation and pharmacology of the gills. In *Fish Physiology, Vol XA*, pp. 185–227 (eds W. S. Hoar & D. J. Randall), Orlando, Fla: Academic Press.

Nilsson, S. (1984b). Adrenergic control systems in fish. *Marine Biol. Lett.* **5**, 127–46.

Nilsson, S. (1985). Filament position in fish gills is influenced by a smooth muscle innervated by adrenergic nerves. *J. Exp. Biol.* **118**, 433–7.

Nilsson, S. & Holmgren, S. (1985). D- and L-isoprenaline have different effects on adrenoceptors in the systemic vasculature of the cod, *Gadus morhua*. *Comp. Biochem. Physiol.* **80C**, 105–7.

Nilsson, S. & Pettersson, K. (1981). Sympathetic nervous control of blood flow in the gills of the Atlantic cod, *Gadus morhua*. *J. Comp. Physiol.* **144**, 157–63.

Nilsson, S., Holmgren, S. & Grove, D. J. (1975). Effects of drugs and nerve stimulation on the spleen and arteries of two species of dogfish, *Scyliorhinus canicula* and *Squalus acanthias*. *Acta. Physiol. Scand.* **95**, 219–30.

Nilsson, S., Abrahamsson, T. & Grove, D. J. (1976). Sympathetic nervous control of adrenaline release from the head kidney of the cod, *Gadus morhua*. *Comp. Biochem. Physiol.* **55C**, 123–7.

Opdyke, D. F., Carroll, G. R. & Keller, N. E. (1982). Catecholamine release and blood pressure changes induced by exercise in dogfish. *Am. J. Physiol.* **242**, R306–10.

Pettersson, K. & Johansen, K. (1982). Hypoxic vasoconstriction and the effects of adrenaline on gas exchange efficiency in fish gills. *J. Exp. Biol.* **97**, 263–72.

Pettersson, K. & Nilsson, S. (1979). Control of branchial blood flow in the Atlantic cod (*Gadus morhua*). *J. Comp. Physiol.* **129**, 179–83.

Pickering, A. D. (1981). Introduction: the concept of biological stress. In *Stress and Fish*, pp. 1–9. (ed. A. D. Pickering). London and New York: Academic Press.

Piiper, J., Meyer, M., Worth, H. & Willmer, H. (1977). Respiration and circulation during swimming activity in dogfish (*Scyliorhinus stellaris*). *Resp. Physiol.* **30**, 221–39.

Priede, I. G. (1974). The effect of swimming activity and section of the vagus nerves on heart rate in rainbow trout. *J. Exp. Biol.* **60**, 305–19.

Rao, G. (1968). Oxygen consumption of rainbow trout (*Salmo gairdneri*) in relation to activity and salinity. *Can. J. Zool.* **46**, 781–6.

Randall, D. J. (1982). The control of respiration and circulation in fish during exercise and hypoxia. *J. Exp. Biol.* **100**, 275–88.

Randall, D. J. & Daxboeck, C. (1982). Cardiovascular changes in the rainbow trout (*Salmo gairdneri* Richardson) during exercise. *Can. J. Zool.* **60**, 1135–40.

Randall, D. J. & Daxboeck, C. (1984). Oxygen and carbon dioxide transfer across fish gills. In *Fish Physiology*, vol. XA, pp. 263–314 (eds W. S. Hoar & D. J. Randall). Orlando, Fla: Academic Press

Roberts, J. L. (1974). Control of ram ventilation: thermal and hypoxic stresses. *Am. Zool.* **14**, 4.

Santer, R. M. (1985). Morphology and innervation of the fish heart. *Adv. Anat. Embryol. Cell Biol.* **89**, 1–102.

Satchell, G. H. (1962). Intrinsic vasomotion in the dogfish gill. *J. Exp. Biol.* **39**, 503–12.

Satchell, G. H. (1971). *Circulation in Fishes.* Cambridge: Cambridge University Press.

Scheuermann, D. W. (1979). Untersuchungen hinsichtlich der Innervation des Sinus

Venosus und des Aurikels von *Protopterus annectens. Acta Morphol. Neerl. Scand.* **17**, 231–2.

Short, S., Butler, P. J. & Taylor, E. W. (1977). The relative importance of nervous, humoral and intrinsic mechanisms in the regulation of heart rate and stroke volume in the dogfish *Scyliorhinus canicula. J. Exp. Biol.* **70**, 77–92.

Smith, D. G. (1977). Sites of cholinergic vasoconstriction in trout gills. *Am. J. Physiol,* **233**, R222–9.

Smith, D. G. (1978). Neural regulation of blood pressure in rainbow trout (*Salmo gairdneri*). *Can. J. Zool.* **56**, 1678–83.

Smith, D. G., Nilsson, S., Wahlqvist, I. & Eriksson, B.-M. (1985). Nervous control of the blood pressure in the Atlantic cod, *Gadus morhua. J. Exp. Biol.* **117**, 335–47.

Smith, L. S., Brett, J. R. & Davis, J. C. (1967). Cardiovascular dynamics in swimming adult sockeye salmon. *J. Fish. Res. Bd Can.* **24**, 1775–90.

Stevens, E. D. (1968). The effect of exercise on the distribution of blood to various organs in rainbow trout. *Comp. Biochem. Physiol.* **25**, 615–25.

Stevens, E. D. & Randall, D. J. (1967a). Changes in blood pressure, heart rate and breathing rate during moderate swimming activity in rainbow trout. *J. Exp. Biol.* **46**, 307–15.

Stevens, E. D. & Randall, D. J. (1967b). Changes in gas concentrations in blood and water during moderate swimming activity in rainbow trout. *J. Exp. Biol.* **46**, 329–37.

Stevens, E. D., Bennion, G. R., Randall, D. J. & Shelton, G. (1972). Factors affecting arterial pressure and blood flow from the heart in intact, unrestrained lingcod, *Ophiodon elongatus. Comp. Biochem. Physiol.* **43A**, 681–95.

Sutterlin, M. A. (1969). Effects of exercise on cardiac and ventilation frequency in three species of freshwater teleosts. *Physiol. Zool.* **42**, 36–52.

Taylor, E. W., Short, S. & Butler, P. J. (1977). The role of the cardiac vagus in the response of the dogfish (*Scyliorhinus canicular L*) to hypoxia. *J. Exp. Biol.* **70**, 57–75.

Wahlqvist, I. (1980). Effects of catecholamines on isolated systemic and branchial vascular beds of the cod, *Gadus morhua. J. Comp. Physiol.* **137**, 139–43.

Wahlqvist, I. (1981). Branchial vascular effects of catecholamines released from the head kidney of the Atlantic cod, *Gadus morhua. Mol. Physiol.* **1**, 235–41.

Wahlqvist, I. & Nilsson, S. (1977). The role of sympathetic fibres and circulating catecholamines in controlling the blood pressure in the cod, *Gadus morhua. Comp. Biochem. Physiol.* **57C**, 65–7.

Wahlqvist, I. & Nilsson, S. (1980) Adrenergic control of the cardiovascular system of the Atlantic cod, *Gadus morhua*, during 'stress'. *J. Comp. Physiol.* **137**, 145–50.

Wardle, C. S. & Kanwisher, D. W. (1974). The significance of heart rate in free swimming cod (*Gadus morhua*). Some observations with ultra-sonic tags. *Mar. Behav. Physiol.* **2**, 311–24.

Wood, C. M. (1974). A critical examination of the physical and adrenergic factors affecting blood flow through the gills of the rainbow trout. *J. Exp. Biol.* **60**, 241–65.

Wood, C. M. (1975). A pharmacological analysis of the adrenergic and cholinergic mechanisms regulating branchial vascular resistance in the rainbow trout (*Salmo gairdneri*). *Can. J. Zool.* **53**, 1569–77.

Wood, C. M., Pieprzak, P. & Trott, J. N. (1979). The influence of temperature and anaemia on the adrenergic and cholinergic mechanisms controlling heart rate in the rainbow trout. *Can. J. Zool.* **57**, 2440–7.

# 6

# GABA and cardiovascular reflexes

C. Kidd[1], J. A. BENNETT[2] and P. N. McWilliam[3]

[1]*Department of Physiology, Marischal College, University of Aberdeen, Aberdeen AB9 1AS, UK;* [2]*Department of Animal Physiology and Nutrition, University of Leeds, Leeds LS9 2JT, UK;* [3]*Department of Cardiovascular Studies, University of Leeds, Leeds LS9 2JT, UK*

## 6.1. GABA and the cardiovascular system

An extensive literature indicates that gamma-aminobutyric acid (GABA) and glycine have roles as inhibitory transmitters in the brain and spinal cord. Evidence that GABA may be involved in the neural control of the cardiovascular system has been provided, very largely by examining the changes in heart rate and blood pressure which follow application of either GABA or its agonists and antagonists, through the vascular system, intracerebroventricularly or directly to nervous tissue (e.g. Gillis *et al.*, 1984). Histochemical evidence for the presence in the brainstem of the synthesising enzyme glutamic acid decarboxylase (GAD) is also available (Massari *et al.*, 1976).

Throughout, little attention has been paid to the potential role of GABA systems in modulating cardiovascular reflexes, and, in particular, their central neural components. Abundant evidence indicates that the central nervous pathways of cardiovascular reflex pathways are open to modulation. For example, the 'defence area' has profound inhibitory influences on carotid sinus reflexes, and stimulation of the fastigial nuclei strongly inhibits the bradycardia mediated by carotid-sinus baroreceptors and the Bezold–Jarish reflex bradycardia evoked by phenyl diguanide (e.g. Hilton, 1963; Smith & Nathan, 1966; Achari & Downman, 1970; Coote 1979). The specific transmitters involved in such actions have not been identified. Several studies (e.g. Barman & Gebber, 1979; Lalley, 1980; Gillis *et al.*, 1980) using indirect approaches have claimed to demonstrate effects on baroreceptor reflexes due to GABA applied to the central nervous system. However, their experimental protocols were not specific, and it is possible to interpret their results in other ways. Thus, we conclude that the potential role of GABA or glycine in modulating cardiovascular reflexes has by no means been adequately established, and that an additional investigation in which specific receptor populations were stimulated is appropriate.

In this respect it has recently been shown (Yamada *et al.*, 1984) that GABA-mediated systems in the superficial areas of the ventral medulla may facilitate baroreceptor reflexes: a pathway thought to be involved in 'defence area' responses. Finally, evidence has been adduced to show, using microion-tophoretic techniques, that local application of GABA may inhibit directly vagal cardiomotor neurones (DiMicco *et al.*, 1979; Gilbey *et al.*, 1985).

Our interest in GABA systems was originally aroused during electro-physiological studies of interneuronal responses in the nucleus tractus solitarius (NTS) following stimulation of myelinated and non-myelinated cardiac and pulmonary vagal afferent fibres (Bennett *et al.*, 1981, 1985; Donoghue *et al.*, 1981). In addition to excitatory actions, profound and long-lasting inhibitory effects on NTS neurones were observed (Bennett *et al.*, 1982).

We decided to investigate the hypothesis that GABA-mediated inhibitory systems exerted powerful effects on the central nervous pathways engaged by cardiovascular reflexes, and this account describes pilot experiments which identified such a system operating in a tonic manner on the vagal efferent pathway mediating the bradycardiac component of some cardiovascular reflexes.

## 6.2. Effect of the GABA autagonist bicuculline on some cardiovascular reflexes

Chloralose-anaesthetised cats were decerebrated initially at the mid-collicular level although other levels of transection were used (see later). Carotid sinus baroreceptors were activated by transient increases in pressure applied through a double lumen catheter inserted into the external carotid artery. Receptors in the lung and heart with non-myelinted vagal afferent fibres were stimulated by injection of small doses (5–25 µg kg) of phenyl biguanide (PBG) into the right atrium. Such doses have been shown to excite pulmonary receptors attached to non-myelinated vagal afferent fibres (see Coleridge & Coleridge, 1984) and to evoke a powerful vagally mediated bradycardia (Fig. 6.1A). Effects of the GABA antagonist bicuculline were examined by infusing small doses 0.25–1.5 mg kg$^{-1}$ intravenously or intracerebroventricularly.

Figure 6.1 shows that an infusion of bicuculline resulted in a striking enhancement of the reflex bradycardia following a right atrial injection of phenyl biguanide. Similarly, the reflex bradycardia in response to an increase in carotid sinus pressure was markedly enhanced (Fig. 6.2). The results from trials on nine animals are summarised in Fig. 6.3. The mean reflex bradycardia following PBG was enhanced from 31 $\pm$ 5 to 105 $\pm$ 12 beats min$^{-1}$ (13 trials), while that in response to a pulsatile increase in carotid sinus pressure was enhanced from 14 $\pm$ 3 to 71 $\pm$ 10 beats min$^{-1}$ (12 trials). Every

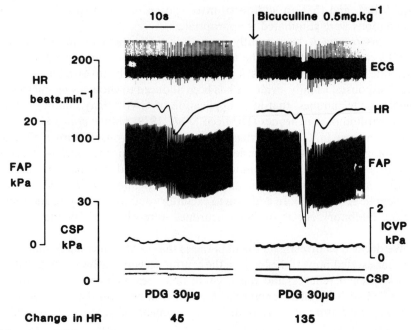

Fig. 6.1.   Effect of bicuculline (0.5 mg kg$^{-1}$) on reflex response to PDG (30 μg i.v.). ECG Electrocardiogram; HR, analogue record of heart rate; FAP, femoral arterial blood pressure; ICVP, intracerebroventricular pressure; CSP, carotid sinus pressure.

infusion of bicuculline resulted in an enhancement of the reflex bradycardia, and the difference is highly significant statistically (paired $t$-test).

In some experiments bicuculline (150–200 μg kg$^{-1}$) was infused in artificial cerebrospinal fluid into the foramen magnum through a double lumen catheter, and in a short time the bradycardiac effects evoked by increases in carotid sinus pressure and PBG injection were also enhanced.

Neuromuscular blocking agents were not employed, and most trials were therefore conducted with subconvulsant doses of GABA; in a minority, convulsions did occur following GABA infusion but the enhancement still occurred.

Immediately after bicuculline there were variable transient changes in heart rate and arterial blood pressure. However, after 3–7 min both blood pressure and heart rate returned to control levels and only at this time were the reflexes examined. The enhanced bradycardia following bicuculline infusion lasted for about 20–40 min, during which time there was a progressive reduction toward control values. In some experiments the magnitude and duration of the enhancement were increased by larger doses of bicuculline but such studies were limited by the onset of convulsions.

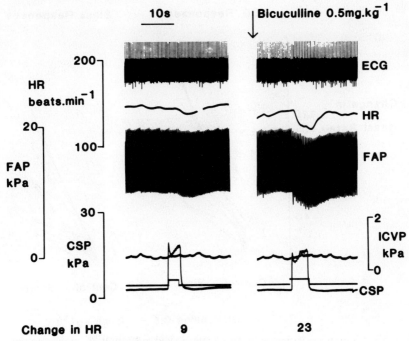

Fig. 6.2. Effect of bicuculline (0.5 mg kg$^{-1}$) on reflex response to increase in carotid sinus pressure. Abbreviations as Fig. 6.1.

Under the conditions of our studies, the reflex bradycardia evoked by carotid sinus baroreceptor stimulation or injection of phenyl biguanide is very largely vagal in origin since little heart rate change remains after infusion of atropine (0.5 μg kg$^{-1}$).

We conclude, therefore, that the vagal efferent component of the reflex responses to both carotid sinus baroreceptor and pulmonary vagal afferent fibres is tonically inhibited in these animals by a GABA-mediated system.

We have also examined, in a preliminary study, the sympathetic efferent component of both reflex responses by recording activity in 'few fibre' strands dissected from the left renal sympathetic nerves. The inhibition of renal sympathetic nerve activity induced by carotid sinus baroreceptor activity and right atrial PBG was enhanced in most trials following subconvulsant doses of bicuculline. The effects of bicuculline on the sympathetic efferent component of both reflex pathways were clearly less consistent than the effect on the vagal bradycardia; nevertheless, the most frequent effect was an enhancement. This was manifested by an increased depression of activity as well as a longer period of inhibition.

Thus both the sympathetic and the vagal components of these powerful

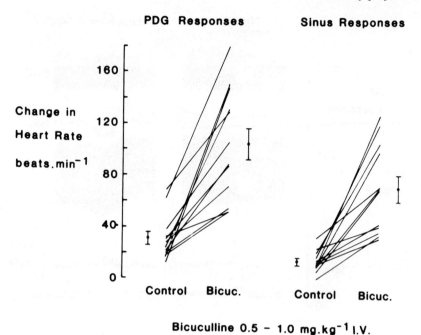

**Bicuculline 0.5 – 1.0 mg.kg⁻¹ I.V.**

Fig. 6.3.    Summary of changes in heart rate evoked in 12 trials. Responses to phenyl
   diguanide (PDG) and carotid sinus distension (sinus) before (control) and after
   (Bicuc.) an intravenous dose of bicuculline.


cardiovascular reflexes are subject to a potent, tonic, GABA-mediated,
inhibitory action which is strongly manifested under the conditions of our
experiments.

### 6.3. Brainstem origin of a tonically active inhibitory system acting on some cardiovascular reflexes

We have carried out pilot experiments to identify possible central nervous
origins for such tonic actions by performing successive transections of the
neuraxis. Essentially, the brainstem was transected at three levels: 'high',
'mid' and 'low', and the results for carotid-sinus-evoked reflex bradycardia
from 13 animals are shown in fig. 6.4. The enhancement of reflex bradycardia
in response to PBG was influenced in a parallel fashion. The 'mid' levels refer
to transections at a midcollicular level, and the enhanced reflex bradycardia
following carotid sinus distension induced by bicuculline is clear. In order to
determine whether rostal areas were the site of origin of the tonic GABA
effect, the brainstem was initially transected at 'high' level in two animals
such that the hypothalamus, and particularly the defence area, were left
intact. In both animals the enhancement by bicuculline of the reflex

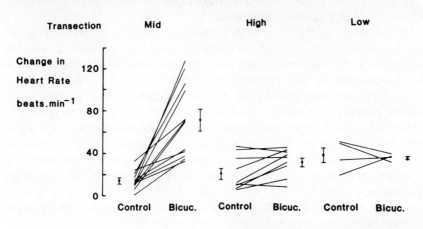

Fig. 6.4. Effect of brainstem transection at three levels, 'mid', 'high' and 'low', on the enhancement by bicuculline of the reflex heart rate change following carotid sinus distension. Control, response before bicuculline; Bicuc., response after i.v. bicuculline.

bradycardia resulting from reflex stimuli was much smaller than in the 'mid' transection animals (Fig. 6.4). In these animals the enhancement of the reflex bradycardias induced by bicuculline became larger and approximated to that in 'mid' collicular animals as the transections were extended caudally to a collicular level. In two animals extension of the transections below the colliculi were without effect until at about the level of the caudal portion of the cerebellar peduncles when the enhancement was abolished. At such levels the control bradycardiac responses to both increases in carotid sinus pressure and PBG were increased. Histological examination confirmed that the transections were complete.

High concentrations of high-affinity GABA receptors have been demonstrated in the cerebellum, particularly the cerebellar nuclei. In six mid-collicularly decerebrate animals, the cerebellum was also removed. In each animal repeated trials showed that the enhancing effect of bicuculline on the carotid sinus and phenyl-diguanide-induced bradycardia was unaffected.

It is clear that the cerebellar pathways that influence these reflex responses were not operating in a tonic fashion and that GABA is not involved. It is also clear that the tonic inhibitory effects on cardiovascular reflexes mediated by the 'defence area' do not involve a tonic GABA system. Although there is a significant extension of the 'defence area' into the lower brainstem, similar transmitters are likely to be involved. On the contrary, since the enhancement of bradycardia induced by bicuculline was smaller in 'high' decerebrate preparations and became larger following caudal transections, one explanation could be that in such 'high' preparations the GABA-mediated inhibitory system was being partially suppressed.

The abolition of the tonic GABA-mediated inhibition by transections of the brainstem at the level of the cerebellar peduncles provides a valuable control in confirming, under conditions where there are brisk reflex responses to carotid-sinus baroreceptor and PBG stimulation, that the bicuculline-induced enhancement results from its effect on central neural pathways and cannot be due to peripheral actions on the heart or autonomic ganglia. The enhanced control responses to both carotid sinus baroreceptor and PBG infusion following the 'low' transection are consistent with the notion of tonic centrally mediated GABA inhibition originating in the brainstem.

In similar studies we have examined the effect of the glycine antagonist strychnine (1.0 mg $kg^{-1}$ i.v.) on the reflex bradycardia induced by carotid sinus baroreceptors and PBG stimulation of cardiac and pulmonary vagal afferent fibres. No enhancement of the bradycardia in response to either stimulus was observed in eight animals. We conclude that it is unlikely that glycine receptors mediate tonic inhibitory effects on reflex vagal systems.

It can be argued that the actions of bicuculline may be non-specific and are not conclusive evidence for GABA actions. However, examination of the literature shows that of the available antagonists bicuculline is one of the most specific (e.g. Andrews & Johnson, 1979; Champagnat et al., 1982); furthermore, a postulated weak alternative mode of action of bicuculline is against glycine receptors which on the basis of our evidence, using the more powerful glycine antagonist, strychnine, are unlikely to play an inhibitory role on these reflexes.

High-affinity GABA receptors have beer demonstrated in several brain-stem areas including the vagal nuclei (Gale et al., 1980); however, further studies are necessary to define the neuronal groups responsible for the tonic actions we have observed.

The system is additional to that involved in the GABA-mediated enhancement of the sympathetic component of the carotid sinus baroreceptor reflex, which originates from areas adjacent to the ventrolateral surface of the medulla (Yamada et al., 1984). It may be that the inconsistent results that we obtained on reflex changes in renal sympathetic efferent fibre activity are explained by interaction of the two systems. The presence of GABA receptors in or close to the vagal cardiomotor neurones (DiMicco et al., 1979; Gilbey et al., 1985) is also compatible with our observations. However, since the enhancement induced by bicuculline in our study was abolished by 'low' brainstem transection at a time when the control reflex bradycardia was enhanced, and since injections of bicuculline were immediately and consistently now followed by a powerful bradycardia, we suggest that yet another tonic GABA-mediated inhibitory system is operating directly upon vagal cardiomotor neurones of the nucleus ambiguus or interneurones in close proximity. Since our studies have shown that a GABA-mediated inhibitory action is also exerted upon renal sympathetic efferent neurones responding to both carotid sinus and vagal pulmonary receptors, an alternative explanation may be that the GABA actions are exerted 'early' in the reflex pathways. Alternatively, a widespread projection from neurones higher in the brainstem would have similar effects.

In summary, we have provided evidence for the existence, under the conditions of our experiments, of a powerful tonic inhibitory action mediated by GABA which is expressed upon vagal and sympathetic components of the central neural reflex pathways activated by stimulation of carotid sinus baroreceptors and cardiac and pulmonary receptors with non-myelinated vagal afferent fibres. Further studies are necessary to identify the sites of origin for these effects. We find no evidence for a tonic inhibitory action mediated by glycine on these reflexes.

## Acknowledgements

It is a pleasure to acknowledge the high-quality technical support of Mrs Jean Kaye. Acknowledgement is also made to the British Heart Foundation and Medical Research Counal for financial support.

## References

Achari, N. K. & Downman, C. B. B. (1970). Autonomic effector responses to stimulation of nucleus fastigius. *J. Physiol.* **210**, 637–50.

Andrews, P. R. & Johnson, G. A. R. (1979). GABA agonists and antagonists. *Biochem. Pharmacol.* **28**, 2697–702.

Barman, S. M. & Gebber, G. L. (1979). Picrotoxin- and bicuculline-sensitive inhibition of cardiac vagal reflexes. *J. Pharmacol. Exp. Therap.* **209**, 67–72.

Bennett, J. A., Goodchild, C. S., Kidd, C. & McWilliam, P. N. (1981). Neurones in the brainstem of the cat activated by myelinated and non-myelinated fibres in the cardiac and pulmonary branches of the vagus. *J. Physiol.* **310**, 64P.

Bennett, J. A., Goodchild, C. S., Kidd, C. & McWilliam, P. N. (1982). Inhibition of evoked and spontaneous activity in the nucleus of the tractus solitarius and dorsal motor vagal nucleus by cardiac and pulmonary vagal afferent fibres in the cat. *J. Physiol.* **332**, 77P.

Bennett, J. A., Goodchild, C. S., Kidd, C. & McWilliam, P. N. (1985). Neurones in the brainstem of the cat excited by vagal afferent fibres from the heart and lungs. *J. Physiol.* **369**, 1–16.

Champagnat, J., Denavit-Saubié, M., Moyanova, S. & Randouin, G. (1982). Involvement of amino acids in periodic inhibitions of bulbar respiratory neurones. *Brain Res.* **237**, 351–65.

Coleridge, J. C. G. & Coleridge, H. M. (1984). Afferent vagal C fibre innervation of the lungs and airways and its functional significance. *Rev. Physiol. Biochem. Pharmacol.* **99**, 1–110.

Coote, J. H., Hilton, S. M. & Perez-Gonzalez, J. F. (1979). Inhibition of the baroreceptor reflex on stimulation in the brainstem defence centre. *J. Physiol.* **288**, 549–60.

DiMicco, J. A., Gale, K., Hamilton, B. & Gillis, R. A. (1979). GABA receptor control of parasympathetic outflow to heart. Characterization and brainstem location. *Science* **204**, 1106–9.

Donoghue, S., Fox, R. E., Kidd, C. & Koley, B. N. (1981). The distribution in the cat brainstem of neurones activated by vagal non-myelinated afferent fibres from the heart and lungs. *Quart. J. Exp. Physiol.* **66**, 391–404.

Gale, K., Hamilton, B. L., Brown, S. C., Norman, W. P., Souza, J. D. & Gillis, R. A. (1980). GABA and specific GABA binding sites in brain nuclei associated with vagal outflow. *Brain Res. Bull.* **5**, Suppl. 2, 325–8.

Gilbey, N. P., Jordan, D., Spyer, K. M. & Wood, L. M. (1985). The inhibitory actions of GABA on cardiac vagal motoneurons in the cat. *J. Physiol.* **361**, 49P.

Gillis, R. A., DiMicco, J. A., Williford, D. J., Hamilton, B. L. & Gale, K. N. (1980). Importance of CNS GABAergic mechanisms in the regulation of cardiovascular function. *Brain Res. Bull.* **5**, Suppl. 2., 303–15.

Gillis, R. A., Yamada, K. A., DiMicco, J. A., Williford, D. J., Segal, S. A., Hamosh, P. & Norman, W. P. (1984). Cortical γ-aminoacidic involvement in blood pressure control. *Fed. Proc.* **43**, 32–8.

Hilton, S. M. (1963). Inhibition of baroreceptor reflexes on hypothalamic stimulation. *J. Physiol.* **165**, 56P.

Massari, V. J., Gottesfeld, Z. & Jacobitz, D. M. (1976). Distribution of glutamic acid decarboxylase in certain thrombocephalic and thalamic nuclei of the rat. *Brain Res.* **118**, 147–53.

Lalley, P. M. (1980). Inhibition of depressor cardiovascular reflexes by a derivative of γ-aminobutyric acid (GABA) and by general anaesthetics with suspected GABA-mimetic effects. *J. Pharmacol. Exp. Therap.* **215**, 418–25.

Smith, A. H. & Nathan, M. A. (1966). Inhibition of the carotid sinus reflex by stimulation of the inferior olive. *Science* **154**, 674–5.

Yamada, K. A., McAllen, R. M. & Loewy, A. D. (1984). GABA antagonists applied to the ventral surface of the medulla oblongata block the baroreceptor reflex. *Brain Res.* **297**, 175–80.

# 7

# Vasopressin and the cardiovascular system

**M. C. Harris**

*Department of Physiology, The Medical School, Vincent Drive, University of Birmingham, Birmingham B15 2TJ, UK*

## 7.1. Introduction

In 1895 Oliver & Schaefer demonstrated that intravenous injection of an aqueous extract of whole pituitary into anaesthetised dogs caused a rapid and prolonged rise in arterial blood pressure. Howell (1898) repeated this but added the significant finding that the pressor principle was confined to the neural lobe. Thus was the foundation laid for the study of the hormone named vasopressin (AVP) by Kamm *et al.* (1928). Although vasopressin was first discovered as a result of its cardiovascular effects, it is only relatively recently that the full import of this influence has been elucidated. In a brief review it is impossible to deal adequately with the interactions between the cardiovascular system and vasopressin. Nevertheless, a short discussion of the cardiovascular influences of the hormone will, I hope, put into context the experimental studies to be discussed later.

## 7.2. Vasopressin and blood pressure

That vasopressin has a physiological role in maintaining arterial blood pressure is now well established. This role is probably achieved in two ways, first, by direct effects on blood vessels, and secondly, by interaction with the cardiovascular reflexes.

### 7.2.1. *Actions on blood vessels*

Frieden & Keller (1954) noted that hypophysectomised dogs show a more rapid fall in blood pressure during haemorrhage than do intact dogs. This has now been demonstrated on numerous occasions in a variety of species, but the best evidence comes from work on the dog where it has been shown that if the influence of vasopressin is eliminated either by preventing release (Errington & Rocha e Silva, 1972), or by blocking its action (Schwartz &

Reid, 1981), then, for the withdrawal of the same volume of blood, the hypotension caused is much greater than in normal dogs. Moreover, if a haemorrhage is performed and the blood pressure is allowed to recover without blood replacement, the return of the pressure to the pre-haemorrhage level has been found to be due almost exclusively to the vasopressin released (Rocha e Silva & Rosenberg, 1969; Cowley *et al.*, 1980). This influence is not, however, confined to the dog, as is shown by Brattleboro' rats which are unable to synthesise vasopressin and also have a labile blood pressure and are more sensitive to haemorrhage than normal rats (Laycock, *et al.*, 1979).

Arterial blood pressure is a rather crude indicator of the cardiovascular influence of vasopressin, however. Better evidence of vasopressin effects is obtained by recording changes of resistance and flow in specific vascular beds. For example, Schmid *et al.* (1974) noted decreased blood flow in superior mesenteric, renal and iliac arteries during vasopressin infusion, with the iliac artery being the most sensitive to the peptide. Pang *et al.* (1979) also observed a fall of blood flow in superior mesenteric artery following vasopressin infusion. They also noted, moreover, that following hypophysectomy not only was the blood flow in that artery greater, but its sensitivity to vasopressin increased fourfold.

Effects of vasopressin on blood flow may be complicated. Jenkins *et al.* (1984) have reported that liver blood flow and hepatic portal venous blood flow show increases as well as decreases which are dependent on the rate of infusion of vasopressin. There is also a report that vasopressin induces concentration-dependent relaxation of dog basilar and coronary artery (Katusic *et al.*, 1984).

Although available evidence suggests that, in normal animals and man, changes in arterial blood pressure do not occur with the usual physiological levels of circulating vasopressin (about 2 $pg/ml^{-1}$ blood), removal of the influence of the cardiovascular reflexes clearly shows up the effects of the hormone (Schmid *et al.*, 1974; Cowley *et al.*, 1980). Even at physiological levels, vasopressin can cause changes in peripheral resistance and heart rate that are not normally reflected in the blood pressure (Montani *et al.*, 1980), and in humans suffering from orthostatic hypotension the pressor effect of the peptide is clearly evident (Wagner & Braunwald, 1956; Mohring *et al.*, 1980).

Even better evidence of the vasoconstrictor action of vasopressin is obtained during dehydration, when large amounts of the hormone are liberated. Injection of a specific vasopressin antagonist will reduce blood pressure in dehydrated rats, but not in hydrated animals (Aisenbury *et al.*, 1981; Andrews & Brenner, 1981), and Brattleboro' rats show a significant fall in blood pressure which is not corrected if their water balance is maintained with a non-pressor analogue of vasopressin (Woods & Johnston, 1984).

## 7.2.2. *Actions on the baroreceptor reflex*

A different although complementary interpretation of the interaction of vasopressin with the cardiovascular system has come from the work of Cowley and his colleagues. This started from a study (Cowley *et al.*, 1974) in which the pressor response curve to infused vasopressin in unanaesthetised dogs was found to shift to the left following baroreceptor denervation. This led these workers to conclude that vasopressin acts in part by increasing the gain of the baroreceptor reflex (Cowley & Barber, 1983). This conclusion has been reinforced by a recent study (Cowley *et al.*, 1984) where it was found in hypophysectomised dogs that elevation of circulating vasopressin gave a big increase in the open-loop baroreflex gain from the isolated perfused carotid sinus, and an increase in total peripheral resistance, without changing blood pressure. This finding suggests that vasopressin has both a direct effect on blood vessels, and an indirect effect through its interaction with the baroreceptor relfex and the sympathetic nervous system (Guo *et al.*, 1982; Hasser *et al.*, 1984).

The means by which vasopressin influences the baroreceptor reflex is still open to dispute, but there is accumulating evidence that at least part of the action is within the central nervous system, in particular in the dorsal medulla oblongata in the region of the nucleus of the tractus solitarius (NTS). Vasopressin has been localised by immunohistochemistry within NTS and surrounding regions (Sofroniew & Schrell, 1981), but perhaps more importantly AVP receptors have been identified within both NTS and the spinal cord (Biegon *et al.*, 1984; Brinton *et al.*, 1984) and there is at least one report of an inhibitory and excitatory interaction of vasopressin on preganglionic sympathetic neurones in the spinal cord (Gilbey *et al.*, 1982). This could account for the changes in blood pressure and heart rate noted following microinjection of vasopressin into the dorsal medulla (Matsuguchi *et al.*, 1982). Whether any vasopressin entering the dorsal medulla arises from the circulation, as suggested by the experiments of Liard *et al.* (1981) or from the neuronal projections from the hypothalamic paraventricular nucleus (PVN), which are known to exist, remains to be elucidated. Certainly, so far as the latter are concerned, there are direct influences of PVN neurones on the NTS, but our own evidence is that the majority of PVN input is to neurones receiving an abdominal innervation, and there is at the moment little evidence for an influence of PVN on NTS neurones with obvious cardiovascular inputs (D. Banks & M. C. Harris, unpublished results).

## 7.2.3. *Cardiovascular reflexes and release of vasopressin*

This problem has been subjected to avid study. There seems to be little doubt that vasopressin is under inhibitory control from the low-pressure atrial receptors of the heart and the high-pressure baroreceptors of the aortic arch and carotid sinus. This subject has recently been succinctly reviewed by Meninger (1985) who points out that the study has been both advanced and slightly confused by the fact that the majority of experiments have been carried out on dogs. There may be a genuine species difference between the dog and other species (including primates), not so much in the existence of reflex controls, but in the relative sensitivities of vasopressin release to the low-pressure and high-pressure reflexes.

In the dog, vasopressin liberation is exquisitely sensitive to inhibition from the atrial receptors, although it is only recently that a clear depression of circulating vasopressin below resting levels at normal hydration has been demonstrated (Ledsome *et al.*, 1983), due largely to the fact that the assays have been at the limit of their sensitivity. Other cardiac receptors may also have an inhibitory influence, since intracoronary injection of veratrum alkaloids depresses the hormone release that normally follows haemorrhage (Thames *et al.*, 1980). The cardiac afferents are carried in the vagi; section of the vagi almost abolishes vasopressin release to haemorrhage in dogs (Share, 1967) and reduces the release in cats (Clark & Rocha e Silva, 1967). The fact that cooling the vagi increases circulating vasopressin (Bishop *et al.*, 1984) suggests also the existence of a tonic inhibition via this route, although there is no electrophysiological evidence for such a tonic influence in the hypothalamus. This reflex system is so sensitive that in dogs increases in vasopressin release can be recorded during slow haemorrhage that reduces left atrial pressure but does not change arterial blood pressure (Gauer *et al.*, 1970). Indeed it was this observation that first signalled the existence of this phenomenon (Rydin & Verney, 1938).

In other species the situation is not so clear. It would appear that in rats, cats and primates a fall in arterial blood pressure is necessary to release the hormone. This was most clearly demonstrated in the experiments of Arnauld *et al.* (1977) who noted in an unanaesthetised monkey that a haemorrhage of 10–20% blood volume which normally resulted in hypotension and vasopressin release did not release the hormone when there was no fall in blood pressure. However, a recent report by Egan *et al.* (1984) indicates that in man a rise in vasopressin will follow manoeuvres that reduce cardiopulmonary blood volume and right atrial pressure but do not change mean arterial blood pressure, pulse pressure or cardiac output. The exact situation may therefore be close to that suggested by Rocha e Silva *et al.* (1978). From their work on dogs they set up a mathematical model of vasopressin release induced by falls in blood pressure and volume, and came to the conclusion that at high arterial pressures (80–170 mmHg) vasopressin release is mainly under the control of the atrial receptors, but that at low pressures (40–79 mmHg) control is mainly via the baroreceptors.

Finally, it should be pointed out that among the early experiments from which many of the later studies have arisen, Share (1965) and Clark & Rocha e Silva (1967) noted that vasopressin is released by bilateral occlusion of the common carotid arteries. This procedure will reduce baroreceptor discharge, but it also increases chemoreceptor discharge. Now the physiological logic behind an interaction between baroreceptor and chemoreceptor reflexes in the control of vasopressin release is not immediately obvious. On a facetious level one might ask, what function is there for a respiratory reflex in releasing an antidiuretic hormone? Later I shall put forward a hypothesis that seeks to rationalise this apparent oddity.

## 7.3. The neurophysiology of baro and chemoreceptor input to the hypothalamus

Our knowledge of the neurophysiology of the baroreceptor and chemoreceptor reflexes falls into two distinct groups, the neurophysiology of the primary afferent pathways and their interactions in the pons and medulla about which an enormous amount is known and which is discussed elsewhere in this book; and the neurophysiology of the reflex influences in the forebrain and hypothalamus about which little is known and where studies of vasopressin control play a large if not exclusive role.

It must be said that studies of the cardiovascular influence on the 'neuroendocrine' hypothalamus have concentrated on the hormone rather than the reflex *per se*. But I hope it will become evident that such studies have already added to our knowledge of the reflexes and are now leading to much wider studies.

Most of the neurophysiological neuroendocrine studies have been performed on rats. The reason for this is because in 1973 Wakerley & Lincoln, while studying the milk-ejection reflex in the rat, noticed an important phenomenon. That is that within the supraoptic (SON) and paraventricular (PVN) nuclei which contain the neurosecretory neurohypophysial neurones, those neurones projecting to the neurohypophysis could be divided into two groups according to their discharge characteristics. One group show a slow (*c*. 1 Hz) fairly continuous discharge. This group was shown to be mainly involved in the suckling reflex (Lincoln & Wakerley, 1974; Poulain *et al.*, 1977), and is thought to secrete oxytocin. The other group showed a distinctive bursting or phasic pattern of discharge. This consisted of bursts of action potentials lasting from a few seconds to a minute or more, alternating with similar periods of almost complete silence. These neurones are not, on the whole, activated by suckling (Lincoln & Wakerley, 1974) but they are exclusively activated by bilateral carotid occlusion (Dreifuss *et al.*, 1976) and (with the non-phasic neurones) by haemorrhage (Poulain *et al.*, 1977), both of which stimulate vasopressin release. Since carotid occlusion probably activates carotid body chemoreceptors while reducing carotid sinus baroreceptor output, and haemorrhage certainly reduces baroreceptor discharge and may activate chemoreceptors, the question arose as to whether the activation of the bursting neurosecretory neurones was influenced from these receptors, and what pathways might be involved. The advantage of this system in the rat is, of course, that there are very few neurones within the hypothalamus whose position and function can be accurately defined during the experiment. With the neurohypophysial neurones it is easy, however, because the neurones can be located within SON or PVN by antidromic invasion following electrical stimulation of the pituitary stalk, and if they show bursting activity they are almost certainly vasopressin secreting.

### 7.3.1. *Baroreceptors*

All the electrophysiological evidence indicates a depressant influence from carotid sinus baroreceptors on the bursting neurosecretory neurones in the rat (Kannan & Yagi, 1978; Harris, 1979). In cats and dogs (which do not seem to show the bursting activity) input from carotid sinus, aortic arch and atrial receptors is generally depressant on most supraoptic neurones (Yamashita, 1977; Meninger, 1979; Yamashita & Koizumi, 1979). As seen in Fig. 7.1, activation of baroreceptors either specifically by inflation of a blind sac of the carotid bifurcation, or generally by intravenous injection of the pure $\alpha$-adrenoceptor stimulant phenylephrine, curtails the bursting discharge of supraoptic neurones. Banks & Harris (1984) have shown that this effect depends upon the ipsilateral locus coeruleus being intact. Another group of neurones, close to locus coeruleus, which receives baroreceptor input and projects directly to the SON, may be part of the same system (Kannan *et al.*, 1981). As a result of these experiments we proposed (Banks & Harris, 1984) that the depressant effect of carotid sinus baroreceptors was carried through a noradrenergic input from the locus coeruleus. This hypothesis was based on the known noradrenergic nature of the locus coeruleus (Swanson, 1976), the removal of the input to SON if the locus coeruleus was destroyed using the neurotoxin 6-hydroxydopamine (6-OHDA; Banks & Harris, 1984), and the available neuropharmacological evidence that direct application of noradrenaline to neurosecretory neurones depressed their discharge (Barker *et al.*, 1971; Moss *et al.*, 1971). This hypothesis is not supported, however, by the elegant experiments of Day & Renaud (1984) and Day *et al.* (1984). They have produced strong evidence, both *in vitro* and *in vivo*, for an excitatory influence of noradrenaline on the neurosecretory neurones. Moreover, when catecholamine terminals around PVN are destroyed with 6-OHDA, baroreceptor inhibition of bursting neurones is still present (Fig. 7.2). The reason for the discrepancy between the results of Day *et al.* (1984) and earlier neuropharmacological results probably lies in the concentrations of catecholamines applied. The early experiments used ionophoresis to apply the catecholamine, a technique which is notoriously inexact in terms of the quantity of drug applied. Day *et al.* (1984) applied different concentrations of noradrenaline by pressure and found that whereas high concentrations did

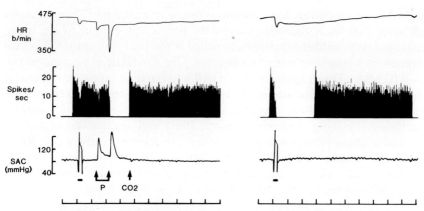

Fig. 7.1. Inhibition of discharge of phasic supraoptic neurone by baroreceptor stimulation in a rat sham-lesioned in the locus coeruleus ipsilateral to the recording site. Carotid sinus baroreceptors were activated by inflation of a blind sac of the carotid bifurcation (bar). All arterial baroreceptors were activated by intravenous injection of 5 μg phenylephrine (P). Left trace shows depression of discharge following inflation of blind sac and after first injection of phenylephrine. A second phenylephrine injection, which increased blood pressure further, stopped neuronal discharge completely. The burst that followed was initiated by stimulation of the ipsilateral carotid body chemoreceptors ($CO_2$). Right trace shows complete inhibition of neurone when sac pressure was increased to 170 mmHg. From Banks & Harris (1984), reproduced with permission.

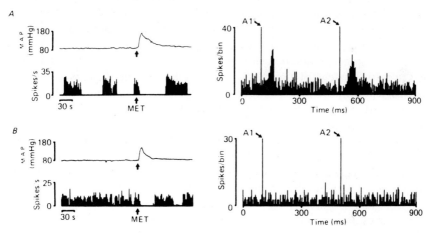

Fig. 7.2. Rate-meter records (left) and peristimulus histograms (right) obtained from two putative VP-secreting PVN neurones, one from a control (saline micro-injection, A) and one from a t-hydroxydopamine-treated (B) subject. Both cells displayed spontaneous pauses in firing, and were thus categorised as phasically active, and both cells were inhibited by baroreceptor activation. The cell recorded in the 6-hydroxydopamine-treated subject, however, was unresponsive to both A1 and A2 stimulation (both stimuli 200 μA, 300 sweeps). From Day *et al.* (1984), reproduced with permission.

indeed cause inhibition, low concentrations were excitatory. Thus, while we all agree that locus coeruleus carries the baroreceptor input to the hypothalamus, it is unlikely that noradrenaline is the final transmitter. The real depressant transmitter remains unknown. One candidate is $\gamma$-aminobutyric acid (GABA). Direct application of GABA to bursting supraoptic neurones does depress them (Bioulac *et al.*, 1978), and GABA applied to the ventral surface of the medulla prevents the release of vasopressin by carotid occlusion (Feldberg & Rocha e Silva, 1981) and antagonists of GABA applied to the same region enhance vasopressin release (Feldberg & Rocha e Silva, 1978), but no convincing connection with the baroreceptor reflex has yet been made. This leaves the question, with what input is noradrenaline involved? The answer may be, with the chemoreceptor input.

### 7.3.2. *Chemoreceptors*

The chemoreceptor input to hypothalamic neurosecretory neurones has been studied in much less detail than that of the baroreceptors. Following the demonstration that bilateral occlusion of the common carotid arteries in rats resulted in activation of bursting supraoptic neurones (Dreifuss *et al.*, 1976), accompanied by a release of vasopressin without oxytocin (Harris *et al.*, 1975), Harris (1979) demonstrated that specific stimulation of carotid body chemoreceptors by injection of $CO_2$-saturated 0.15m NaCl solution into the internal carotid artery was followed by activation of the bursting neurones of the ipsilateral supraoptic nucleus. Later Harris *et al.* (1984) found that the chemoreceptor afferents were confined to the ipsilateral brain, and reached the supraoptic nucleus by taking a lateral path to a region rostral to SON and then turning medial and descending through the medial hypothalamus. The exact rostral extent of the pathway is not known, but lesions within the lateral septum abolish the release of vasopressin by carotid occlusion and lesions within the preoptic area abolish chemoreceptor-evoked activation of supraoptic neurones.

Speculation as to the transmitter at the SON has taken an interesting new turn in the last year. Previously many, including the author, would have suggested acetylcholine (ACh) as the transmitter. Its injection to the hypothalamus released vasopressin (Pickford & Watt, 1951). Direct application of ACh to bursting SON neurones activated them, whereas there was no effect or a depression of the non-bursting neurones (Bioulac *et al.*, 1978). Moreover, recently Hatton *et al.* (1983) identified a group of cholinergic neurones in the periphery of the SON whose stimulation specifically activated the bursting neurones. Now, however, following the finding of Day *et al.* (1984), noradrenaline must be considered a strong candidate. There is a large noradrenergic input to both SON and PVN from the ventrolateral medullary A1 group of neurones (Sawchenko & Swanson, 1982) and electrical stimulation within the A1 region activates supraoptic neurones

(Day & Renaud, 1984). Lesions of A1 with 6-OHDA also abolish the chemoreceptor-induced activation of SON neurones (Harris *et al.*, 1984), and Caverson & Ciriello (1984) have electrophysiologically identified single neurones in the ventrolateral medulla which send axons to both the supraoptic and paraventricular nuclei, some of which are activated by electrical stimulation of the carotid sinus and aortic depressor nerves. Since the anatomical links between NTS and the ventrolateral medulla are known to exist (Errington & Dashwood, 1972), this must be a strong candidate for the chemoreceptor pathway to the rostral brain.

## 7.4. General chemoreceptor and baroreceptor influences on the brain

Earlier in this chapter I suggested that although the neuroendocrine studies had been directed towards studying the influences of cardiovascular reflexes on vasopressin release rather than the reflexes *per se*, the results have given some interesting indications of the more general effects that these reflexes might have on the central nervous system. For the baroreceptor reflex, the involvement of the locus coeruleus indicates a widespread influence. Locus coeruleus has a wide distribution throughout the forebrain (Jones & Moore, 1977) including the cerebral cortex (Waterhouse *et al.*, 1983). The actions of the baroreceptor reflex so far studied have been depressant, and it may be that the major function of this input to the forebrain is to depress it. The lowering of blood pressure and release of vasopressin may be just two manifestations of this role.

The chemoreceptor reflex may be the other side of this coin, that is, its major role may be as a general activation of the central nervous system. This latter contention is supported by some recent experiments from my laboratory. Making use of the ipsilateral nature of the chemoreceptor input to the forebrain, we have looked at the extent of cerebral activation by this input using $^{14}$C-2-deoxyglucose (2DG) autoradiography (Sokoloff, 1981). In urethane-anaesthetised rats 2DG was injected intravenously, and one carotid body was stimulated at 1-min intervals for 45 min. The brain was then removed, frozen 20-μm coronal sections were cut, and alternate sections were subjected to autoradiography. The results, illustrated by the diagram in Fig. 7.3, showed a profound activation of the forebrain, as well as of the expected regions of the hindbrain. In the hindbrain increased $^{14}$C uptake was seen in NTS, the reticular formation and the ventrolateral medulla. In the midbrain periventricular grey was particularly noticeable. In the forebrain, however, increased uptake was largely confined to the stimulated side and involved large areas of the amygdala, the hippocampus, the lateral septum, the caudate putamen, the thalamus (some of which was bilateral) and the piriform cortex. On the other hand, apart from the ipsilateral supraoptic nucleus, the hypothalamus was unaffected. Even the paraventricular nuclei were not activated.

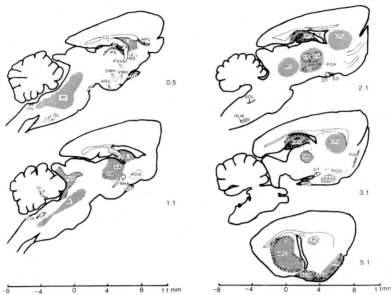

Fig. 7.3. Influence of carotid body chemoreceptor stimulation on $^{14}$C-2-deoxyglucose uptake in the brain of the urethane-anaesthetised rat. Diagrammatic representations of parasagittal sections of the rat brain adapted from the stereotaxic atlas of Pellegrino *et al.* (1979). Hatching shows those areas with a prominent increase in $^{14}$C-uptake following activation of the carotid body chemoreceptors of that side. The number alongside each section gives the position of that section in millimetres lateral to the midline. *Abbreviations*: AAA, anterior amygdaloid area; ACO, cortical amygdaloid nucleus; AHA, anterior hypothalamic area; ARC, arcuate nucleus of the hypothalamus; CC, corpus callosum; CPU, caudate putamen; DMH, dorsomedial nucleus of the hypothalamus; FX, fornix; HPC, hippocampus; IP, nucleus inter-positus; LS, lateral septum; MS, medial septum; NF, fastigial nucleus; OL, inferior olivary nuclei; OT, optic tract; PIR, piriform cortex; POA, preoptic area; PV, paraventricular nucleus of the thalamus; PVH, paraventricular neucleus of the hypothalamus; RF, reticular formation; RLM, lateral reticular nucleus; SO, supraop-tic nucleus; SOL, solitary nucleus; V, ventriclc; VA, anterior ventral nucleus of the thalamus; VB, basal ventral nucleus of the thalamus; VM, medial ventral nucleus of the thalamus; VMH, ventromedial nucleus of the hypothalamus; ZI, zona incerta.

These results indicate that the chemoreceptor reflex does indeed have a very wide influence within the CNS, even in an anaesthetised animal. But, although there is ample evidence that descending influences passing through the hypothalamus have a profound effect on the cardiovascular system, and that these are sensitive to chemoreceptor stimulation (Marshall, 1981; Hilton, 1982), from these experiments it must be concluded that the hypothalamus itself plays little or no part in this influence. It must be pointed out, however, that the present experiments were performed on rats under urethane anesthesia, and it is notoriously difficult, if not impossible, to achieve some of the cardiovascular effects of chemoreceptor stimulation which are thought to be regulated from the hypothalamic level using this anaesthetic (Marshall, 1981). Repetition of the experiments using a different anaesthetic or without anaesthesia will probably answer this question.

Thus, it appears that research into the role of vasopressin has not only provided more insight into cardiovascular function at the periphery, but is providing the basis at least for further studies into the central influences of the cardiovascular reflexes.

## References

Aisenbury, G. A., Handelman, W. A., Arnold, P., Manning, M. & Schrier, R. W. (1981). Vascular effects of arginine vasopressin during fluid deprivation in the rat. *J. Clin. Invest.* **67**, 961–8.

Andrews, C. E. Jr & Brenner, B. M. (1981). Relative contributions of arginine vasopressin and angiotensin II to maintenance of systemic arterial blood pressure in the anaesthetised water-deprived rat. *Circ. Res.* **48**, 254–8.

Arnauld, E., Czernichow, P., Fumoux, F. & Vincent, J. D. (1977). The effects of hypotension and hypovolemia on the liberation of vasopressin during hae-morrhage in the unanaesthetised monkey (*Macaca mulatta*). Pflügers Arch. **37**, 193–200.

Banks, D. & Harris, M. C. (1984) Lesions of the locus coeruleus abolish baroreceptor-induced depression of supraoptic neurones in the rat. *J. Physiol.* **355**, 383–98.

Barker, J. L., Crayton, J. W. & Nicoll, R. A. (1971). Noradrenaline and acetylcholine responses of supraoptic neurosecretory cells. *J. Physiol.* **218**, 19–32.

Biegon, A., Terlou, M., Voorhuis, Th. D. & De Kloet, E. R. (1984). Arginine–vasopressin binding sites in rat brain: a quantitative autoradiographic study. *Neurosci. Lett.* **44**, 229–34.

Bioulac, B., Gaffori, O., Harris, M. C. & Vincent, J. D. (1978). Effects of acetylcholine, sodium glutamate and GABA on the discharge of supraoptic neurones in the rat. *Brain Res.* **15**, 159–62.

Bishop, V. S., Thames, M. D. & Schmid, P. S. (1984). Effects of bilateral vagal cold block on vasopressin in conscious dogs. *Am. J. Physiol.* **24**, R566–9.

Brinton, R. E., Gee, K. W., Walmsley, J. K., Davis, T. P. & Yamamura, H. I. (1984). Regional distribution of putative vasopressin receptors in rat brain and pituitary by quantitative autoradiography. *Proc. Nat. Acad. Sci.* **81**, 7248–52.

Caverson, M. M. & Ciriello, J. (1984). Electrophysiological identification of neurones in ventrolateral medulla sending collateral axons to paraventricular and supraoptic nuclei in the cat. *Brain Res.* **30**, 375–9.

Clark, B. J. & Rocha e Silva, M. Jr (1967). An afferent pathway for the selective release of vasopressin in response to carotid occlusion and haemorrhage in the cat. *J. Physiol.* **19**, 529–42.

Cowley, A. W. Jr & Barber, B. J. (1983). Vasopressin vascular and reflex effects — a theoretical analysis. *Progr. Brain Res.* **60**, 415–24.

Cowley, A. W. Jr, Merrill, D., Osborn, J. & Barber, B. J. (1984). Influence of vasopressin and angiotensin on baroreflexes in the dog. *Circ. Res.* **54**, 163–73.

Cowley, A. W., Monos, E. Jr & Guyton, A. C. (1974). Interaction of vasopressin and the baroreceptor reflex system in the regulation of arterial blood pressure in the dog. *Circ. Res.* **34**, 505–14.

Cowley, A. W. Jr, Switzer, S. J. & Guinn, M. M. (1980). Evidence and quantification of the vasopressin arterial pressure control system in the dog. *Circ. Res.* **46**, 58–67.

Day, T. A., Ferguson, A. V. & Renaud, L. P. (1984). Facilitatory influence of noradrenergic afferents on the excitability of rat paraventricular nucleus neuro-secretory cells. *J. Physiol.* **355**, 237–49.

Day, T. & Renaud, L. P. (1984). Electrophysiological evidence that noradrenergic afferents selectively facilitate the activity of supraoptic neurons. *Brain Res.* **30**, 233–40.

Dreifuss, J. J., Harris, M. C. & Tribollet, E. (1976) Excitation of phasically firing hypothalamic supraoptic neurones by carotid occlusion in rats. *J. Physiol* **257**, 337–54.

Egan, B., Grekin, R., Ibsen, H., Osterziel, K. & Stevo, J. (1984). Role of cardio-pulmonary mechanoreceptors in ADH release in normal humans. *Hypertension* **6**, 832–6.

Errington, M. L. & Dashwood, M. R. (1979). Projections to the ventral surface of the cat brain demonstrated by horseradish peroxidase. *Neurosci. Lett.* **12**, 153–8.

Errington, M. L. & Rocha e Silva M. Jr (1972). Vasopressin clearance and secretion during haemorrhage in normal dogs and in dogs with experimental diabetes insipidus. *J. Physiol.* **227**, 395–418.

Feldberg, W. & Rocha e Silva Jr, M. (1978). Vasopressin release in anaesthetised cats by antagonists of γ-aminobutyric acid and glycine. *Br. J. Pharmacol.* **62**, 99–106.

Feldberg, W. & Rocha e Silva Jr, M. (1981). Inhibition of vasopressin release to carotid occlusion by γ-aminobutyric acid and glycine. *Br. J. Pharmacol.* **72**, 17–24.

Frieden, J. & Keller, A. D. (1954). Decreased resistance to hemorrhage in neurohypo-physectomised dogs. *Circ. Res.* **2**, 214–20.

Gauer, O. H., Henry, J. P. & Behn, C. (1970). The regulation of extracellular fluid volume. *Ann. Rev. Physiol.* **32**, 547–95.

Gilbey, M. P., Coote, J. H., Fleetwood-Walker, S. & Peterson, D. F. (1982). The influence of the paraventriculo-spinal pathway, oxytocin and vasopressin on sympathetic preganglionic neurones. *Brain Res.* **251**, 283–90.

Guo, G. B., Sharabi, F. M., Abboud, F. M. & Schmid, P. G. (1982). Vasopressin augments baroreflex inhibition of lumbar sympathetic nerve activity in rabbits. *Circulation* **66**, Suppl. II–34.

Harris, M. C. (1979). Effects of chemoreceptor and baroreceptor stimulation on the discharge of hypothalamic supraoptic neurones in rats. *J. Endocrinol.* **82**, 115–25.

Harris, M. C., Dreifuss, J. J. & Legros, J. J. (1975). Excitation of phasicaly firing supraoptic neurones during vasopressin release. *Nature, London* **25**, 80–2.

Harris, M. C., Ferguson, A. V. & Banks, D. (1984). The afferent pathway for carotid body chemoreceptor input to the hypothalamic supraoptic nucleus in the rat. *Pflügers Arch.* **400**, 80–7.

Hasser, E. M., Haywood, J. R., Johnson, A. K. & Bishop, V. S. (1984). The role of vasopressin and the sympathetic nervous system in the cardiovascular response to vagal cold block in the conscious dog. *Circ. Res.* **55**, 454–62.

Hatton, G. I., Ho, Y. W. & Mason, W. T. (1983). Synaptic activation of phasic bursting in rat supraoptic nucleus neurones recorded in hypothalamic slices. *J. Physiol.* **34**, 297–317.

Hilton, S. M. (1982). The defence-arousal system and its relevance for circulatory and respiratory control. *J. Exp. Biol.* **100**, 159–74.

Howell, W. H. (1898). The physiological effects of extracts of the hypophysis cerebri and infundibular body. *J. Exp. Med.* **3**, 246–58.

Jenkins, S. A., Mooney, B., Taylor, I. & Shields, R. (1984). Effect of vasopressin on liver blood flow in the hypophysectomised rat. *Digestion*, **29**, 177–82.

Jones, B. E. & Moore, R. Y. (1977). Ascending projections of the locus coeruleus in the rat. II Autoradiographic study. *Brain Res.* **127**, 23–53.

Kamm, O. Aldrich, T. B., Grote, I. W., Rowe, L. W. & Bugbee, E. P. (1928). The active principles of the posterior lobe of the pituitary gland. I. Demonstration of the presence of two active principles. II. Separation and concentration of the two principles. *J. Am. Chem. Soc.* **50**, 573–601.

Kannan, H. & Yagi, K. (1978). Supraoptic neurosecretory neurons: evidence for the existence of converging inputs both from carotid baroreceptors and osmoreceptors. *Brain Res.* **14**, 385–90.

Kannan, H., Yagi, K. & Sawaki, Y. (1981). Pontine neurones: electrophysiological inputs to supraoptic neurones in rats. *Expl. Br. Res.* **42**, 362–70.

Katusic, Z. S., Shepherd, J. T. & Vanhoutte, P. M. (1984). Vasopressin causes endothelium-dependent relaxations of the canine basilar artery. *Circ. Res.* **55**, 575–9.

Laycock, J. F., Penn, W., Shirley, D. G. & Walter, S. J. (1979). The role of vasopressin in blood pressure regulation immediately following acute haemorrhage in the rat. *J. Physiol.* **29**, 267–75.

Ledsome, J. R., Ngsee, J. & Wilson, N. (1983). Plasma vasopressin concentration in the anaesthetised dog before, during and after atrial distension. *J. Physiol.* **338**, 413–21.

Liard, J. F., Deriaz, O., Tschopp, M. & Schoun, J. (1981). Cardiovascular effects of vasopressin infused into the vertebral circulation of conscious dogs. *Clin. Sci.* **61**, 345–7.

Lincoln, D. W. & Wakerley, J. B. (1974). Electrophysiological evidence for the activation of supraoptic neurones during the release of oxytocin. *J. Physiol.* **24**, 533–54.

Marshall, J. M. (1981). Interaction between the responses to stimulation of peripheral chemoreceptors and baroreceptors: the importance of chemoreceptor activation of the defence areas. *J. Auton. Nerv. Syst.* **3**, 389–400.

Matsuguchi, H., Sharabi, F. M., Gordon, F. J., Johnson, A. K. & Schmid, P. G. (1982). Blood pressure and heart rate responses to microinjection of vasopressin into the nucleus tractus solitarius region of the rat. *Neuropharmacology* **21**, 687–93.

Meninger, R. P. (1979). Response of supraoptic neurosecretory cells to changes in left atrial distension. *Am. J. Physiol.* **236**, R261–7.

Meninger, R. P. (1985). Current concepts of volume receptor regulation of vasopressin release. *Fed. Proc.* **44**, 55–8.

Mohring, J., Glanzer, K., Maciel, J. A., Dusing, R., Kramer, H. J., Arbogast, R. & Koch-Weser, J. (1980). Greatly enhanced pressor response to antidiuretic hormone in patients with impaired cardiovascular reflexes due to idiopathic hypotension. *J. Cardiovasc. Pharmacol.* **2**, 367–76.

Montani, J.–P., Liard, J. F., Schoun, J. & Mohring, J. (1980). Haemodynamic effects of exogenous and endogenous vasopressin at low plasma concentratons in conscious dogs. *Circ. Res.* **47**, 346–55.

Moss, R. L., Dyball, R. E. J. & Cross, B. A. (1971). Responses of antidromically identified supraoptic and paraventricular units to acetylcholine, noradrenaline and glutamate applied iontophoretically. *Brain Res*, **35**, 573–5.

Oliver, G. & Schaefer, E. A. (1895). On the physiological action of extracts of pituitary body and certain other glandular organs. *J. Physiol.* **18**, 278–9.

Pang, C. C. Y., Wilcox, W. C. & McNeill, J. R. (1979). Hypophysectomy and saralasin on mesenteric vasoconstrictor response to vasopressin. *Am. J. Physiol.* **23**, H200–5.

Pellegrino, L. J., Pellegrino, A. S. & Cushman, A. J. (1979). *A Stereotaxic Atlas of the Rat Brain.* New York: Plenum Press.

Pickford, M. & Watt, J. A. (1951). A comparison of the effect of intravenous and intracarotid injections of acetylcholine in the dog. *J. Physiol.* **114**, 333–5.

Poulain, D. A., Wakerley, J. B. & Dyball, R. E. J. (1977). Electrophysiological differentiation of oxytocin- and vasopressin-secreting neurones. *Proc. R. Soc. Lond. (Biol.)* **196**, 367–84.

Rocha e Silve, M. Jr, Celso de Lima, W. & Castro de Souza, E. M. (1978). Vasopressin secretion in response to haemorrhage: mathematical modelling of the factors involved. *Pflügers Arch.* **376**, 185–90.

Rocha e Silva, M. Jr & Rosenberg, M. (1969). The release of vasopressin in response to haemorrhage and its role in the mechanism of blood pressure regulation. *J. Physiol.* **202**, 535–57.

Rydin, H. & Verney, E. B. (1938). The inhibition of water diuresis by emotional stress and by muscular exercise. *Quart. J. Exp. Physiol.* **27**,343–73.

Sawchenko, P. E. & Swanson, L. W. (1982). The organisation of noradrenergic pathways from the brain stem to the paraventricular and supraoptic nuclei in the rat. *Brain Res. Revs* **4**, 275–325.

Schmid, P. G., Abboud, F. M., Wendling, M. G., Ramberg, E. S., Mark, A. L., Heistad, D. D. & Eckstein, J. W. (1974). Regional vascular effects of vasopressin: plasma levels and circulatory responses. *Am. J. Physiol.* **227**, 998–1004.

Schwartz, J. & Reid, I. (1981). Effect of vasopressin blockade on blood pressure regulation during hemorrhage in conscious dogs. *Endocrinology* **109**, 1778–80.

Share, L. (1965). Effects of carotid occlusion and left atrial distension on plasma vasopressin. *Am. J. Physiol.* **208**, 219–23.

Share, L. (1967). Role of peripheral receptors in the increased release of vasopressin in response to haemorrhage. *Endocrinology* **81**, 1140–6.

Sofroniew, M. V. & Schrell, U. (1981). Evidence for a direct projection from oxytocin and vasopressin neurones to the medulla oblongata: immunohistochemical visualisation of both the horseradish peroxidase transported and the peptide produced by the same neurons. *Neurosci. Lett.* **22**, 211–17.

Sokoloff, L. (1981). The deoxyglucose method for the measurement of local glucose utilization and the mapping of local functional activity in the central nervous system. *Int. Rev. Neurobiol.* **22**, 287–333.

Swanson, L. W. (1976). The locus coeruleus: a cytoarchitectonic, golgi and immuno-histochemical study in the albino rat. *Brain Res.* **110**, 39–56.

Thames, M. D., Petersen, M. G. & Schmid, P. G. (1980). Stimulation of cardiac receptors with veratrum alkaloids inhibits ADH secretion. *Am. J. Physiol.* **239**, H784–8.

Wagner, H. N. & Braunwald, E. (1956). The pressor effect of the antidiuretic principle of the posterior pituitary in orthostatic hypotension. *J. Clin. Invest.* **35**, 1412–18.

Wakerley, J. B. & Lincoln, D. W. (1973). The milk-ejection reflex of the rat: a 20- to 40-fold acceleration in the firing of paraventricular neurones during oxytocin release. *J. Endocrinol.* **57**, 477–93.

Waterhouse, B. D., Lin, C.-S., Burne, R. A. & Woodward, D. J. (1983). The distribution of neocortical projection neurones in the locus coeruleus. *J. Comp. Neurol.* **217**, 418–31.

Woods, R. L. & Johnston, C. I. (1984). Contribution of vasopressin to the maintenance of blood pressure during dehydration. *Am. J. Physiol.* **245**, F615–21.

Yamashita, H. (1977). Effect of baro- and chemoreceptor activation on supraoptic nuclei neurons in the hypothalamus. *Brain Res.* **126**, 551–6.

Yamashita, H. & Koizumi, K. (1979). Influence of carotid and aortic baroreceptors on neurosecretory neurons in supraoptic nuclei. *Brain Res.* **170**, 259–77.

# 8

# Localisation and biological function of angiotensin in the nervous system

**Christopher Suter**[†]

*Department of Physiology, The Medical School, Vincent Drive, University of Birmingham, Birmingham B15 2TJ, UK*

## Abbreviations

| | |
|---|---|
| ACTH | adrenocorticotrophic hormone |
| AII | angiotensin II |
| CNS | central nervous system |
| CSF | cerebrospinal fluid |
| iv | intravenous |
| ivt | intracerebroventricular |

## 8.1. Introduction

Angiotensin II is well known as a circulating octapeptide hormone formed by the pathway shown in Fig. 8.1. The enzyme renin, formed in the juxtaglomerular cells of the kidney, acts upon the 453 amino acid renin substrate (also called angiotensinogen), released into the bloodstream from the liver, to form the decapeptide angiotensin I. This in turn is cleaved by converting enzyme, principally in the lungs but also in plasma, kidney and testis, to form angiotensin II. Angiotensin II is the most potent naturally occurring pressor substance known, causing vasoconstriction in arterial smooth muscle (Regioli *et al.*, 1974) and stimulating the heart, causing an increase in heart rate and myocardial activity (Peach, 1977). Angiotensin II also enhances vasoconstrictor responses to direct stimulation or reflex activation of sympathetic nerves by facilitating release of adrenergic transmitter (Hughes & Roth, 1971) and by increasing the responsiveness of smooth muscle to noradrenaline (Zimmerman, 1978). Angiotensin can block re-uptake of transmitter at sympathetic nerve endings (Davila & Khairallah, 1970) but it seems that this

---

[†]*Present address:* Department of Biological Sciences, North East Surrey College of Technology, Reigate Road, Ewell, Surrey KT17 3DS, UK.

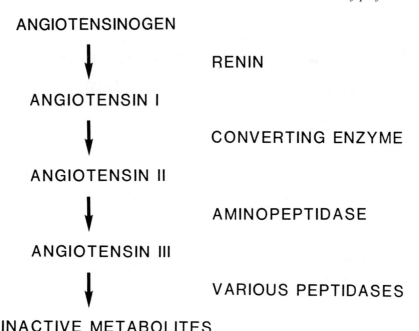

ANGIOTENSINOGEN

RENIN

ANGIOTENSIN I

CONVERTING ENZYME

ANGIOTENSIN II

AMINOPEPTIDASE

ANGIOTENSIN III

VARIOUS PEPTIDASES

INACTIVE METABOLITES

Fig. 8.1. Biosynthetic pathway for the formation and catabolism of angiotensin II in the peripheral circulation.

does not cause the potentiation of sympathetic actions on smooth muscle (Hughes & Roth, 1970; Zimmerman, 1978).

### 8.2. Actions of intravenous and intraventricular angiotensin on the central nervous system

In 1961 Bickerton & Buckley published the results of their cross-circulation experiments. In these the cerebral circulation of an anaesthetised dog (the recipient) was disconnected from the rest of the circulation and was instead joined up to the systemic circulation of a second anaesthetised dog (the donor). Administration of angiotensin II to the cross-circulating blood caused systemic hypertension in both animals. Since the cross-circulating blood entered only the cerebral circulation of the recipient dog, they concluded that the pressor response of that animal was due to an action of the peptide on the central nervous system. Since that time a great deal of evidence has been gathered for direct actions of circulating angiotensin II on specific receptors within the brain which bring about a variety of effects, including an elevation of blood pressure, increases in drinking and sodium appetite, and secretion from the pituitary of vasopressin and ACTH. These actions are mediated by receptors of angiotensin II within some circumventricular organs (area postrema, subfornical organ, organum vasculosum laminae terminalis) which are penetrated by fenestrated capillaries that make the neurones accessible to blood-borne factors (for reviews see Phillips, 1978; Ramsay, 1982).

Until about 18 years ago angiotensin was thought of as being purely a classical circulating hormone which could also have actions on the circumventricular organs. Since that time a considerable amount of evidence has been accumulating for a separate renin–angiotensin system functioning within the central nervous system, although this evidence cannot yet be regarded as being complete (see Reid, 1977, 1979; Ramsay, 1979, 1982).

In 1967 Severs *et al.* showed that injection of angiotensin II into the cerebral ventricles evoked increases in blood pressure, and Booth (1968) showed that AII injection into rat brains also caused the animals to drink. Mouw *et al.* (1971) demonstrated that angiotensin acts on the brain to release vasopressin, this being earlier implied by Severs *et al.* (1970), Olsson (1970) and Anderson (1971). Phillips (1983) believed that these effects are due to actions of angiotensin II on receptors within the blood–brain barrier and he presented evidence to suggest that substances injected into the cerebral ventricles cannot penetrate to the circumventricular organs except under conditions where the blood–brain barrier is breached, for example during large increases in blood pressure brought about by large doses of AII injected intravenously. Ganong (1984), on the other hand, presented evidence to suggest that angiotensin II injected into the cerebral ventricles can penetrate to the circumventricular organs where it acts upon receptors also accessible to circulating AII to bring about increases in blood pressure, water intake and vasopressin secretion. Of course, this finding would not preclude the possibility that angiotensin II synthesised in the CNS, presumably in smaller quantities than those infused ivt and acting in more restricted areas than those reached by ivt infusion, acts purely on receptors within the blood–brain barrier.

Angiotensin II, administered by both intravenous and intraventricular routes, also increases ACTH secretion from the anterior pituitary, possibly due in both cases to direct actions on the pituitary. The ivt AII may reach this organ via the hypophyseal portal vessels (see Ganong, 1984). Its action on the anterior pituitary may mimic the effect of a proposed angiotensinergic pathway from the paraventricular nucleus of the hypothalamus to the anterior pituitary (see Lind *et al.*, 1985). Both intraventricular and intravenous AII inhibit the secretion of renin from the kidneys, but whereas the ivt AII acts by increasing vasopressin secretion (Ganong *et al.*, 1982) and by depressing activity in the renal nerve (Fukijama, 1972), the circulating AII acts directly on the kidney.

There are some effects of ivt AII that cannot be produced by systemic administration and have therefore been presumed to be due to actions on receptors located inside the blood–brain barrier. These effects include increased turnover of dopamine in the hypothalamus, of noradrenaline in the supraoptic nuclei and preoptic area (Alper *et al.*, 1982) and a biphasic effect on serotonin release (Nahmod *et al.*, 1978). Ivt AII also causes increased secretion of luteinising hormone (Steele *et al.*, 1981, 1982a) and decreased secretion of prolactin (Steele *et al.*, 1981; Alper *et al.*, 1982) possibly as a consequence of its actions on amine turnover (Weiner & Ganong, 1978; Steele *et al.*, 1982b).

### 8.3. Synthesis and localisation of angiotensin in central nervous tissue

Some years before the demonstration of those effects of ivt AII presumed to be mediated by receptors located within the blood–brain barrier, Ganten *et al.* (1971) and Fischer-Ferraro *et al.* (1971) had reported the existence of renin-like activity in the brain. These results were confirmed in different animal species by several groups (see Ganten *et al.*, 1981, for references). However the optimal pH for the activity of this enzyme was 4·5–5·5, with very little activity above pH 6 (Ganten *et al.*, 1971; Daul *et al.*, 1975; Day & Reid, 1976), thus casting doubt on whether this renin-like activity could function in the brain under *in vivo* conditions. Day & Reid (1976) have in fact presented convincing evidence that this brain renin-like activity having a low pH optimum can be accounted for by the lysozomal enzyme cathepsin D. However, it has more recently been demonstrated that the brain also contains an angiotensin-generating enzyme that closely resembles renal renin (Hirose *et al.*, 1978, 1980; Inagami *et al.*, 1980, 1982), being active at pH 7·4, the pH of the extracellular fluid of the brain, and neutralised by antibodies to renal renin. Hirose *et al.* (1980) have also presented evidence that the brain contains an inactive prorenin that is activated by trypsin.

Since the first demonstration of the presence of renin-like activity in the CNS, the other components of the renin–angiotensin system have been demonstrated within the CNS using immunohistochemistry or bioassay or by both techniques, and the capacity of the brain to generate angiotensin II has also been demonstrated. This has been reviewed by Ganten *et al.* (1981), Ganong (1983, 1984), Deboben *et al.* (1983) and Phillips (1983).

### 8.3.1. *Renin substrate (angiotensinogen)*

The presence of angiotensinogen-like material in mammalian (dog) brain was first demonstrated by Ganten *et al.* (1971) and it has since been shown that both CSF and brain tissue contain renin substrate. Since its molecular weight and electrophoretic characteristics are similar to those of plasma renin substrate (Reid 1976), it is possible that this angiotensinogen is derived from plasma rather than synthesised in the brain (see Reid, 1977). However, the discoveries that its carbohydrate structure differs from that of plasma angiotensinogen (Reid *et al.*, 1978), that the level in CSF is regulated independently of that in plasma (Schelling *et al.*, 1982) and that the substrate extracted from brain tissue differs immunologically from that in plasma (Morris & Reid, 1979; Ito *et al.*, 1980) make it unlikely that the brain substrate is of peripheral origin.

Intraventricular injection of renin causes formation of AII in the CNS (Reid *et al.*, 1978), suggesting that the CNS contains angiotensinogen upon which the renin acts to form angiotensin I which in turn is cleaved to make angiotensin II. Angiotensinogen is released by brain slices *in vitro*, although this release is unaffected by inhibitors of protein synthesis which prevent the release of substrate from liver slices (Sernia & Reid, 1980; Reid & Brownfield, 1982). Campbell *et al.* (1984) have presented evidence for the presence of angiotensinogen mRNA in rat brain, and have demonstrated synthesis of angiotensinogen precursors, identical to those found in the liver, by cell-free translation of brain RNA. These precursors are cleaved by renin to give angiotensin I identical to that shown for liver.

### 8.3.2. *Converting enzyme*

Angiotensin I converting enzyme activity is present in high concentrations in brain tissue. Much of this is concentrated in the brush border of the choroid plexus (Rix *et al.*, 1981) and in the vacular network of the CNS (Brecher *et al.*, 1978). However, it is also found in cultured neuroblastoma cells (see Deboben *et al.*, 1983), and unilateral chemical lesions of the striatum, which destroy only nerve cells, reduce converting enzyme activity in the ipsilateral substantia nigra and striatum (Arregui *et al.*, 1978; Fuxe *et al.*, 1980), thus providing good evidence for its intraneuronal presence. Small but measurable amounts of converting enzyme activity are found in CSF.

Converting enzyme immunoreactivity has been found in brush-border and endothelial cells throughout the brain (Rix *et al.*, 1981; Brownfield *et al.*, 1982; Defendini *et al.*, 1983) but, with the exception of the subfornical organ, there is very little staining in nervous tissue. This is odd in view of the good evidence for intraneuronal localisation of converting enzyme obtained from biochemical studies. Ganong (1983) suggested that the biochemical method may be more sensitive than the immunological method or that the antibodies raised against lung converting enzyme do not cross-react fully with brain converting enzyme. However, Ganong (1983) considered this latter possibility to be unlikely because rat brain converting enzyme is neutralised by antibodies to lung converting enzyme (Polsky-Cynkin & Fanburg, 1979). A further possibility is that the biochemical assay is less specific than the immunocytochemical method (Brownfield *et al.*, 1982).

### 8.3.3. *Angiotensin*

Angiotensin was first reported to be present in extracts of brain tissue of dogs and rats (Fischer-Ferraro *et al.*, 1971; Ganten *et al.*, 1971). Angiotensin I has since been demonstrated in CSF (see Ganong, 1981, 1983, 1984) and, despite some early disagreement, angiotensins II and III are probably also present in CSF (see Deboben *et al.*, 1983; Ganong, 1983, 1984). Since Hermann *et al.* (1982) used HPLC in combination with radioimmunoassay to demonstrate the presence of (Ile$^5$)Ang I and (Ile$^5$)Ang II in rat and human CSF, a variety of techniques — bioassay, HPLC and radioimmunoassay — have been employed to measure the amounts of angiotensins I, II and III in brain tissue. The techniques used have sometimes been criticised (Horvarth *et al.*, 1977; Reid *et al.*, 1977) but the results of Sirett *et al.* (1981) and Hermann *et al.* (1982) provide reasonable evidence for the presence of these compounds in brain tissue. Raizada *et al.* (1983) have suggested that AII is synthesised in cultures of fetal rat brain.

The localisation of angiotensin II or III within central nervous tissue has been examined by various groups using immunohistochemistry (see Ganong, 1983, 1984, for references). Most of this immunoreactivity is in nerve endings rather than cell bodies, although staining was seen in cell bodies of neurones following inhibition of axoplasmic flow with colchicine. No staining was seen in glia or ependyma. Lind *et al.* (1985) have demonstrated angiotensin-II-like materia in cell bodies and fibres in various areas of the CNS with and without colchicine treatment. It was preferentially found in brainstem, hypothalamic and limbic areas involved in control of homeostatic functions.

### 8.3.4. *Angiotensinase*

Brain tissue contains high levels of peptidase enzymes which break down angiotensin II into inactive fragments (Schelling *et al.*, 1980; Sirett *et al.*, 1981). CSF contains little or no angiotensinase activity but AII is slowly removed from CSF *in vivo*, presumably by contact with peptidases in brain tissue.

### 8.3.5. *Angiotensin receptors*

Saturable binding of AII to receptors of high affinity and specificity has been demonstrated in many parts of the brain (Bennett & Snyder, 1976, 1980; Baxter *et al.*, 1980; Harding *et al.*, 1981; Sirett *et al.*, 1977). Systemically administered saralasin (a competitive antagonist of AII) does not affect this binding (Baxter *et al.*, 1980), indicating that these binding sites are within the blood-brain barrier. Mendelsohn *et al.* (1984) used the technique of *in vitro* autoradiography followed by computerised densitometry and colour coding to show that AII receptors are located in localised areas of rat CNS.

## 8.4. Effects of angiotensin II on electrical activity of central neurones

It has been shown that iontophoretic application of AII to individual neurones in various areas of the CNS causes excitation of spiking activity in those neurones. This was first demonstrated in neurones in the supraoptic region (Nicholl & Barker, 1971) and has since been seen in subfornical organ (Felix & Akert, 1974; Felix & Schlegel, 1978; Nicholaidis *et al.*, 1983), hypothalamus (Wayner *et al.*, 1973) and cerebral cortex (Phillis & Limacher, 1974; Sudakov *et al.*, 1976) and on sympathetic preganglionic neurones in the spinal cord (C. Suter & J. H. Coote, unpublished observations). Excitation by AII of neurones in hypothalamic and hippocampal brain slices (Knowles & Phillips, 1980; Haas *et al.*, 1980) and of hypothalamic and spinal neurones in culture (Gahwiler & Dreifuss, 1980; Phillips *et al.*, 1980; Legendre *et al.*, 1984) has also been demonstrated.

The excitation of neurones *in vivo* by AII could be due to local ischaemia caused by vasoconstriction in the region of the neurones. In fact Rosendorf *et al.* (1970) have shown that iv AII causes an increase in cerebrovascular resistance, but that despite this the cerebral blood flow remained constant. It therefore appears that the resistance change negates the effects of the pressor response to angiotensin. Also Simmonet & Vincent (1980) have presented evidence to indicate that in neostriatum AII binds to neuronal membranes rather than blood vessels. Furthermore, the responsiveness of the *in vitro* slices and cultures would suggest that angiotensin has a direct excitatory effect on nervous tissue. It is therefore unlikely that the neuroexcitatory actions of AII are due to local ischaemia.

The mechanisms of these excitatory actions have been studied using isolated tissues (slices of nervous tissue and isolated ganglia) since such preparations permit long-term intracellular recordings to be made and drugs to be applied to restricted areas or even to single neurones. Dun *et al.* (1978) demonstrated that AII stimulated sympathetic ganglia isolated from cats by acting postsynaptically to depolarise the neurones. They showed that this change in membrane potential was due to an increase in the sodium conductance of the postsynaptic membrane. In 1980 Brown *et al.* (1980) showed that AII could also depolarise neurones in rat isolated superior cervical ganglion by reducing their membrane conductance.

Haas *et al.* (1980) obtained evidence from experiments on hippocampal slices to suggest that AII excites CA1 pyramidal cells by disinhibition; however, the data they present do not completely rule out the possibility that AII also has direct excitatory actions on these cells on areas of membrane some distance from the somal recording sites.

In mouse spinal cord cultures Phillips *et al.* (1980) demonstrated that AII stimulated phasic firing of cells identified as neurones. AII also hyperpolarised these cells but a similar effect was obtained in control experiments. More recently Legendre *et al.* (1984) have demonstrated that the effect of AII on mouse spinal cord neurones in culture depends on the concentration of the drug. At low concentrations ($10^{-6}$M) AII depolarised the cells by an ionic mechansim which involved a reduction in chloride conductance, whereas at higher concentrations ($10^{-4}$ M) depolarisations due to increased sodium conductance were seen. Interestingly Simmonet & Vincent (1980) had previously shown that two pharmacologically distinct classes of receptor exist on membranes of CNS neurones in rats, one recognised by a low concentration of AII and the other composed of sites poorly recognised by AII. Legendre *et al.* (1984) speculated that the two classes of high- and low-affinity receptors correspond to the two distinct electrophysiological actions of AII on mouse spinal cord cultures seen at low and high concentrations.

### 8.5. **Biological role of angiotensin in the central nervous system**

The results outlined above provide strong evidence for the synthesis and location of AII in the CNS and for actions of this compound on the activity of central neurones, in a few cases this having been shown to be due to direct actions of the peptide upon the cell from which recordings were being made. In this section the consequences for the animal of these central actions of AII will be considered. It should be remembered, however, that although the experimental demonstration of an action of AII in the brain provides evidence for a role for that compound in evoking the response in the animal, it does not actually prove that AII has such a role in non-experimental situations. This is so even when the effect can be elicited by application in areas of the brain where AII is known to be present, since the synthesis of AII in neurones and its release subsequent to the application of appropriate external or internal stimuli must also first be demonstrated. Since this information is at present lacking, the suggested roles discussed here are to some extent speculative.

#### 8.5.1. *Blood pressure*

Angiotensin II immunoreactivity has been demonstrated in cell bodies and nerve endings in the nucleus of the solitary tract and in the intermedio-lateral cell column of the spinal cord (Lind *et al.*, 1985); these structures are involved in the nervous control of the cardiovascular system.

An increase in blood pressure can be brought about by injection of AII into the ventricles of the brain, causing release of vasopressin from the posterior pituitary and altering autonomic activity (see above for references). Infusion of AII into the spinal subarachnoid space also causes a dose-dependent increase in blood pressure and an increase in activity in sympathetic outflows from the spinal cord (Coote & Suter, 1985; Suter & Coote, 1987). These results support the proposal that brain AII has a role in the nervous control of blood pressure. However, whereas intraventricular infusion of saralasin and converting enzyme inhibitors cause a reduction of blood pressure in spontaneously hypertensive rats, they have no effect on the blood pressure of normal animals (Ganten *et al.*, 1978; Crofton *et al.*, 1981). Also, Suter & Coote (1987) have shown that infusion of saralasin into the spinal subarachnoid space has little effect on sympathetic activity recorded from the splanchnic nerve of anaesthetised rats, but it reduces the increase in activity brought about by lowering the blood pressure with iv acetylcholine. Therefore it may be that angiotensin does not act as a transmitter in the nervous control loops involved in blood-pressure regulation but it may be involved in setting the level at which the blood pressure is maintained or in regulating the sensitivity of the baroreceptor reflex.

### 8.5.2. *Dipsogenic effects*

Drinking is stimulated by increased effective osmotic pressure of the plasma, by decreases in extracellular fluid volume and also by psychological factors. Fitzsimmons (1969) demonstrated that a factor from the kidneys was involved in hypovolaemic thirst, and Fitzsimmons & Simons (1969) subsequently showed that AII caused drinking in the water-replete animal when administered systemically. It now seems likely that reduced circulating blood volume leads to the release of renin from the kidneys and hence to increased circulating AII levels. The AII acts on the subfornical organ, and possibly also on the organum vasculosum of the lamina terminalis, of the brain, leading to increased drinking. This was first demonstrated by Booth (1968) in rats and has since been shown to be the case in many species of vertebrate, even when water-replete (Epstein *et al.*, 1970; Ramsay, 1982). Malvin *et al.* (1977) reduced the water intake of water-deprived rats by ivt infusion of saralasin, thus providing evidence for a central role for angiotensin in thirst. It did not reduce the food intake of fasted rats. However, previous studies had failed to achieve such a result (see Malvin *et al.*, 1977, for references), and these authors only obtained a positive result following prolonged (75 min) ivt infusion of saralasin. Further work is needed to ensure that the antagonist was not acting on peripherally raised angiotensin levels. There is no information on the effect on dehydration of levels on components of the renin–angiotensin system in the brain, and it must be emphasised that although the demonstration of a dipsogenic response to centrally administered angiotensin is consistent with a role for AII in thirst and drinking, it is only a part of the necessary evidence and much more work remains to be done. The centrally administerd AII could in fact be penetrating to the angiotensin receptors in the circumventricular organs which are involved in the dipsogenic response to circulating angiotensin. There are several mechanisms involved in the central control of water intake, one of which is probably the level of blood-borne angiotensin (see Fitzsimmons, 1980), and so it is a difficult task to assess the possible contribution made by the central renin–angiotensin system.

### 8.5.3. *Sodium appetite*

It is well established that intracranial administration of AII stimulates sodium appetite (see Fitzsimmons, 1980, for references), and increased sodium appetite seen following ivt injection of renin can be blocked with converting enzyme inhibitors or angiotensin receptor antagonists administered by the same route (Avrith & Fitzsimmons, 1980). Furthermore, spontaneously hypertensive rats, which are believed to have elevated levels of brain AII (see Phillips, 1983), possess an exaggerated salt appetite which can be decreased by ivt administration of the converting enzyme inhibitor captopril (Di Nicolantonio *et al.*, 1982). However, ivt captopril or saralasin did not block increased salt uptake by sodium-deprived sheep (Coghlan *et al.*, 1981). Ivt administration of AII stimulates ACTH release from anterior pituitary (Sobel, 1983). This could possibly lead to an elevation in the levels of circulating aldosterone, thereby causing decreased sodium loss in the kidney. As with the dipsogenic effect of angiotensin, it is probable that several mechansims operate to control sodium appetite and to mediate the response to angiotensin administration. Further work is clearly necessary to prove that the brain renin–angiotensin system has a role in controlling this.

### 8.5.4. *Memory*

Conditioned avoidance responses in rats are disrupted by ivt injection of AII (Köller *et al.*, 1979) and injection of AII into the neostriatum has been reported to produce amnesia (Morgan & Routtenberg, 1977). This may correlate with the high level of angiotensin in the hippocampus and its excitatory effect on hippocampal neurones (Felix *et al.*, 1982) but these results must be regarded as preliminary and do not yet signify a role for brain angiotensin.

### 8.6. **Concluding remarks**

There is now good, if incomplete, evidence for a renin–angiotensin system in the CNS separate from that in the periphery. Several approaches have demonstrated that the components of such a system (or substances that closely resemble them) are present in the CNS, and the synthesis of AII by brain tissue has been demonstrated. There are also physiological results, obtained by administering components of the renin–angiotensin system to the CNS, which are consistent with a role for brain angiotensin in the control of water and salt intake and control of blood pressure. Many of these results could also be explained in terms of the centrally injected material reaching the circumventricular organs where there are angiotensin receptors which may normally be targets for circulating AII. However, since there is evidence that not all the angiotensin-like material found in he circumventricular organs is derived from the circulation (Lind *et al.*, 1985), it is possible either that the angiotensin receptors are normally acted upon by both circulating and brain angiotensin or that the particular location of each receptor determines whether it is a target for circulating or for brain angiotensin.

Although AII has been shown to excite neurones directly *in vitro*, it is not yet clear whether it acts *in vivo* as a transmitter or as a modulator of transmission. The latter may well tie in well with the role, proposed above, in altering the set point at which blood pressure is regulated by the nervous system.

Before it can be concluded that the brain renin–angiotensin system has any role, further evidence is required. In particular, appropriate physiological stimuli must be shown to evoke the release of AII from nerve terminals in areas of the brain which are involved in salt and water balance or blood-pressure control and which are known to be responsive to exogenous AII. Also required is a clear demonstration of effects of AII application to regions of the CNS receiving AII-containing nerve terminals. So far most of the work of this nature has involved application to the circumventricular organs, and indeed evidence is accumulating to suggest that the brain renin–angiotensin system is particularly active in these regions. However, at this stage it is not completely certain that the angiotensin, or angiotensin-like material, found in these regions is not derived from the circulation, and so there is a possibility, although perhaps a slight one, that the application of the peptide to these regions may be mimicking the effects of circulating rather than brain AII. Coote & Suter (1985) and Suter & Coote (1987) have recently demonstrated pressor and sympathoexcitatory effects following the application of AII to the spinal cord. The intermediolateral cell column of the cord, the site of the cell bodies of the sympathetic preganglionic neurones, has a high density of nerve terminals containing AII-like material (Ganten *et al.*, 1977). This is the first demonstration of an effect of AII on an area of the CNS in which AII-containing nerve terminals are believed to be present, yet which is not accessible to circulating angiotensin.

### Acknowledgements

The author's work reported here was supported by a grant from the British Heart Foundation to Professor J. H. Coote.

## References

Alper, R. H., Steele, M. K. & Ganong, W. F. (1982). Angiotensin II increases catecholamine synthesis in selected hypothalamic nuclei. *Neurosci. Abst.* **8**, 421.

Anderson, B., (1971). Thirst and the control of water balance. *Am. Sci.* **59**, 405–15.

Arregui, A., Emson, P. C. & Spokes, E. (1978). Angiotensin converting enzyme in substantia nigra: reduction of activity in Huntingdon's disease and after intrastriatal kainic acid in rats. *Eur. J. Pharmacol.* **52**, 121–4.

Avrith, D. & Fitzsimmons, J. T. (1980). Increased sodium appetite in the rat induced by intracranial administration of components of the renin–angiotensin system. *J. Physiol.* **301**, 349–64.

Baxter, C. R. Horvarth, J. S., Duggin, C. G. & Tiller, D. J. (1980). Effect of age on specific AII binding sites in rat brain. *Endocrinology* **100**, 995–9.

Bennett, J. P. & Snyder, S. M. (1976). Angiotensin II binding to mammalian brain membranes. *J. Biol. Chem.* **251**, 7423–30.

Bennett, J. P. & Snyder, S. M. (1980). Receptor binding interactions of the angiotensin II antagonist [125]I [sarcosine[1], leucine[8]] angiotensin II with mammalian brain and peripheral tissues. *Eur. J. Pharmacol.* **67**, 11–25.

Bickerton, R. K. & Buckley, J. P. (1961). Evidence for a central mechanism in angiotensin induced hypertension. *Proc. Soc. Exp. Biol. Med.* **106**, 834–6.

Booth, D. A. (1968). Mechanism of the action of nor-epinephrine in eliciting an eating response on injection in the rat hypothalamus. *J. Pharmacol. Exp. Therap.* **160**, 336–48.

Brecher, P. I., Tercyak, A., Gavras, H. & Chobanian, A. V. (1978). Peptidyl dipeptidase in rabbit brain microvessels. *Biochim. Biophys. Acta* **526**, 537–46.

Brown, D. A., Constanti, A. & Marsh, S. (1980). Angiotensin mimics the action of muscarinic agonists on rat sympathetic neurones. *Brain Res.* **193**, 614–19.

Brownfield, M. S., Reid, I. A., Ganten, D. & Ganong, W. F. (1982). Differential distribution of immunoreactive angiotensin and converting enzyme in rat brain. *Neuroscience* **7**, 1759–69.

Campbell, D. J., Bouhnik, J., Menard, J. & Corvol, P. (1984). Identity of angiotensinogen precursors of rat brain and liver. *Nature, London* **308**, 206–8.

Coghlan, J. P., Considine, P. J., Denton, D. A., Fei, D. W., Leskell, L. G., McKinley, M. J., Muller, A. F., Tarjan, E., Weisinger, R. S. & Bradshaw, R. A. (1981). Sodium appetite in sheep induced by cerebral ventricular infusion of angiotensin: comparison with sodium deficiency. *Science* **214**, 195–7.

Coote, J. H & Suter, C. (1985). Excitatory actions of angiotensin II on sympathetic preganglionic neurones in the rat. *J. Physiol.* **367**, 49P.

Crofton, J. T., Rockhold, R. W., Share, L., Wang, B. C., Horovitz, Z. P., Manning, M. & Sawyer, W. H. (1981). Effect of intracerebroventricular captopril on vasopressin and blood pressure in spontaneously hypertensive rats. *Hypertension* **3**, II. 71–4.

Daul, C. B., Heath, R. G. & Garey, R. E. (1975). Angiotensin-forming enzyme in humans. *Neuropharmacology* **14**, 75–8.

Davila, D. & Khairallah, P. A. (1970). Effects of ions on inhibition of norepinephrine uptake by angiotensin. *Arch. Int. Pharmacodyn.* **192**, 357–64.

Day, R. P. & Reid, I. A. (1976). Renin activity in dog brain: enzymological similarity to cathepsin D. *Endocrinology* **99**, 93–100.

Deboben, A., Inagami, T. & Ganten, D. (1983). Tissue renin. In *Hypertension Physiopathology and Treatment*, pp. 194–209 (eds J. Genest, O. Kuchol, p. Hamet & M. Cantin). New York: McGraw-Hill.

Defendini, R., Zimmerman, E. A., Weare, J. A., Alhenc-Gelas, F. & Erdös, E. G. (1983). Angiotensin converting enzyme in epithelial and neuroepithelial cells. *Neuroendocrinology* **37**, 32–40.

Di Nicolantonio, R., Hutchinson, J. S. & Mendelsohn, F. A. O. (1982). Exaggerated salt appetite of spontaneously hypertensive rats is decreased by central angiotensin-converting enzyme blockade. *Nature, London* **298**, 846–8.

Dun, N. J. Nishi, S. & Karczmar, A. G. (1978). An analysis of the effect of angiotensin II on mammalian ganglion cells. *J. Pharmacol. Exp. Therap.* **204**, 669–75.

Epstein, A. N., Fitzsimmons, J. T. & Rolls, J. (1970). Drinking induced by injection of angiotensin into the brain of the rat. *J. Physiol.* **210**, 457–74.

Felix, D. & Akert, K. (1974). The effect of angiotensin II on neurones of the cat subfornical organ. *Brain Res.* **76**, 350–3.

Felix, D., Schelling, P. & Haas, H. L. (1982). Angiotensin and single neurones. In *The Renin Angiotensin System: a Model for the Synthesis of Peptides in the Brain*, pp. 225–69 (eds D. Ganten, M. P. Printz, M. I. Phillips & B. A. Schölkens). Berlin: Springer-Verlag.

Felix, D. & Schlegel, W. (1978). Angiotensin receptive neurones in the subfornical organ. Structure–activity relations. *Brain Res.* **149**, 107–16.

Fischer-Ferraro, C., Nahmod, V. E., Goldstein, D. J. & Finkielman, S. (1971). Angiotensin and renin in dog and rat brain. *J. Exp. Med.* **133**, 353–61.

Fitzsimmons, J. T. (1969). The role of a renal thirst factor in drinking induced by extracellular stimuli. *J. Physiol.* **201**, 349–68.

Fitzsimmons, J. T. (1980). Angiotensin II in the control of hypovolaemic thirst and sodium appetite (8th J. A. F. Stevenson memorial Lecture). *Can. J. Physiol. Pharmacol.* **58**, 441–4.

Fitzsimmons, J. T. & Simons, B. J. (1969). The effect on drinking in the rat of intravenous angiotensin, given alone or in combination with other stimuli of thirst. *J. Physiol.* **203**, 45–7.

Fukijama, K. (1972). Central action of angiotensin and hypertension-increased central vasomotor outflow by angiotensin. *Jpn. Circ. J.* **36**, 599–602.

Fuxe, K., Ganten, D., Hökfelt, T., Locatelli, V. & Speck, G. (1980). Evidence for differential localisation of angiotensin I-converting enzyme and renin in the corpus striatum of the rat. *Acta Physiol. Scand.* **110**, 321–3.

Gahwiler, B. H. & Dreifuss, J. J. (1980). Transition from random to phasic firing induced in neurones cultured from the hypothalamic supraoptic area. *Brain Res.* **193**, 415–25.

Ganong, W. F. (1981). The brain and the renin angiotensin system. In *Central Nervous System Mechanisms in Hypertension*, pp. 283–92 (eds J. P. Buckley & C. M. Ferraro). New York: Raven Press.

Ganong, W. F. (1983). The brain renin–angiotensin system. In *Brain Peptides* (eds D. T. Krieger & M. Brownstein), pp. 805–26. New York: Wiley-Interscience.

Ganong, W. F. (1984). The brain renin–angiotensin system. *Ann. Rev. Physiol.* **46**, 17–31.

Ganong, W. F., Shinsako, J., Reid, I. A., Keil, L. C. & Hoffman, D. L. (1982). Role of vasopressin in the renin and ACTH responses to intraventricular angiotensin II. *Ann. NY Acad. Sci.* **394**, 619–24.

Ganten. D., Fuxe, K., Ganten, U., Hökfelt, T. & Bolme, P. (1977). The brain isorenin–angiotensin system: localisation and biological function. *Progr. Brain Res.* **47**, 155–9.

Ganten, D., Fuxe, K., Phillips, M. I., Mann, J. F. E. & Ganten, U. (1978). The brain isorenin–angiotensin system: biochemistry, localisation and possible role in drinking and blood pressure regulation. In *Frontiers in Neuroendocrinology*, vol. 5, pp. 61–100 (eds W. F. Ganong & L. Martini). New York: Raven Press.

Ganten, D., Marquez-Julio, A., Granger, D., Hayduk, K., & Karsunky, K. P. (1971). Renin in dog brain. *Am. J. Physiol.* **221**, 1733–7.

Ganten, D., Minnich, J. E., Granger, P., Hayduk, K., Brecht, H. M., Barbeau, A., Boucher, R. & Genest, J. (1971). Angiotensin-forming enzyme in brain tissue. *Science* **173**, 64–5.

Ganten, D., Speck, G., Schelling, P. & Unger, T. (1981). The brain renin–angiotensin system. In *Neurosecretion and Brain Peptides*, pp. 359–72 (eds J. B. Martin, S. Reichlin & K. L. Bick). New York: Raven Press.

Haas, H. L., Felix, D., Celio, M. R. & Inagami, T. (1980). Angiotensin II in the hippocampus. A histochemical and electrophysiological study. *Experientia* **36**, 1394–5.

Harding, J. W., Stone, L. P. & Wright, J. W. (1981). The distribution of angiotensin II binding sites in rodent brain. *Brain Res.* **205**, 265–74.

Hermann, K., Ganten, D., Bayer, C., Unger, Th., Lang, R. E. & Rascher, W. (1982). Definite evidence for the presence of (Ile$^5$) angiotensin I and (IIe$^5$) angiotensin II in the brain of rat. In *The Renin–Angiotensin System: a Model for the Synthesis of Peptides in the Brain*, pp. 192–207 (eds D. Ganten, M. P. Printz, M. I. Phillips & B. A. Schölkens). Berlin: Springer-Verlag.

Hirose, S., Yokosawa, H. & Inagami, T. (1978). Immunochemical identification of renin in rat brain and distinction from acid proteases. *Nature, London* **274**, 392–3.

Hirose, S., Yokosawa, A., Inagami, T. & Workman, R. S. (1980). Renin and prorenin in the hog brain: ubiquitous distribution and high concentration in the pituitary and pineal. *Brain Res.* **191**, 489–99.

Horvarth, J. S., Baxter, C.R., Furby, F. & Tiller, D. J. (1977). Endogenous angiotensin in brain. *Progr. Brain Res.* **47**, 161–9.

Hughes, J. & Roth, R. H. (1971). Evidence that angiotensin enhances transmitter release during sympathetic nerve stimulation. *Br. J. Pharmacol.* **41**, 239–55.

Inagami, T., Celio, M. R., Clemens, D. L., Lau, D., Takii, Y. (1980). Renin in rat and mouse brain: immunohistochemical identification and localisation. *Clin. Sci.* **59**, 49s–51s.

Inagami, T., Okamura, T., Hirose, S., Clemens, D. L., Celio, M. R., Naruse, K., Takii, Y. & Yokosawa, H. (1982). Identification, characterisation and evidence for intraneuronal function of renin in the brain and neuroblastoma cells. In *The Renin–Angiotensin System: a Model for the Synthesis of Peptides in the Brain*, pp. 64–75 (eds D. Ganten, M. P. Printz, M. I. Phillips & B. A. Schölkens). Berlin: Springer-Verlag.

Ito, T., Eggenn, P., Barnett, J. D., Katz, D., Metter, J. & Sambhi, M. P. (1980). Studies on angiotensinogen of plasma and cerebrospinal fluid in normal and hypertensive human subjects. *Hypertension* **3**, 432–6.

Knowles, W. D. & Phillips, M. I. (1980). Angiotensin II cells in the organum vasculosum lamina terminalis (OVLT) recorded in hypothalamic brain slices. *Brain Res.* **197**, 256–9.

Köller, M., Krause, H. P., Hoffmeister, F. & Ganten, D. (1979). Brain angiotensin II (ang II) disrupts avoidance learning. *Neurosci. Lett.* Suppl. 3 S327 (Abstr.)

Legendre, P., Simonnet, G. & Vincent, J. D. (1984). Electrophysiological effects of angiotensin II in cultured mouse spinal cord neurones. *Brain Res.* **297**, 287–96.

Lind, R. W., Swanson, L. W. & Ganten, D. (1985). Organisation of angiotensin II immunoreactive cells and fibres in the rat central nervous system. *Neuroendocrinology* **40**, 2–24.

Malvin, R. L., Mouw, D. & Vander, A. J. (1977). Angiotensin: physiological role in water-deprivation-induced thirst of rats. *Science* **197**, 171–3.

Mendelsohn, F. A. O., Quirion, R., Saavedra, J. M., Aguilera, G. & Catt, K. J. (1984). Autoradiographic localisation of angiotensin-II receptors in rat brain. *Proc. Nat. Acad. Sci.* **81**, 1575.

Morgan, J. M. & Routtenberg, A. (1977). Angiotensin injected into the neostriatum after learning disrupts retention performance. *Science* **196**, 87–9.

Morris, B. J. & Reid, I. A. (1979). Difference in immunochemical properties of dog angiotensinogens in plasma and cerebrospinal fluid. *IRCS Med. Sci.* **7**, 194.

Mouw, D., Bonjour, J. P., Malvin, R. L. & Vander, A. J. (1971). Central actions of angiotensin in stimulating ADH release. *Am. J. Physiol.* **220**, 239–42.

Nahmod, V. E., Finkielman, S., Benaroch, E. E. & Pirola, C. J. (1978). Angiotensin regulates release and synthesis of serotonin in brain. Science **202**, 1091–3.

Nicholaidis, S., Ishibashi, S., Gueguen, B., Thornton, S. N. & de Beaurepaire, R. (1983). Iontophoretic investigation of identified SFO angiotensin responsive neurones firing in relation to blood pressure changes. *Brain Res. Bull.* **10**, 357–63.

Nicholl, R. A. & Barker, J. L. (1971). Excitation of supraoptic neurosecretory cells by angiotensin II. *Nature, London* **233**, 172–4.

Olsson, K. (1970). Effects on water diuresis of infusion of transmitter substances into the third ventricle. *Acta Physiol. Scand.* **79**, 133–5.

Peach, M. J. (1977). Renin–angiotensin system: biochemistry and mechanisms of action. *Physiol. Rev.* **57**, 313–70.

Phillips, M. I. (1978). Current review. Angiotensin in the brain. *Neuroendocrinology* **25**, 354–77.

Phillips, M. I. (1983). New evidence for brain angiotensin and for its role in hypertension. *Fed. Proc.* **42**, 2667–72.

Phillips, M. I., Nelson, P. G., Neal, E. & Quinlan, J. (1980). Angiotensin induced phasic firing of spinal cord neurones in culture. *Soc. Neurosci. Abstr.* **6**, 619.

Phillis, J. W. & Limacher, J. J. (1974). Excitation of cerebral cortical neurons by various polypeptides. *Exptl Neurol.* **43**, 414–23.

Polsky-Cynkin, R. & Fanburg, B. (1979). Immunochemical comparison of angiotensin I converting enzyme from different rat organs. *Int. J. Biochem.* **10**, 669–74.

Raizada, M. K., Phillips, M. I. & Gerndt, J. S. (1983). Primary cultures from total rat brain incorporate [$^3$H]-isoleucine and [$^3$H]-valine into immunoprecipitable angiotensin II. *Neuroendocrinology* **36**, 64–7.

Ramsay, D. J. (1979). The brain renin angiotensin system: a re-evaluation. *Neuroscience* **4**, 313–21.

Ramsay, D. J. (1982). Effects of circulating angiotensin II on the brain. In *Frontiers in Neuroendocrinology*, vol. 7, pp. 263–86 (eds W. F. Ganong & L. Martini). New York: Raven Press.

Regioli, D., Park, W. K. & Rioux, F. (1974). Pharmacology of angiotensin. *Pharmacol. Rev.* **26**, 69–123.

Reid, I. A. (1976). The brain renin–angiotensin system: new observations. In *Regulation of Blood Pressure by the Central Nervous System*, pp. 161–73 (eds G. Onesti, M. Fernandez & K. E. Kim) New York: Grune & Stratton.

Reid, I. A. (1977). Is there a brain renin–angiotensin system? *Circ. Res.* **41**, 147–53.

Reid, I. A. (1979). The brain renin–angiotensin system: a critical analysis. *Fed. Proc.* **38**, 2255–9.

Reid, I. A. & Brownfield, M. S. (1982). The brain renin–angiotensin system. Some unsolved problems. In *The Renin–Angiotensin System: a Model for the Synthesis of Peptides in the Brain*, pp. 284–94 (eds D. Ganten, M. P. Printz, M. I. Phillips & B. A. Schölkens). Berlin: Springer-Verlag.

Reid, I. A., Day, R. P., Moffat, B. & Hughes, H. G. (1977). Apparent angiotensin immunoreactivity in dog brain resulting from angiotensinase. *J. Neurochem.* **28**, 435–8.

Reid, I. A., Moffat, B. & Morris, B. J. (1978). Two forms of angiotensinogen in dog cerebrospinal fluid. *IRCS Med. Sci.* **6**, 383.

Rix, F., Ganten, D., Schüll, B., Unger, T. & Taugner, R. (1981). Converting enzyme in the choroid plexus, brain and kidney: immunocytochemical and biochemical studies in rats. *Neurosci. Lett.* **22**, 125–30.

Rosendorf, F. C., Lowe, R. D., Lavery, H. & Chanston, W. I. (1970). Cardiovascular effects of angiotensin mediated by the central nervous system of the rabbit. *Cardiovasc. Res.* **4**, 36–43.

Schelling, P., Felix, D. & Liard, J. F. (1982). Regulation of angiotensinogen in cerebrospinal fluid and plasma. In *The Renin–Angiotensin System: a Model for the Synthesis of Peptides in the Brain* (eds D. Ganten, M. P. Printz, M. I. Phillips & B. A. Schölkens). Berlin; Springer-Verlag.

Schelling, P., Ganten, U., Sponer, G., Unger, T. & Ganten, D. (1980). Components of the renin–angiotensin system in the CSF of rats and dogs with special considera-tion of the origin and fate of angiotensin II. *Neuroendocrinology*, **31**, 297–308.

Sernia, C. & Reid, I. A. (1980). Release of angiotensinogen by rat brain *in vivo*. *Brain Res.* **192**, 217–25.

Severs, W. G., Daniels, A. E. & Buckley, J. P. (1967). On the central hypertensive effect of angiotensin II. *Int. J. Pharmacol.* **6**, 199–205.

Severs, W. B., Summy-Long, J., Taylor, J. S. & Connor, J. D. (1970). A central effect of angiotensin: release of pituitary pressor material. *J. Pharmacol. Exp. Therap.* **174**, 27–34.

Simmonet, G. & Vincent, J. D. (1980). Characteristics of angiotensin II binding sites in neostriatum of rat brain. *Neurochem. Int.* **4**, 149–55.

Sirett, N. F., Bray, J. J. & Hubbard, J. I. (1981). Localisation of immunoreactive angiotensin II in the hippocampus and striatum of rat brain. *Brain Res.* **217**, 405–11.

Sirett, N. E., McLean, A. S., Bray, J. J. & Hubbard, J. R. (1977). Distribution of angiotensin II receptors in rat brain. *Brain Res.* **122**, 299–312.

Sobel, D. O. (1983). Characterisation of angiotensin-mediated ACTH release. *Neuroendocrinology* **36**, 249–53.

Steele, M. K., Brownfield, M. S., Reid, I. A. & Ganong, W. F. (1982a). A possible role for the renin–angiotensin system in the regulation of LH secretion. *Endocrinology* **110**, 387A.

Steele, M. K., Negro-Vilar, A. & McCann, S. M. (1981). Effects of angiotensin II on *in vivo* and *in vitro* release of anterior pituitary hormones in the female rat. *Endocrinology* **109**, 893–9.

Steele, M. K., Negro-Vilar, A. & McCann, S. M. (1982b). Modulation by dopamine and estradiol of central effects of angiotensin II on anterior pituitary hormone release. *Endocrinology* **111**, 722–9.

Sudakov, K. V., Sherstnev, V. V. & Osipovskii, S. D. (1976). Direct action of angiotensin II on central neurones. *Byulleten Eksperimental noi Biologii i Meditsiny* **82**, 899–902.

Suter, C. & Coole, J. H. (1987). Intrathecally administered angiotensin II increases sympathetic activity in the rat. *J. Auton. Nerv. Syst.* In press.

Wayner, M. J., ONO, T. & Nolley, D. (1973). Effects of angiotensin II on central neurones. *Pharmacol. Biochem. Behav.* **1**, 679–91.

Weiner, R. I. & Ganong, W. F. (1978). The role of brain monoamines and histamine in the regulation of anterior pituitary secretion. *Physiol. Rev.* **58**, 905–76.

Zimmerman, B. G. (1978). Actions of angiotensin on adrenergic nerve endings. Fede. Proc. **37**, 199–202.

# 9

# The functional role of noradrenaline and 5-hydroxytryptamine terminals in the thoracic spinal cord

**J. H. Coote**

*Department of Physiology, The Medical School, Vincent Drive, University of Birmingham, Birmingham B15 2TJ, UK*

## 9.1. Noradrenergic projections to the spinal cord

### 9.1.1. *Anatomy*

There is a wealth of anatomical evidence demonstrating that catecholamine — containing neurones project to the spinal cord (Dahlstrom & Fuxe, 1964; Westlund *et al.*, 1982). These neurones are arranged in groups located in quite different regions of the brainstem (Fig. 9.1). They were originally identified in the rat and classified as $A_1$ to $A_{13}$ (Dahlstrom & Fuxe, 1964; Palkovits & Jacobowitz, 1974). Similar groups are present in the cat (Dahlstrom & Fuxe, 1964; Pin *et al.*, 1968; Coote & Macleod, 1974; Poitras & Parent, 1978; Lackner, 1980), in dog (Ishikawa *et al.*, 1975), in rabbit (Blessing *et al.*, 1978), in primates (Felten *et al.*, 1974; Hubbard & Di Carlo, 1974a; Garver & Sladek, 1975; Demirjian *et al.*, 1976), in humans (Nobin & Björklund, 1973), in birds (Fuxe & Ljunggren, 1965; Ikeda & Gotah, 1971; Dube & Parent, 1981) and probably reptiles and amphibians (Parent, 1973, 1975, 1978). Terminals of these neurones are to be found throughout the grey matter at all levels of the spinal cord, but the sympathetic lateral cell column (IML) in the thoracic cord receives a particularly dense innervation. Several studies have attempted to identify the group or groups of catecholamine neurones which contribute to this innervation. Dahlstrom & Fuxe (1965) noted that following spinal cord transection neurones in the $A_1$ and $A_2$ cell groups displayed swelling and accumulation of fluorescent material, indicating that spinally projecting axons had been cut: a finding that seemingly was confirmed in the more recent studies of Nygren & Olsen (1977). A surprising feature, however, was that Dahlstrom & Fuxe (1965) could find no evidence for descending projections from other catecholamine cell groups which recent experiments have shown quite clearly (Satoh *et al.*, 1977; Loewy *et al.*, 1979; Westlund *et al.*, 1983). In the experiments of Loewy *et al.* (1979)

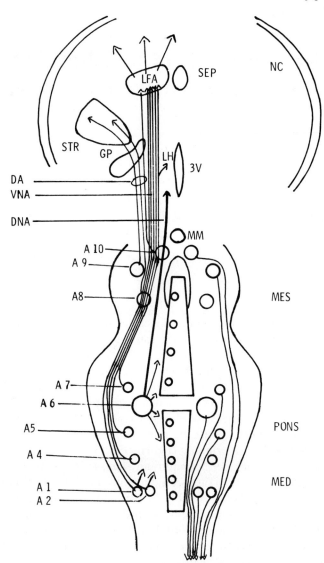

Fig. 9.1. Diagram showing the catecholamine cell groups $A_1$–$A_{10}$ and their projections. Abbreviations: DA, dopamine pathways; DNA, doral noradrenergic pathway;
GP, globus pallidus; LFA, limbic forward area; LH, lateral hypothalamic area;
MED, medulla oblongata; MES, mesencephalon; MM, mamillary nuclei; NC,
neocortex; SEP, septal area; STR, striatum; 3V, third ventricle; VNA, ventral
noradrenaline pathway. Modified from Morgane & Stern (1978).

injections of $^3H$ amino acid restricted to the $A_5$ region of the pons resulted in quite dense labelling of terminals in IML, and this was not present if these injections had been preceded by the catecholamine neurotoxin 6-hydroxy-tryptamine (6OHDA) given intraventricularly. Cells in the $A_5$ region containing catecholamine could also be labelled following injections of horseradish peroxidase (HRP) into the thoracic spinal cord. Westlund *et al.* (1983) injected HRP into the thoracic spinal cord at unidentified locations and convincingly showed cells in the $A_7$ group doubly labelled for HRP and catecholamine. However, in contrast to Satoh *et al.* (1977) and Loewy *et al.* (1979), there were very few labelled cells in $A_5$ and there were no doubly labelled cells in $A_1$. This latter observation has been interpreted as indicating that the $A_1$ catecholamine neurones in the rat do not project to the spinal cord. Such an absolute conclusion should be looked at with caution since the anatomical techniques are not foolproof (Heuser & Reese, 1973; Nauta *et al.*, 1974; Jones, 1975; Hedreen & McGrath, 1977). It is also clearly incorrect according to the data presented in Figs 2, 4 and 5 of McKellar & Loewy (1982).

Therefore the anatomical evidence leads us to the conclusion that in the rat there are spinally projecting catecholamine neurones in $A_7$, $A_6$, $A_5$, $A_2$ and $A_1$ but there is only clear evidence of an innervation of IML from $A_5$ and perhaps to a lesser extent from $A_1$.

In general, electrophysiological experiments are in agreement with this. Small spinally projecting neurones in the $A_1$, $A_5$ and $A_6$ regions have been identified by an antidromic activation of their axons in the spinal cord, and their location has been correlated with the position of catecholamine-containing cells (Guyenet, 1980; Andrade & Aghajanian, 1982; Fleetwood-Walker *et al.*, 1983; Coote & West, unpublished observations). No similar studies have so far been conducted on the $A_7$ group.

In the rabbit, catecholamine-fluorescent cells containing retrogradely transported HRP from the spinal cord are located mainly in $A_7$, $A_6$, $A_5$ and the rostral part of $A_1$ in the medulla (Blessing *et al.*, 1981).

Similar double labelling studies in the chick show that $A_6$ and $A_1$ project to the thoracic spinal cord but that $A_1$ provides the main catecholamine innervation of the grey matter dorsal to the central canal, presumably because the autonomic nucleus dominates this region in the bird (Smolen *et al.*, 1979).

In the cat we have used a somewhat different approach to determine which group of spinal projecting catecholamine neurones innervate IML. Following electrolytic lesions placed to destroy separate catecholamine cell groups in the medulla and pons of different cats, biochemical analysis of discrete regions in the third thoracic segment of the spinal cord was performed. Bilateral lesions in the ventrolateral medulla, to destroy $A_1$ neurones, caused a marked and very selective depletion of noradrenaline in the IML: whereas lesions of $A_2$, $A_5$ and $A_6$ had no or only a small effect on catecholamine levels in this nucleus. A contribution from $A_7$ cannot be excluded because the ventrolateral medullary lesion was quite extensive and could have destroyed $A_7$ fibres if they passed through this region on their way to the spinal cord (Fleetwood-Walker & Coote, 1981).

Electrophysiological studies on the cat have shown that spinally projecting neurones with slowly conducting axons are located in the region occupied by $A_1$ cells (Caverson *et al.*, 1983; Coote, unpublished observations), but evidence that these are catecholamine cells is lacking.

In summary the IML in the third thoracic segment of the cat receives a dense and highly specific noradrenergic innervation which originates from cell bodies in the $A_1$ region or from axons passing through this ventrolateral medullary area possibly from cells in $A_7$.

The terminals of these spinally projecting noradrenaline cells appear to make axo-dendritic synaptic contact with sympathetic preganglionic neurones (Wong & Tan, 1974). These authors showed that there was a degeneration of nerve terminals in the IML following 6OHDA given systemically. Some caution is required in interpreting this interesting result because of possible non-specific action of the neurotoxin, particularly when given by the systemic route. It would be very useful to repeat this ultrastructural study using gold-labelled antibodies to the catecholamines.

There have been some suggestions that the IML receives a specific innervation from spinally projecting adrenaline-containing neurones located at the rostral extent of $A_1$ (Blessing *et al.*, 1981; McKellar & Loewy, 1982). This group of neurones designated as $C_1$ was originally described by Hokfelt *et al.* (1974) using an immunohistofluorescence technique based on an antibody to phenylethanolamine *n*-methyl transferase (PNMT), the adrenaline-synthesising enzyme. Terminal projections were identified in the IML of the rat. Quantitative biochemical methods estimating adrenaline in IML have been less convincing. Reid *et al.* (1975) using mass fragmentography showed that adrenaline was present in rat spinal cord in small amounts, but Van der Guyten *et al.* (1976) could not demonstrate its presence in IML. In the rabbit the presence of adrenaline in the IML has only been inferred indirectly as the difference between total catecholamine and amounts of noradrenaline and dopamine (Zivin *et al.*, 1975). In the cat adrenaline levels in the thoracic cord were too low to allow a reliable interpretation of the data obtained from a highly sensitive radioenzymatic assay (Fleetwood-Walker & Coote, 1981). It must therefore be concluded that the adrenaline innervation of IML if it exists is very sparse.

### 9.1.2. *Actions of catecholamine pathways*

The influence of this catecholamine innervation on sympathetic activity is likely to be an inhibitory one, although this again is an area surrounded by controversy.

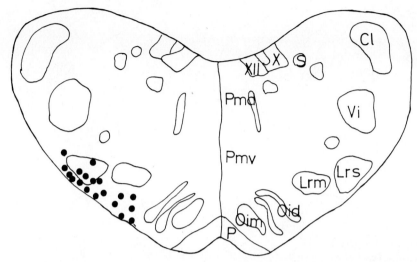

Fig. 9.2. Transverse section of medulla oblongata of anaesthetised cat 1.5 mm rostral to obex, showing points (filled circles) from which electrical stimulation (10 s train, 100 Hz, 100–300 μA) inhibited sympathetic activity in splanchnic and renal nerves and lower thoracic white rami. Abbreviations: Lrm, Lrs, subnuclei of nucleus lateralis reticularis; Oim, Oid, nucleus of inferior olive complex; P, tractus pyramidalis; S, nucleus tractus solitarius; Vi, nucleus spinalis nervi trigemini; X, nucleus nervi vagi dorsalis motorius; XII, nucleus nervi hypoglossi; Pmd, Pmv, subnuclei of nucleus paramedian reticularis; CI, nucleus cuneatus. (From Coote &Macleod, 1984a.)

Electrical stimulation of fibres of passage or cells via electrodes accurately located among catecholamine neurones in the ventrolateral medulla (as judged by fluorescence histochemistry of the brains of experimental animals) produced inhibition of sympathetic activity in white rami or in vasomotor postganglionic fibres in renal nerve (Coote & Macleod, 1974; Fig. 9.2). This inhibition was abolished after damaging a limited region of the dorsolateral funiculus of the cervical spinal cord whereas inhibition or excitation from other brainstem sites was unaffected (Coote & Macleod, 1975. Fig. 9.3). This suggested that the inhibition was produced by stimulating a descending pathway to the IML, a supposition which appeared to be supported by the demonstration in spinal animals of sympatho-inhibitory sites confined to that part of the dorsolateral funiculus where the lesions abolished the effects of stimulating in the ventrolateral medulla. In addition the calculated conduction velocities for medullary sites to sympathetic outflow and spinal sites to sympathetic outflow were similar, having a mean of $<2$ m.s.$^{-1}$ (Coote & Macleod, 1974; 1975), which is consistent with the effect being mediated by small unmyelinated catecholamine fibres. Further support for such a conclusion comes from the observation that the $\alpha_2$ adrenoreceptor antagonist piperoxane ($< 2$ mg kg$^{-1}$) given intravenously reduced the inhibitory effect of

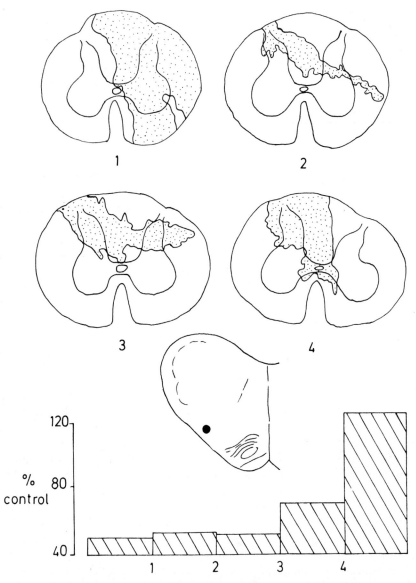

Fig. 9.3. Effect of spinal cord lesions (anaesthetised cat) on the inhibition of reflex discharge in the 10th thoracic white ramus ($T_{10}$ WR) elicited by stimulation of the 9th intercostal nerve ($IC_9$, $IC_9-T_{10}$ WR) produced by electrical stimulation in he ventrolateral medulla at the point shown (filled circle). In the bar graph the size of the $IC_9-T_{10}$ WR reflex elicited after medullary stimulation expressed as a percentage of the size of the control reflex responses is shown after each of four lesions (1, 2, 3, 4) had been made in the spinal cord at $C_3$. The extent of these lesions is illustrated by the stippled areas in the four TS of spinal cord. (From Coote & Macleod, 1975.)

stimulating in the ventrolateral medulla by some 70% in three animals Coote & Macleod, unpublished observations). However, it is conceded that great weight cannot be placed on this result since the drug given by the intravenous route may be acting at many sites in the nervous system to produce its effect. Another study claimed that stimulation of the $A_1$ region of the medulla of the cat caused excitation of sympathetic preganglionic neurones (Franz *et al.*, 1975). It is difficult to take this claim seriously since the published location of tested sites shows that they were much too dorsal in the medulla, and no evidence is provided that catecholamine neurones were present in this region; in any case the latency to onset of the effect was far too short to be dependent on a slowly conducting catecholamine pathway. The authors then go on to presume that the depressant action of chlorpromazine on these responses was due to an α-adrenoreceptor antagonist property of the drug, yet it has several other non-adrenergic actions.

### 9.1.3. *Microiontophoresis*

Iontophoretic administration of the catecholamines noradrenaline, dopamine and adrenaline into the vicinity of sympathetic preganglionic neurones or antecedent neurones inhibits their activity (Fig. 9.4; DeGroat & Ryall, 1967; Coote *et al.*, 1981a; Kadzielawa, 1983a), an effect which in the cat (Kadzielawa, 1983a), and in the bird is blocked by $\alpha_2$-adrenoreceptor antagonists such as yohimbine or piperoxane (Guyenet & Cabot, 1981; Guyenet & Stornetta, 1982). A full interpretation of this result is of course dependent on whether the catecholamine fibres terminate directly on to sympathetic neurones, and at present this is still not proven (but see Wong & Tan, 1974). However, what is quite clear from these studies is that each of the catecholamines has a similar action, i.e. inhibition, and that the adrenoreceptor in the IML is exclusively of the $\alpha_2$ type (Coote *et al.*, 1979; Unnerstall *et al.*, 1984; Dashwood *et al.*, 1985). These facts must limit the scope of any interpretation.

### 9.1.4. *Pharmacological studies*

Pharmacological studies are again more strongly supportive of an inhibitory role for the catecholamine pathways. Perfusion of the subarachnoid space of the thoracic spinal cord of the rat with noradrenaline (0.30 μmol) inhibits sympathetic nerve activity (LoPachin & Rudy, 1983). Intravenous administration of *L*-dihydroxyphenylalamine (*L*-dopa 40–100 mg kg$^{-1}$) in the majority of laboratories causes a decrease in both pre- and post ganglionic sympathetic activity (Sinha *et al.*, 1973; Coote & Macleod, 1974) — an action present in spinal animals and presumed to be due to its being taken up by monoamine nerve terminals in the spinal cord and the subsequent release of

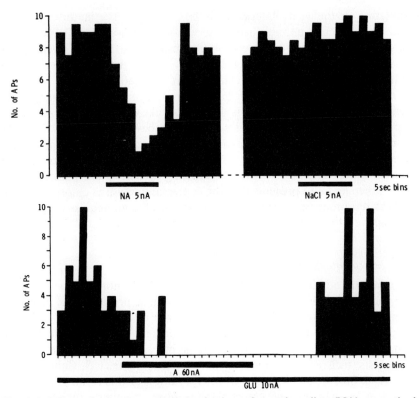

Fig. 9.4. Effect of microiontophoretic ejection of noradrenaline (NA) on a single spontaneously active SPN (top) and of adrenaline (A) on a glutamate (GLU) driven SPN, bottom. NaCl, current control. $T_3$ segment, anaesthetised cat. (Partly from Coote *et al.*, 1981a.)

endogenous transmitter. Although there is little doubt that such an action occurs, the result should be viewed with some caution because *L*-dopa still has similar effects on spinal reflexes, although to a lesser degree, even following degeneration of descending monoaminergic fibres in chronically spinalised cats (Baker & Anderson, 1970; Kirchner *et al.*, 1975). Also *L*-dopa may exert a direct action on certain central neurones (Ohye *et al.*, 1970). At variance with these results is the interesting observation by Hare *et al.* (1972), that intravenous *L*-dopa in spinal cats had a biphasic effect on somato-sympathetic reflexes recorded in upper thoracic white rami. There was an initial decrease followed by a prolonged marked enhancement. Surprisingly, intraspinal evoked responses in the white rami were only depressed. Pretreatment with *p*-chlorophenylalanine (*p*CPA) eliminated the depressant action of *L*-dopa, as did tolazoline. The assumption made by these investigators was that *p*CPA and tolazoline were having specific effects on a 5-hydroxytryptamine system in the IML, for which they carried out no controls. The fact that tolazoline by itself enhanced both reflex evoked and intraspinal evoked sympathetic responses and that the *L*-dopa enhancement of the somato-sympathetic reflexes was reduced following *p*CPA treatment would appear to justify this criticism.

In contrast to his conclusions that noradrenaline is a sympatho-excitatory transmitter in the spinal cord, Franz provided evidence that adrenaline may be a sympatho-inhibitory transmitter (Franz *et al.*, 1982). It was shown that inhibition of adrenaline synthesis using a selective inhibitor of the enzyme PNMT caused a gradual enhancement of the sympathetic response to intraspinal stimulation.

Other pharmacological evidence supports a sympatho-inhibitory role for the descending catecholamine pathway. Haeusler (1977) demonstrated in the cat that discharges in splanchnic nerve evoked by intraspinal stimulation are reduced by clonidine ($< 25$ mg kg$^{-1}$) and $\alpha$-methyl-dopa ($< 100$ mg kg$^{-1}$), this effect being blocked by $\alpha$-adrenoceptor antagonists phentolamine and piperoxane. Clonidine (10–25 mg kg$^{-1}$ i.v.) also blocks somato-sympathetic reflexes in white rami or ongoing activity in renal nerves in spinal animals (Franz *et al.*, 1975; Coote & Macleod, unpublished observations). Franz *et al.* (1975) attributed the depression of sympathetic outflow by clonidine to stimulation of 5-hydroxytryptamine receptors on sympathetic preganglionic neurones mainly on the evidence that its effect was antagonised by tolazoline. Yet this drug, as well having some antagonism to 5-hydroxytryptamine, is a more effective antagonist at $\alpha$-adrenoceptors.

In addition, 5-hydroxytryptamine applied in the vicinity of sympathetic preganglionic neurones has a clear excitatory action (DeGroat & Ryall, 1967; Coote *et al.*, 1981a).

The conclusion that the bulbospinal catecholamine pathway is inhibitory is further reinforced by the enhancement of the spinal component of the somato-sympathetic reflex in $T_3$ white ramus following intravenous yohimbine (0.45 mg kg$^{-1}$), the $\alpha_2$-adrenoceptor antagonist. This indicates that the bulbospinal catecholamine neurones to IML are tonically active. This suggestion is supported by the fact that either cooling the dorsolateral funiculus or a small lesion in the dorsolateral funiculus of the cervical cord where catecholamine fibres descend (which abolishes the inhibitory effect of stimulating in the ventrolateral medulla from which or through which catecholamine neurones destined for IML descend, see earlier section) causes enhancement of somato-sympathetic reflexes (Coote & Macleod, 1975; Dembowkey *et al.*, 1980).

In contrast Taylor & Brody (1976) considered that the descending noradrenergic pathway might be excitatory to IML. They stimulated the lateral funiculus in spinal cats caudal to the transection and found that they could attenuate a pressor response or vasoconstriction in a perfused hind limb by infusing large doses of the α-adrenoreceptor antagonist phentolamine (up to 900 mg) into the subarachnoid space. No controls for the specificity of action of the antagonist were performed, and in view of the large doses it is difficult to take this result seriously.

Others have considered that adrenaline-synthesising neurones in the rostral ventrolateral medulla (Howe *et al.*, 1980) project selectively to sympathetic preganglionic neurones and carry the important tonic excitatory drive to these cells (Ross *et al.*, 1983). However, although these authors stimulated cell bodies in the rostal ventrolateral medulla, no evidence was provided that the sympatho-excitatory effects were mediated by adrenaline. In fact this same group of cells is thought by others to cause sympatho-excitation by the release of substance P (Helke *et al.*, 1982; Loewy & Sawyer, 1982; Takano *et al.*, 1984), although this needs substantiating.

### 9.1.5. *Function of noradrenaline pathway*

With regard to the sympathetic function of the spinally projecting noradrenergic neurones it has been suggested that they might be involved in mediating the baroreceptor inhibition that occurs directly on sympathetic preganglionic neurones (Coote *et al.*, 1981b). Inflation of an isolated blind sac preparation of a carotid sinus strongly inhibited a response in $T_3$ white ramus elicited by stimulating descending excitatory fibres. This inhibition was reversibly abolished on application of phentolamine (2 μg) to the surface of the $T_3$ segment of the spinal cord. In other experiments the inhibition induced by electrical stimulation of a carotid sinus nerve on the somato-sympathetic reflex in $T_{10}$ white ramus was markedly reduced by intraspinal injections of the catecholamine neurotoxin 6-hydroxydopamine (Coote & Macleod, 1977) but not by the 5-hydroxytryptamine neurotoxin 5,6-dihydroxytryptamine or by systemic administration of *p*CPA (Coote *et al.*, 1978). Seemingly at variance with these findings are those by Dembowsky *et al.* (1980) which showed that baroreceptor denervation did not alter the spinal cold block induced increase in amplitude of a spinal somato-sympathetic reflex. This suggests that descending tonic inhibition (which was sensitive to yohimbine) was not dependent on baroreceptor drive. In addition Haeusler & Lewis (1975) found that after depletion of central catecholamines with either intraventricular injections of 6-hydroxydopamine or reserpine and α-methyl-*p*-tyrosine pretreatment there was no reduction in the inhibitory response seen in sympathetic activity during baroreceptor activation. Inasmuch as these experiments did not examine directly the spinal arm of the baroreceptor reflex inhibition of sympathetic preganglionic neurones, the findings still leave the question open.

## 9.2. **5-Hydroxytryptaminergic projections to the spinal cord**

### 9.2.1 *Anatomy*

The terminals of nerve cell bodies containing 5-hydroxytryptamine (5HT) are probably present in most parts of the central nervous system of mammals, birds, reptiles and amphibians (Broughton, 1972; Fuxe & Jonsson, 1973; Saavedra *et al.*, 1973, 1974; Tauber, 1974; Parent, 1975, 1978; Bobillier *et al.*, 1976; Kuypers & Martin, 1982). The cell bodies are only found in the brainstem localised to midline nuclei or closely associated regions extending from the decussation of the pyramids to the mesencephalon (Fig. 9.5). Similar groups of neurones have been identified in birds, opossum, mouse, rat, rabbit, cat, dog, monkey and man (Nobin & Bjorklund, 1973; Hubbard & DiCarlo, 1974b; Lackner, 1980; Cabot *et al.*, 1982; Kuypers & Martin, 1982) and these have been labelled $B_1-B_9$ (Dahlstrom & Fuxe, 1964). Spinally projecting 5HT neurones lie mainly in the $B_1-B_3$ cell group and an associated ventral medullary group sometimes referred to as the arcuate group or the nucleus interfascicularis hypoglossi (Dahlstrom & Fuxe, 1965; Loewy, 1981; Loewy & McKellar, 1981; Steinbusch, 1981; Bowker *et al.*, 1982). According to Bowker *et al.* (1982) some 5HT neurones in the pontine cell group $B_5$ and midbrain group $B_7$, also project to the spinal cord, the latter rather interestingly only to the cervical spinal cord.

Axons of these spinally projecting neurones are small, 1–2 μm in diameter, and probably unmyelinated (Dahlstrom & Fuxe, 1965; Loizou, 1972; Coote & Macleod, unpublished observations). They descend in the lateral and ventral funiculi, concentrated towards the outer margin of the spinal cord at least from the thoracic levels onwards (Dahlstrom & Fuxe, 1964; Coote & Macleod, 1974; Loewy, 1981). It has been shown in the opossum, rat, cat, dog and bird that the sympathetic cell groups in the spinal cord receive a dense 5HT innervation (Dahlstrom & Fuxe, 1965; Konishi, 1968; Coote & Macleod, 1974; Coote *et al.*, 1978; Cabot *et al.*, 1979; Loewy, 1981; Loewy & McKellar, 1981; Martin *et al.*, 1982) although whether the terminals end pre- or postsynaptically on sympathetic preganglionic nerones or on interneurones is unclear. This innervation arises at least in part from nucleus raphe pallidus and obscurus of the medulla. Dahlstrom & Fuxe (1965) treated rats with nialamide and were able to trace 5HT-containing neurones from their location in the nucleus raphe pallidus ($B_1$) and raphe obscurus ($B_2$) into the dorsal and lateral funiculus to their termination in the IML. Lesions in the dorsolateral funiculus abolished the 5HT-formaldehyde-induced fluorescence in IML. More substantive evidence for this 5HT projection to IML from the $B_1$ and $B_2$ groups of cells has come from recent double-labelling studies in the rat which also confirm that the general course of the 5HT axons is in the lateral and dorsolateral funiculi (Loewy, 1981; Loewy & McKellar, 1981). In the cat and opposum, 5HT axons innervating

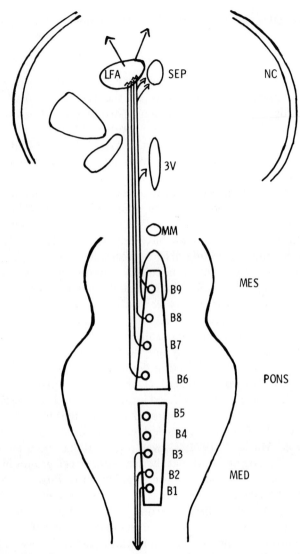

Fig. 9.5. Diagram showing the location of the indolamine cell groups $B_1$–$B_9$ and their projections. Abbreviations as in Fig. 9.1. (Modified from Morgane & Stern, 1978.)

IML also descend in the dorsolateral funiculus since lesions (either local injection of 5, 6-dihydroxytryptamine or cuts) here abolish 5HT fluorescence in the IML (Coote *et al.*, 1978; Martin *et al.*, 1982). Some of these axons may well originate from cell bodies in nucleus raphe pallidus and obscurus since injection of horseradish peroxidase more or less confined to the IML is found in cells in these brainstem nuclei (Amendt *et al.*, 1979) and since electrical stimulation in the dorsal quadrant of spinal cord of cat antidromically excites slowly conducting axons with cell bodies in these nuclei (Morrison & Gebber, 1984). There is also clear evidence in the rat for a 5HT projection from a ventral medullary group of cells lying lateral to $B_1$ (Loewy & McKellar, 1981) and close to the surface of the ventral medulla. These have been termed the arcuate group of 5HT neurones or nucleus interfascicularis hyperglossi, although it is difficult to consider them as a nucleus because the cells are so scattered and diffuse.

Neurones in nucleus raphe magnus also project to IML but there is no clear evidence as yet that these are 5HT-containing cells. In the cat and opossum there is a dense labelling of terminals in the IML following injections of $^3$H-leucine in the region of nucleus raphe magnus (see Fig. 10, Holstege & Kuypers, 1982; Martin *et al.*, 1979, 1982). In the rat, Bowker *et al.* (1982) have shown that many 5HT-containing cells in nucleus raphe magnus project to the spinal cord, and the majority send their axons via the lateral and dorsolateral funiculus. Since the 5HT innervation of the IML appears to come mainly from fibres in the lateral funiculus, it was natural for these authors to conclude that many of the raphe magnus or $B_3$ 5HT cells were destined for the IML. This was reinforced when Basbaum & Fields (1979) confirmed this and in addition reported in the cat that many neurones in raphe pallidus and obscurus send spinal projections via the ventrolateral and ventral funiculi. However, on closer examination the data presented by Bowker *et al.* (1982) are not so conclusive. These authors found that the number of 5HT cell bodies in raphe magnus taking up horseradish per-oxidase (HRP) was considerably reduced (81%) following section of the dorsal quadrant of the spinal cord above the level of an HRP injection site. However, there was nearly as marked a reduction in the number of HRP-stained 5HT neurones in raphe obscurus (71%) and raphe pallidus (41%). These percentages refer to my own calculations, based on the data shown in Fig. 9 of Bowker *et al.* (1982).

### 9.2.2. *Actions of 5HT pathways*

Progress in establishing the role of spinally projecting 5HT neurones in sympathetic regulation has been slow. Inadequacies in the design of the experiments and in the techniques have been partly to blame for this. For example, recording of blood pressure and heart rate while electrically stimulating with electrodes placed in raphe nuclei is too imprecise to allow the conclusion that spinally projecting neurones are involved. Similarly the action of drugs which deplete brain 5HT, in most cases, has not been confined to the spinally projecting neurones. As a consequence the data are conflicting (see Kuhn *et al.*, 1980a, b). None the less such approaches have quite clearly indicated that the raphe nuclei are not homogeneous in function. There are distinct regions from which pressor responses and increases in heart rate can be obtained, whereas, at other locations in the raphe nuclei, depressor responses and heart-rate decreases predominate (Coote & Macleod, 1974; Neumayr *et al.*, 1974; Gillis *et al.*, 1976; Adair *et al.*, 1977; Smits *et al.*, 1978; Cabot *et al.*, 1979; Yen *et al.*, 1983). By far the most compelling evidence regarding the influence on sympathetic activity of spinally projecting 5HT neurones has come from electrophysiological studies. It has been shown that inhibition of sympathetic activity, together with falls in blood pressure, results from stimulation in the nucleus raphe pallidus of cat and bird, possibly including cells of the nucleus inter-fascicularis hyperglossi (Coote & Macleod, 1974; Neumayr *et al.*, 1974; Cabot *et al.*, 1979). The inhibition was likely to be occuring at a spinal site since spinal sympathetic reflexes were depressed together with supraspinal sympathetic reflexes and spontaneous sympathetic activity (Coote & Macleod, 1974; Neumayr *et al.*, 1974). The effect on the spinal reflexes could not have been due to a disfacilitation because removal of all descending excitatory inputs to sympathetic neurones by spinal cord transection had little effect on the size or threshold of the particular sympathetic reflexes studied (Coote & Macleod, 1974). It was argued by Coote & Macleod (1974, 1975) that small indolamine neurones were activated in these experiments because the stimulus threshold for eliciting the sympatho-inhibitory effects was markedly higher than needed to elicit sympatho-inhibitory or excitatory effects from the classical pressor and depressor regions of the medulla. Furthermore, the fact that the stimulating electrodes were well correlated with electrode placements close to 5HT neurones appears to support the conclusions. Other circumstantial evidence, suggesting that small spinally projecting 5HT neurones are involved in the sympatho-inhibition, is difficult to disregard. Thus the inhibitory effect was preferentially abolished by small cuts in the dorsolateral cervical spinal cord (Coote & Macleod, 1975), descending sympatho-excitatory pathways and a ventromedial sympatho-inhibitory pathways still being patent (Fig. 9.6). The lesions were placed in part of the spinal cord from which inhibition of sympathetic activity can be obtained in spinal cats (Illert & Gabriel, 1970, 1972; Coote & Macleod, 1974, 1975), suggesting that an inhibitory pathway descends in this region. A comparison of the latency to onset of the sympatho-inhibition obtained from the dorsolateral funiculus in the mid-cervical spinal cord ($> 40$ ms) and raphe pallidus of the medulla ($> 100$ ms) suggests that neurones with similar axonal conduction velocities are involved — that is, of course, assuming a fairly direct influence on the IML from both regions (Coote & Macleod, 1974; 1975). Clear evidence that the inhibitory effect of stimulating elements in raphe pallidus was due to an action close to or on sympathetic preganglionic neurones was provided in a further paper by Gilbey *et al.* (1981). In this study the excitability of sympathetic neurones was also tested by intraspinal stimulation of descending excitatory pathways in addition to reflexly activating these neurones. Stimulation in raphe pallidus inhibited

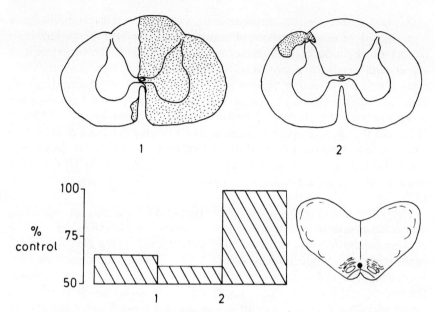

Fig. 9.6. Effect of spinal cord lesions (anaesthetised cat) on the inhibition of $IC_9-T_{10}$ WR reflex by stimulation in the nucleus raphe pallidus (filled circle in TS of medulla). In the bar graph the size of the $IC_9-T_{10}$ WR reflex following medullary stimulation is plotted as a percentage of control reflex before and after each of two lesions (1 and 2) were made in the spinal cord at $C_4$. The extent of these lesions is shown by the stippled areas in the TS of spinal cord (1 and 2). (From Coote & Macleod 1975.)

activity elicited by either means, so it is unlikely that the effect of raphe stimulation was mediated via an action on dorsal horn transmission. Recently Morrison & Gebber (1984) recorded neurones in raphe pallidus which were antidromically activated following stimulation in the dorsolateral funiculus of the upper thoracic spinal cord. Many of these had latencies greater than 100 ms, supporting the idea that the axons of raphe spinal sympatho-inhibitory neurones are located in this region of the spinal cord. Sympatho-inhibitory effects elicited from some regions of raphe obscurus are probably also mediated via small spinal projecting neurones travelling in the dorsolateral funiculus (Coote & Macleod, 1974; Gilbey *et al.*, 1981).

### 9.2.3. *Pharmacological studies*

These suggest that the inhibition of sympathetic activity elicited from stimulating sites in raphe pallidus and obscurus is mediated by spinally projecting 5HT neurones.

The first piece of evidence concerns the effects on sympathetic activity of systemically administered 5-hydroxytryptophan (5HTP) the precursor of

5HT which passes into the central nervous system where it is metabolised and is presumed to cause overflow of transmitter from 5HT nerve terminals (Anderson & Shibuya, 1966; Baker & Anderson, 1970). This treatment in spinal cats produces a profound inhibition of pre- and postganglionic sympathetic nerve activity (Hare *et al.*, 1972; Coote & Macleod, 1974); Neumayr *et al.*, 1974). The onset and time course of the inhibition are consistent with the kinetics of precursor uptake, synthesis and release of 5HT, and the effect of 5HTP is prevented by blocking synthesis of 5HT with a central decarboxylase inhibitor RO 4-4602 (Franz *et al.*, 1978). Amitriptyline and chlorimipramine, tricyclic antidepressants selective for 5HT, rapidly and markedly enhance the depression produced by 5HTP (Sangdee & Franz, 1979).

The involvement of spinally projecting 5HT neurones in inhibiting sympathetic neurones was tested more directly in anaesthetised cats by examining the effect of a variety of 5HT antagonists on long latency to onset raphe-spinal inhibition (Gilbey *et al.*, 1981). Sympathetic responses were evoked in $T_3$ or $T_{10}$ white rami either reflexly or by intraspinal stimulation at the midcervical level. In seven cats, lysergic acid diethylamide (LSD) in a dose range 25–50 µg kg$^{-1}$ i.v., or 0.6 µg applied topically to a spinal cord segment, reversibly reduced the raphe spinal inhibition by 40–100%, topical application being more effective than i.v. administration (Fig. 9.7) In five of these cats, stimulating within the classical inhibitory region of the ventromedial reticular formation at sites unlikely to contain 5HT neurones produced a short latency to onset inhibition of sympathetic activity which was unaffected by LSD. The relatively low concentration of LSD and its selective action in antagonising the raphe spinal inhibition argue against LSD's acting as a 5HT agonist since this characteristic of the drug is only manifest at high concentration (0.5–2.0 mg kg$^{-1}$) and is accompanied by non-specificity (Haigler & Aghajanian, 1974). The putative 5HT antagonists methysergide, cinanserin and cyproheptadine all depressed sympathetic discharge in the absence of brain stimulation, both in cats with intact central nervous systems and in spinal cats, so ruling out the possibility that the effect of these drugs in the intact cat was due to their antagonising a tonically active 5HT excitatory system.

An inhibitory role for a bulbospinal 5HT pathway is also supported by studies on sympathetic preganglionic neurones in the pigeon (Cabot *et al.*, 1979). However, the results of the latter study should be interpreted cautiously. It is unclear whether stimulating electrodes located rostrally in the medullary raphe were in raphe magnus or pallidus, and this could have some bearing on the meaning of the rather fast conduction velocities (4–12.0 m.s.$^{-1}$) reported for the inhibitory fibres. It seems unlikely that the small unmyelinated axons of 5HT neurones would conduct at such speeds. In the cat, as well as the larger, faster-conducting neurones more numerous in raphe magnus there is also a population of slow, small neurones (Wessendorf

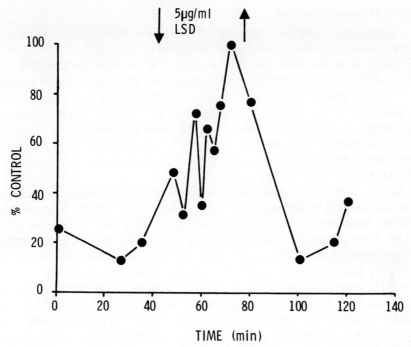

Fig. 9.7. Effect of topically applied LSD on raphe spinal inhibition of intraspinally ($C_4$) evoked sympathetic discharge in $T_3$ WR. Filled circles show the size of the $T_3$ WR response (average × 8) following raphe stimulation and plotted as a percentage of the mean value of the 'bracketing' (average × 8), $T_3$ WR response in the absence of raphe stimulation (ordinate), at various times (abscissa) during the pre-drug, drug and post-drug periods. Time of drug application indicated by distance between arrows. Raphe stimulation commenced 400 ms prior to spinal cord (intra-spinal) stimulation. (From Gilbey *et al.*, 1981).)

& Anderson, 1983; Morrison & Gebber, 1984) which are likely to be 5HT containing. Unfortunately Cabot *et al.* (1979) presented no further evidence in favour of a 5HT identity of the neurones, neither was there evidence indicating that the sympatho-inhibitory effects were taking place at a spinal as opposed to a medullary site.

Despite these reservations, the evidence is still much in favour of an inhibitory action on sympathetic preganglionic neurones of raphe spinal 5HT neurones. Therefore, since Dahlstrom & Fuxe (1965) implied that 5HT terminals could end directly on sympathetic preganglionic neurones (although there is no direct evidence as yet for this), we might expect that the direct cellular action of 5HT would be inhibitory.

### 9.2.4. *Microiontophoresis*

In studies employing the technique of microiontophoresis, 5HT has been found to excite the majority of sympathetic preganglionic neurones (DeGroat & Ryall, 1967; Coote *et al.*, 1981a; Kadzielawa, 1983b; McCall, 1983). Excitation occurred irrespective of whether the neurones were quiescent, spontaneously active or induced to discharge with excitatory amino acids such as *L*-glutamate or *DL*-homocysteic acid. Distinct receptors appear to mediate the excitatory response to 5HT, since iontophoretic or systemic administration of methysergide, metergoline or cinanserin attenuates the response to 5HT without affecting the excitatory response to amino acids (Kadzielawa, 1983b; McCall, 1983).

In two studies 5HT applied microiontophoretically inhibited 14% of the thoracic preganglionic neurones tested (Coote *et al.*, 1981a; Kadzielawa, 1983b). Inhibition was usually limited only to the period of ejection after which firing increased rapidly to reach or even exceed the previous control level. Coote *et al.* (1981a) concluded that neuronal inhibition was most probably the result of an action of creatinine which was ejected along with the 5HT, since the inhibition was never observed when the bimaleate salt of 5HT was used. However, this argument would seem to be dismissed because Kadzielawa (1983b) observed inhibition in precisely similar proportion of sympathetic preganglionic neurones when using the hydrochloride salt of 5HT. The receptor mediating this 5HT inhibition or that elicited by stimulating raphe spinal neurones remains undefined, but the lack of effect of cinanserin, cyproheptadine, methysergide and the blocking effect of LSD suggest that they could be of the $5HT_1$ type (see Fozard, 1984).

### 9.2.5. *Sympatho-inhibition vs sympatho-excitation by 5HT neurones*

In view of the foregoing, it is possible that spinally projecting 5HT neurones have direct excitatory or inhibitory influences on sympathetic preganglionic neurones depending on the type of postsynaptic receptor associated with the 5HT release site. However, in view of the facts that most neurones are excited by directly applied 5HT and yet are inhibited by raphe stimulation, it seems more likely that the latter is due to an inhibitory interneurone in the IML interspersed between the 5HT terminal and the preganglionic neurone.

Notwithstanding this, direct excitatory actions of raphe stimulation (particularly raphe magnus) have been claimed (McCall, 1984). However, whether the observed excitatory effects were due to release of 5HT and its action on specific receptors on preganglionic neurones was not clearly established. McCall (1984) showed that stimulation at various sites in nucleus raphe magnus, pallidus and obscurus excited or inhibited activity in the inferior cardiac nerve of anaesthetised cats. The excitations were blocked by intravenous methysergide and by metergoline and very slightly potentiated by the 5HT uptake inhibitor chlorimipramine, whereas the inhibitions were unaffected by these drugs. Similarly an excitatory response elicited from stimulation of a lateral pressor area was unaffected by the drug treatment. This evidence again needs cautious interpretation since unfortunately no proof was provided that the raphe stimulus was exciting spinally projecting pathways. Even if it had been, the calculated conduction velocities of 3.3 m.s.$^{-1}$, a figure that contains a number of assumptions and approximations, still seems somewhat fast for small unmyelinated 5HT axons. The conduction velocities of axons of raphe spinal neurones reported by Wessendorf *et al.* (1981) and by Morrison & Gebber (1984) can be divided into three groups, those units conducting between 0.7 and 1.0 m.s.$^{-1}$, those conducting between 3.1 and 6.0 m.s.$^{-1}$ and those conducting between 6.1 and 3.2 m.s.$^{-1}$. Wessendorf *et al.* (1981) considered that the first two groups were serotonergic neurones since the number of units located for each electrode penetration was markedly reduced following, 5,7-dihydroxytryptamine. However, there were also marked reductions in units with considerably higher conduction velocities which might make suspect the specificity of the 5HT neurotoxin. An additional problem with the study by McCall (1984) was that the 5HT antagonists were administered intravenously, and therefore we have no way of knowing whether their ability to block the raphe-sympathetic responses wad due to an action at a 5HT excitatory synapse in the brainstem or in the spinal cord. If the interpretation by McCall (1984) proves to be correct, then it also suggests the possibility that some spinally projecting 5HT neurones synapse directly with sympathetic preganglionic neurones. Such evidence is clearly lacking at present. A properly designed histological study at the ultrastructural level with specific labelling of the 5HT terminals is very much needed.

### 9.2.6. *Functions of the 5HT pathways*

With regard to the functional role of the spinally projecting 5HT neurones, it is interesting to consider which particular aspects of the central control of sympathetic outflow this system is involved with. In a study by Coote *et al.* (1978) following a number of drug treatments to damage 5HT neurones no differences were observed in a number of sympatho-excitatory and inhibitory responses, neither was blood pressure changed. These authors concluded that the influence of the 5HT was masked by anaesthesia.

Subsequent experiments in unanaesthetised decerebrate cats indicate that spinally projecting 5HT neurones of the raphe obscurus are necessary for the inhibition of sympathetic activity that accompanies a paradoxical sleep-like state in these preparations (Coote *et al.*, 1985). Earlier Futuro-Neto & Coote (1982a) showed that during paradoxical sleep there is repatterning of sympathetic vasoconstrictor activity, that to most vascular beds being inhibited while that to skeletal muscle vascular bed was excited. This pattern could also be obtained from a restricted region of the nucleus raphe obscurus of cat (Futuro-Neto & Coote, 1982b) and rat (Coote & Yusof, 1985). The interesting question is whether the excitation of vasoconstrictor neurones to skeletal muscle is similarly dependent on spinally projecting 5HT neurones or on the non-5HT type of neurone found in the raphe nuclei.

The caudal raphe nuclei are not only anatomically but also functionally inhomogenous. Whereas, at many sites in raphe obscurus and in raphe pallidus, inhibition of activity in all sympathetic outflows was obtained, at some sites excitation of all sympathetic outflows was obtained although the extent to which this was dependent on spinally projecting neurones was not ascertained (Futuro-Neto & Coote, 1982b; Coote & Yusof, 1985). The significance of the profound sympatho-inhibitory influence that can be exerted by neurones in raphe pallidus remains to be determined, as does the functional influence of the dense projection to the IML of neurones in raphe magnus.

## References

Adair, J. R., Hamilton, B. L., Scappaticci, K. A., Helke, C. J. & Gillis, R. A. (1977). Cardiovascular responses to electrical stimulation of the medullary raphe area of the cat. *Brain Res.* **128**, 141–5.

Amendt, K., Czachurski, J., Dembowsky, K. & Seller, H. (1979). Bulbospinal projections to the intermediolateral cell column; a neuroanatomical study. *J. Auton. Nerv. Syst.* **1**, 103–17.

Anderson, E. G. & Shibuya, T. (1966). The effects of 5-hydroxytryptophan and L-tryptophan on spinal synaptic activity. *J. Pharmacol. Exp. Therap.* **153**, 352–60.

Andrade, R. & Aghajanian, G. K. (1982). Single cell activity in the noradrenergic $A_5$ region. Responses to drugs and peripheral manipulations of blood pressure. *Brain Res.* **242**, 125–35.

Baker, R. G. & Anderson, E. G. (1970). The effects of 1–3,4-dihydroxyphenylalamine on spinal reflex activity. *J. Pharmacol. Exp. Therap.* **173**, 212–23.

Basbaum, A. I. & Fields, H. L. (1979). The origin of descending pathways in the dorsolateral funiculus of the spinal cord of the cat and rat: further studies on the anatomy of pain modulation. *J. Comp. Neurol.* **187**, 513–32.

Blessing, W. W., Chalmers, J. P. & Howe, P. R. C. (1978). Distribution of catecholamine containing cell bodies in the rabbit central nervous system. *J. Comp. Neurol.* **179**, 407–24.

Blessing, W. W., Goodchild, A. K., Dampney, R. A. L. & Chalmers, J. P. (1981). Cell groups in the lower brainstem of the rabbit projecting to the spinal cord, with special reference to catecholamine-containing neurones. *Brain Res.* **221**, 35–55.

Bobillier, P., Sequin, S., Petitjean, F., Salvert, D., Touret, M. & Jouvet, M. (1976). The raphe nuclei of the cat brainstem: a topographic atlas of their afferent projections as revealed by autoradiography. *Brain Res.* **113**, 449–86.

Bowker, R. M., Westlund, K. N., Sullivan, M. C. & Coulter, J. D. (1982). Organisation of descending serotonin projections to the spinal cord. *Progr. Brain Res.* **57**, 239–65.

Broughton, R. (1972). Phylogenetic evolution of sleep systems. In *The Sleeping Brain. Perspectives in the Brain Sciences*, vol. 1, pp. 2–7 (ed. M. H. Chase). Brain

Information Service, Brain Research Institute, University of California, Los Angeles.

Cabot, J. B., Reiner, A. & Bogan, N. (1982). Avian bulbospinal pathways: anterograde and retrograde studies of cells of origin, funicular trajectories and laminar terminations. *Progr. Brain Res.* **57**, 79–108.

Cabot, J. B., Wild, J. M. & Cohen, D. H. (1979). Raphe inhibition of sympathetic preganglionic neurones. *Science* **203**, 184–6.

Caverson, M.M., Ciriello, J. & Calaresu, F. R. (1983). Cardiovascular afferent inputs to neurones in the ventrolateral medulla projecting to the central autonomic area of the thoracic cord in the cat. *Brain Res.* **274**, 354–8.

Coote, J. H., Fleetwood-Walker, S. M. & Mitchell, P. R. (1979). Catecholamine receptors in thoracic spinal cord. *Br. J. Pharmacol.* **68**, 137P.

Coote, J. H., Futuro-Neto, H. A. & Logan, S. D. (1985). The involvement of serotonin neurones in the inhibition of renal nerve activity during desynchronised sleep. *Brain Res.* **340**, 277–84.

Coote, J. H. & Macleod, V. H. (1974). The influence of bulbospinal monoaminergic pathways on sympathetic nerve activity. *J. Physiol.* **241**, 453–75.

Coote, J. H. & Macleod, V. H. (1975). The spinal route of sympatho-inhibitory pathways descending from the medulla oblongata. *Pflügers Arch.* **359**, 335–47.

Coote, J. H. & Macleod, V. H. (1977). The effect of intraspinal microinjections of 6-hydroxydopamine on the inhibitory influence exerted on spinal sympathetic activity by the baroreceptors. *Pflügers Arch.* **371**, 271–77.

Coote, J. H., Macleod, V. H., Fleetwood-Walker, S. M. & Gilbey, M. P. (1981a). The response of individual sympathetic preganglionic neurones to microiontophoretically applied endogenous monoamines. *Brain Res.* **215**, 135–45.

Coote, J. H., Macleod, V. H., Fleetwood-Walker, S. M. & Gilbey, M. P. (1981b). Baroreceptor inhibition of sympathetic activity at a spinal site. *Brain Res.* **220**, 81–93.

Coote, J. H., Macleod, V. H. & Martin, I. L. (1978). A search for the role of bulbospinal tryptaminergic neurones in the control of sympathetic activity. *Pflügers Arch.* **379**, 109–16.

Coote, J. H. & Yusof, A. P. (1985). The responses of vasoconstrictor neurones to skeletal muscle and kidney, to stimulation of the medullary raphe area of the rat. *J. Physiol.* **365**, 112P.

Dahlstrom, A. & Fuxe, K. (1964). Evidence for the existence of monoamine-containing neurones in the CNS. 1. Demonstration of monoamines in the cell bodies of brainstem neurones. *Acta Physiol. Scand.* **62**, Suppl. 232, 1–55.

Dahlstrom, A. & Fuxe, K. (1965). Evidence for the existence of monoamine-containing neurones in the CNS. II. Experimentally induced changes in the intraneuronal amine levels of bulbospinal neurone systems. *Acta Physiol. Scand.* **64**, Suppl. 247, 5–36.

Dashwood, M. R., Gilbey, M. P. & Spyer, K. M. (1985). The localisation of adrenoreceptors and opiate receptors in regions of the cat central nervous system involved in cardiovascular control. *Neuroscience* **15**, 537–51.

DeGroat, W. C. & Ryall, R. W. (1967). An excitatory action of 5-hydroxytryptamine on sympathetic preganglionic neurones. *Exptl Brain Res.* **3**, 299–303.

Dembowsky, K., Czachurski, J., Amendt, K. & Seller, H. (1980). Tonic descending inhibition of the spinal somato-sympathetic reflex from the lower brainstem. *J. Auton. Nerv. Syst.* **2**, 157–82.

Demirjian, C. R., Grossman, R., Meyer, R. & Katzman, R. (1976). The catecholamine pontine cellular groups locus coeruleus A4, sub coeruleus in the primate *Cebus apella. Brain Res.* **115**, 395–411.

Dube, L. & Parent, A. (1981). The monoamine-containing neurone in the avian brain: 1. A study of the brainstem of the chicken (*Gallus domesticus*) by means of fluorescence and acetylcholinesterase histochemistry. *J. Comp. Neurol.* **196**, 695–708.

Felten, D. P., Laities, A. M. & Carpenter, M. B. (1974). Monoamine-containing cell bodies in the squirrel monkey brain. *Am. J. Anat.* **139**, 153–66.

Fleetwood-Walker, S. M. & Coote, J. H. (1981). The contribution of brainstem catecholamine cell groups to the innervation of the sympathetic lateral cell column. *Brain Res.* **205**, 141–55.

Fleetwood-Walker, S. M., Coote, J. H. & Gilbey, M. P. (1983). Identification of spinally projecting neurones in the $A_1$ catecholamine cell group of the ventrolateral medulla. *Brain Res.* **273**, 25–33.

Fozard, J. R. (1984). Neuronal 5-HT receptors in the periphery. *Neuropharmacol.* **23**, 1473–86.

Franz, D. N., Hare, B. D. & Neumayr, R. J. (1975). Reciprocal control of sympathetic preganglionic neurones by monoaminergic bulbospinal pathways and a selective effect of clonidine. In *Recent Advances in Hypertension*, vol. 1, pp. 85–96 (eds P. Milliez and M. Safar). Ingelheim: Boehringer.

Franz, D. N., Hare, B. D. & Neumayr, R. J. (1978). Depression of sympathetic preganglionic neurones by clonidine: evidence for stimulation of 5-HT receptors. *Clin. Exp. Hypert.* **1**, 115–40.

Franz, D. N. Madsen, P. W., Peterson, R. G. & Sangdee, C. (1982). Functional roles of monoaminergic pathways to sympathetic proganglionic reurone. *Clin. Exp. Hypert.* **A4** (4 α 5), 543–62.

Futuro-Neto, H. A. & Coote, J. H. (1982a). Changes in sympathetic activity to heart and blood vessels during desynchronised sleep. *Brain Res.* **252**, 259–68.

Futuro-Neto, H. A. & Coote, J. H. (1982b). Desynchronised sleep-like pattern of sympathetic activity elicited by electrical stimulation of sites in the brainstem. *Brain Res.* **252**, 269–76.

Fuxe, K. & Jonsson, G. (1973). Further mapping of central 5-hydroxytryptamine neurones; studies with neurotoxin dihydroxytryptamine. *Adv. Biochem. Psychopharmacol.* **10**, 1–12.

Fuxe, K. & Ljunggren, L. (1965). Cellular localisation of monoamines in the upper brain stem of the pigeon. *J. Comp. Neurol.* **148**, 61–90.

Garver, D. L. & Sladek, J. R. (1975). Monoamine distribution in primate brain. 1. Catecholamine-containing perykarya in the brain stem of *Macaca speciosa*. *J. Comp. Neurol.* **159**, 289–304.

Gilbey, M. P., Coote, J. H., Macleod, V. H. & Peterson, D. F. (1981). Inhibition of sympathetic activity by stimulating in the raphe nuclei and the role of 5-hydroxytryptamine in this effect. *Brain Res.* **226**, 131–42.

Gillis, R. A., Helke, C. J., Hamilton, B. L. & Morgenroth, U. H. (1976). Cardiac arrhythmias produced by electrical stimulation of the mid brain raphe in the cat. *Neurosci. Abst.* **2**, 74.

Guyenet, P. G. (1980). The coeruleospinal noradrenergic neurones: anatomical and electrophysiological studies in the rat. *Brain Res.* **189**, 121–33.

Guyenet, P. G. & Cabot, J. B. (1981). Inhibition of sympathetic preganglionic neurones by catecholamines and clonidine: mediation by an α-adrenergic receptor. *J. Neurosci.* **1**, 908–17.

Guyenet, P. G. & Stornetta, R. L. (1982). Inhibition of sympathetic preganglionic discharges by epinephrine and α methyl epinephrine. *Brain Res.* **235**, 271–83.

Haeusler, G. (1977). Neuronal mechanisms influencing transmissions in the baroreceptor reflex arc. *Progr. Brain Res.* **47**, 95–109.

Haeusler, G. & Lewis, P. (1975). The baroreceptor reflex and its relation to central adrenergic mechanisms. In *Recent Advances in Hypertension*, vol. 2, pp. 17–26. (eds P. Milliez & M. Safar). Ingelheim: Boehringer.

Haigler, H. J. & Aghajanian, G. K. (1974). Lysergic acid diethylamide and serotonin. A comparison of effects on serotonin neurones and neurones receiving a serotonin input. *J. Pharmacol. Exp. Neurol.* **188**, 688–99.

Hare, B. D., Neumayr, R. J. & Franz, D. N. (1972). Opposite effects of L-dopa and 5-HTP on spinal sympathetic reflexes. *Nature, London* **239**, 336–7.

Hedreen, J. C. & McGrath, S. (1977). Observations of labelling of neuronal cell bodies, axons and terminals after injection of horseradish peroxidase into rat brain. *J. Comp. Neurol.* **176**, 225–46.

Helke, C. A., Neil, J. J., Massari, V. J. & Loewy, A. D. (1982). Substance P neurones project from the ventral medulla to the intermediolateral cell column and ventral horn in the rat. *Brain Res.* **243**, 147–52.

Heuser, J. E. & Reese, T. S. (1973). Evidence for recycling of synaptic vesicle membrane during transmitter release at the frog neuromuscular junction. *J. Cell. Biol.* **57**, 315–44.

Hokfelt, T., Fuxe, K., Goldstein, M. & Johansson, O. (1974). Immunohistochemical evidence for the existence of adrenaline neurones in the rat brain. *Brain Res.* **66**, 235–51.

Holstege, G. & Kuypers, H. G. J. M. (1982). The anatomy of brain stem pathways to the spinal cord in cat. A labelled amino acid tracing study. *Progr. Brain Res.* **57**, 145–75.

Howe, P. R. C., Costa, M., Furness, J. B. & Chalmers, J. P. (1980). Simultaneous demonstration of phenylethanolamine *N*-methyl transferase immunofluorescent and catecholamine fluorescent nerve cell bodies in the rat medulla oblongata. *Neuroscience* **5**, 2229–38.

Hubbard, J. E. & Di Carlo, V. (1974a). Fluorescence histochemistry of monoamine containing cell bodies in the brainstem of the squirrel monkey (*Siamiri sciureus*) II. Catecholamine-containing groups. *J. Comp. neurol.* **153**, 369–84.

Hubbard, J. E. & Di Carlo, V. (1974b). Fluorescence histochemistry of monoamine-containing cell bodies in the brainstem of the squirrel monkey (*Saimiri sciureus*) III. Serotonin containing groups. *J. Comp. Neurol.* **153**, 385–98.

Ikeda, H. & Gotah, J. (1971). Distribution of monoamine-containing cells in the central nervous system of the chicken. *Jpn. J. Pharmacol.* **21**, 763–84.

Illert, M. & Gabriel, M. (1970). Mapping the cord of the spinal cat for sympathetic and blood pressure responses. *Brain Res.* **23**, 274–6.

Illert, M. & Gabriel, M. (1972). Descending pathways in the cervical cord of cats affecting blood pressure and sympathetic activity. *Pflügers Arch.* **335**, 109–24.

Ishikawa, M., Shimada, S. & Tanaka, C. (1975). Histochemical mapping of catecholamine neurones and fiber pathways in the pontine tegmentum of the dog. *Brain Res.* **86**, 1–16.

Jones, E. G. (1975). Possible determinants of the degree of retrograde neuronal labelling with horseradish peroxidase. *Brain Res.* **85**, 249–54.

Kadzielawa, K. (1983a). Inhibition of the activity of sympathetic preganglionic neurones and neurones activated by visceral afferents by alpha-methyl noradrenaline and endogenous catecholamines. *Neuropharmacol.* **22**, 3–17.

Kadzielawa, K. (1983b). Antagonism of the excitatory effects of 5-hydroxytryptamine on sympathetic preganglionic neurones and neurones activated by visceral afferents. *Neuropharmacol.* **22**, 19–27.

Kirchner, F., Wyszogrodski, I. & Polosa, C. (1975). Some properties of sympathetic neurone inhibition by depressor area and intraspinal stimulation. *Pflügers Arch.* **357**, 349–60.

Konishi, M. (1968). Fluorescence microscopy of the spinal cord of the dog with special reference to the autonomic lateral horn cells. *Arch. Histol. Japan.* **30**, 33–44.

Kuhn, D. M., Wolf, W. A. & Lovenberg, W. (1980a). Pressor effects of electrical stimulation of the dorsal and median raphe nuclei in anaesthetised rats. *J. Pharmacol. Exp. Therap.* **214**, 403–9.

Kuhn, D. M., Wolf, W. A. & Lovenberg, W. (1980b). Review of the role of central serotonergic neuronal system in blood pressure regulation. *Hypertension* **2**, 243–55.

Kuypers, H. G. J. M. & Martin, G. F. (1982). Anatomy of descending pathways to the spinal cord. *Progr. Brain Res.* **57**, 1–411.

Lackner, K. J. (1980). Mapping of monoamine neurones and fibres in the cat lower brainstem and spinal cord. *Anat. Embryol.* **161**, 169–95.

Loewy, A. D. (1981). Raphe pallidus and raphe obscurus projections to the intermediolateral cell column in the rat. *Brain Res.* **222**, 129–33.

Loewy, A. D. & McKellar, S. (1981). Serotonergic projections from the ventral medulla to the intermediolateral cell column in the rat. *Brain Res.* **211**, 146–52.

Loewy, A. D., McKellar, S. & Saper, C. B. (1979). Direct projections from the A$_5$ catecholamine cell group to the intermediolateral cell column. *Brain Res.* **174**, 309–14.

Loewy, A. D. & Sawyer, W. B. (1982). Substance P antagonists inhibit vasomotor responses elicited from ventral medulla in rat. *Brain Res.* **245**, 379–83.

Loizou, L. A. (1972). The postnatal ontogeny of monoamine-containing neurones in the central nervous system of the albino rat. *Brain Res.* **40**, 395–418.

Lopachin, R. M. & Rudy, T. A. (1983). Sites and mechanism of action for the effects of intrathecal noradrenaline on thermoregulation in the rat. *J. Physiol.* **341**, 527–44.

McCall, R. B. (1983). Serotonergic excitation of sympathetic preganglionic neurones: a microiontophoretic study. *Brain Res.* **289**, 121–7.

McCall, R. B. (1984). Evidence for a serotonergically mediated sympatho-excitatory response to stimulation of medullary raphe nuclei. *Brain Res.* **311**, 131–9.

McKellar, S. & Loewy, A. D. (1982). Efferent projections of the A$_1$ catecholamine cell groups in the rat: an autoradiographic study. *Brain Res.* **241**, 11–29.

Martin, G. F., Cabana, T., DiTirro, F. J., Ho, R. H. & Humberston, A. O., (1982). Reticular and raphe projections to the spinal cord of the North American opossum. Evidence for connectional heterogeneity. *Progr. Brain Res.* **57**, 109–29.

Martin, G. F., Humberston, A. O., Laxson, C. & Panneton, W. M. (1979). Evidence for direct bulbospinal projections to laminae IX, X and the intermediolateral cell column. Studies using axonal transport techniques in the North American opossum. *Brain Res.* **170**, 165–71.

Morgane, P. J. & Stern, W. C. (1978). Serotonin in the regulation of sleep. In *Serotonin in Health and Disease, vol. 11. Physiological Regulation and Pharmacological Action.* pp. 205–45 (ed. B. W. Essman). New York: Spectrum.

Morrison, S. F. & Gebber, G. L. (1984). Raphe neurones with sympathetic-related activity: baroreceptor responses and spinal connections. *Am. J. Physiol.* **243**, R49–59.

Nauta, H. J. W., Pritz, M. B. & Lusek, R. J. (1974). Afferents to the rat caudoputamen studied with horseradish peroxidase. An evaluation of a retrograde neuronanatomical research method. *Brain Res.* **67**, 219–38.

Neumayr, J. J., Hare, B. D. & Franz, D. N. (1974). Evidence for bulbospinal control of sympathetic preganglionic neurones by monoaminergic pathways. *Life Science* **14**, 793–806.

Nobin, A. & Björkluand, A. (1973). Topography of monoamine systems in the human brain as revealed in fetuses. *Acta Physiol. Scand.* **88**, Suppl. 388, 1–40.

Nygren, O. G. & Olsen, L. (1977). Intracisternal neurotoxins and monoamine neurones innervating the spinal cord: acute and chronic effects on cell and axon counts and nerve terminal densities. *Histochemistry* **52**, 281–306.

Ohye, C., Bouchard, R., Boucher, R. & Poirier, L. J. (1970). Sponaneous activity of the putamen after chronic interruption of the dopaminergic pathway: effect of L-dopa. *J. Pharmacol. Exp. Therap.* **175**, 700–8.

Palkovits, M. & Jacobowitz, D. M. (1974). Topographical atlas of catecholamines and acetylcholinesterase-containing neurones in the rat brain. II. Hindbrain (mesencephalon, rhombencephalon). *J. Comp. Neurol.* **157**, 29–42.

Parent, A. (1973). Demonstration of a catecholamine pathway from the midbrain to the strio amygdaloid complex in the turtle (*Chrysemys picta*). *J. Anat (Lond.)* **114**, 379–87.

Parent, A. (1975). The monoaminergic innervation of the telencephalon of the frog, *Rana pipiens. Brain Res.* **99**, 35–47.

Parent, A. (1978). Monoaminergic systems of the brain. In *Biology of the Reptilia*, pp. 247–85. (ed. C. Gans) London: Academic Press.

Pin, C., Jones, B. & Jouvet, M. (1968). Topographie des neurones monoaminergiques du tronc cerebral du chat: étude par histofluorescence. *C. R. Soc. Biol. (Paris)* **162**, 21–36.

Poitras, D. & Parent, A. (1978). Atlas of the distribution of monoamine-containing nerve cell bodies in the brainstem of the cat. *J. Comp. Neurol.* **179**, 699–718.

Reid, J. L., Zivin, J. A., Foppen, F. & Kopin, I. J. (1975). Catecholamine neurotransmitters and synthetic enzymes in the rat spinal cord. *Life Sciences* **16**, 975–84.

Ross, C. A., Ruggiero, D. A., Joh, T. H., Park, D. H. & Reis, D. J. (1983). Adrenaline-synthesising neurones in the rostral ventrolateral medulla: a possible role in tonic vasomotor control. *Brain Res.* **273**, 356–61.

Saavedra, J. M., Brownstein, M. & Axelrod, J. (1973). A specific and sensitive enzymatic isotopic microscopy for serotonin in tissues. *J. Pharmacol. Exp. Therap.* **186**, 508–515.

Saavedra, J. M., Palkovits, M., Brownstein, M. & Axelrod, J. (1974). Serotonin distribution in the nuclei of the rat hypothalamus and preoptic region. *Brain Res.* **77**, 157–65.

Sangdee, C. & Franz, D. N. (1979). Enhancement of central norepinephrine and 5-hydroxytryptamine transmission by tricyclic antidepressants: a comparison. *Psychopharmacology* **62**, 9–16.

Satoh, K., Tohyama, M., Yamamoto, K., Sukumoto, T. & Shimizu, N. (1977). Noradrenaline innervation of the spinal cord studied by the horseradish peroxidase method combined with monoamine oxidase staining. *Exp. Brain Res.* **30**, 175–86.

Sinha, J. N., Atkinson, J. M. & Schmidt, H. (1973). Effects of clonidine and L-dopa on spontaneous and evoked splanchnic nerve discharges. *Eur. J. Pharmacol.* **24**, 113–19.

Smits, J. F. M., van Essen, H. & Struyker-Boudier, H. A. J. (1978). Serotonin mediated cardiovascular responses to electrical stimulation of the raphe nuclei in the rat. *Life Sciences* **23**, 173–8.

Smolen. A. J., Glazer, E. J. & Ross, L. L. (1979). Horseradish peroxidase histochemistry combined with glyoxylic acid induced fluorescence used to identify brainstem catecholaminergic neurones which project to the chick thoracic spinal cord. *Brain Res.* **160**, 358–7.

Steinbusch, H. W. M. (1981). Distribution of serotonin-immunoreactivity in the central nervous system of the rat — cell bodies and terminals. *Neuroscience* **6**, 557–618.

Takano, Y., Martin, J. E., Leeman, S. E. & Loewy, A. D. (1984). Substance P immunoreactivity released from rat spinal cord after kainic acid excitation of the ventral medulla oblongata: a correlation with increases in blood pressure. *Brain Res.* **291**, 168–72.

Tauber, E. S. (1974). Physiology of sleep. *Adv. Sleep Res.* **1**, 133–72.

Taylor, D. G. & Brody, M. J. (1976). Spinal adrenergic mechanisms regulating sympathetic outflow to blood vessles. *Circ. Res.* **38**, Suppl. 11, 10–20.

Unnerstall, J. R., Kopajtic, T. A. & Kuhar, M. J. (1984). Distribution of $\alpha_2$ agonist binding sites in the rat and human central nervous system: analysis of some functional anatomic correlates of the pharmacological effects of clonidine and related adrenergic agents. *Brain Res. Rev.* **7**, 69–101.

Van der Guyten, J., Palkovits, M., Wijnen, H. L. J. M. & Versteeg, D. H. G. (1976). The regional distribution of adrenaline in the rat brain. *Brain Res.* **107**, 171–5.

Wessendorf, M. V., Proudfit, H. K. & Anderson, E. G. (1981). The identification of serotonergic neurones in the nucleus raphe magnus by conduction velocity. *Brain Res.* **214**, 168–73.

Wessendorf, M. V. & Anderson, E. G. (1983). Single unit studies of identified bulbospinal serotonergic units. *Brain Res.* **279**, 93–103.

Westlund, K. N., Bowker, R. M., Ziegler, M. G. & Coulter, J. D. (1982). Descending noradrenergic projections and their spinal terminations in descending pathways to the spinal cord. *Progr. Brain Res.* **57**, 219–38.

Westlund, K. N., Bowker, R. M., Ziegler, M. G. & Coulter, J. D. (1983). Noradrenergic projections to the spinal cord of the rat. *Brain Res.* **203**, 15–32.

Wong, W. C. & Tan, C. K. (1974). Degeneration in the adult rat spinal cord following systemic treatment with 6-hydroxydopamine. Electron microscopic study. *Experientia* **30**, 1455–9.

Yen, C. T., Blum, P. S. & Spath, J. A. (1983). Control of cardiovascular function by electrical stimulation within the medullary-raphe region of the cat. *Exp. Neurol.* **79**, 666–79.

Zivin, J. A., Reid, J. L., Saavedra, J. M. & Kopin, I. J. (1975). Quantitative localisation of biogenic amines in the spinal cord. *Brain Res.* **99**, 293–301.

# 10

# Cardiovascular control from neurones in the ventrolateral medulla

**T. A. Lovick**

*Department of Physiology, The Medical School, Vincent Drive, University of Birmingham, Birmingham B15 2TJ, UK*

## 10.1. Introduction

For over a century it has been recognised that the brainstem plays a vital role in maintaining arterial blood pressure at its normal resting level. Even so, in his review of the anatomical organisation of that part of the central nervous system concerned with control of the heart and blood vessels, published in 1960, Bard (1960) was able to conclude only that the region that maintains the tonic drive to the sympathetic outflow lay somewhere in the medulla between the level of the caudal pons and the obex. In more recent years, rapid progress has been made towards localising and understanding the function and connections of the medullary neurones which provide the tonic sympatho-excitatory drive. The impetus for much of the latest work stems from the observation by Feldberg & Guertzenstein (1972) that blood pressure fell precipitously when sodium pentobarbitone was applied bilaterally to a restricted area on the ventral surface of the medulla. Guertzenstein & Silver (1974) later found that application of glycine to a similar region of the medullary surface was just as effective, and that bilateral electrolytic lesions of this so-called 'glycine-sensitive area' reduced arterial blood pressure to the level seen in the spinal animal. These latter findings have recently been confirmed by Dampney & Moon (1980) and by Lebedev *et al.* (1984b).

## 10.2. Nucleus paragigantocellularis lateralis (PGL) and cardiovascular control

The region of the ventral medullary surface where glycine exerted its hypotensive effect lay lateral to the pyramidal tract, caudal to the trapezoid body and rostral to the hypoglossal rootlets. As shown in Fig. 10.1, a number of fibre tracts run superficially through the ventral medulla at this site but there is also an area in the ventral part of nucleus paragigantocellularis lateralis (PGL) where neuronal perikarya lie in close proximity to the surface

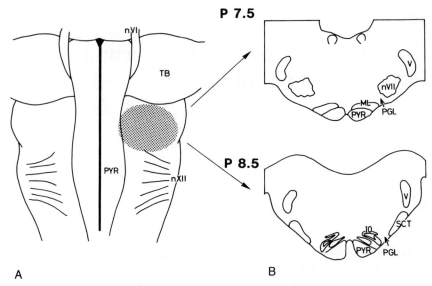

A                                                                B

Fig. 10.1. A. Schematic drawing of the ventral surface of the medulla of the cat to show the location of the 'glycine-sensitive area' (hatching). B. Outline drawings of transverse sections through the medulla at the level of the 'glycine-sensitive area'. Neuronal cell bodies lie in close proximity to the medullary surface in nucleus paragigantocellularis lateralis. Abbreviations: IO, inferior olive; ML, medial lemniscus; PGL, nucleus paragigantocellularis lateralis; PYR, pyramidal tract; SCT, spinocerebellar tract; TB, trapezoid body; nVII, facial nucleus; V, spinal trigeminal tract; nXII, hypoglossal nerve rootlets.

of the neuropil (Taber, 1961; Andrezik *et al.*, 1981a). These cells are obviously readily accessible to most substances diffusing from the medullary surface, and in recent years a number of compounds have been shown to produce cardiovascular changes when applied directly to the neuropil which underlies the nucleus. For example, topical application of the excitotoxic agent kainic acid or the GABA antagonist bicuculline has been reported to evoke pressor responses (Loewy & Sawyer, 1982; McAllen *et al.*, 1982; Yamada *et al.*, 1982, 1984), and the inhibitory amino acids GABA and glycine produced hypotension (Hilton *et al.*, 1983; Keeler *et al.*, 1984), presumably due to suppression of ongoing sympatho-excitatory drive. More detailed interpretation of such findings as these is limited because of the inability to localise the precise site of action of drugs when applied topically to the medullary surface. This problem can largely be overcome by making microinjections of small, nanomolar quantities of D, L-homocysteic acid or sodium glutamate, which selectively stimulate cell bodies but not fibres of passage (Goodchild *et al.*, 1982). By using this technique it has been possible to localise a group of neurones in the ventrolateral medulla of the cat which can initiate cardiovascular responses, and a functional nucleus has now been defined which lies immediately lateral to the pyramidal tract and medial lemniscus and extends from the level of the caudal third of the facial nucleus to the level of the most rostral hypoglossal rootlets (Fig. 10.2). This region corresponds closely to nucleus paragigantocellularis lateralis (PGL) as described by Taber (1961). A similarly located pressor area has also been described in the rabbit and rat (Dampney *et al.*, 1982; Howe *et al.*, 1983; Ross *et al.*, 1984b). Dampney *et al.* (1984) concluded that the rise in blood pressure was due to an undifferentiated, generalised increase in sympathetic activity. However, more recent evidence suggests that the nucleus is not functionally homogeneous since it appears to contain distinct but overlapping subpopulations of neurones which are dedicated to controlling different components of the sympathetic outflow.

## 10.3. Functional specitivity of neurones within PGL

In these experiments regional blood flow to the renal, splanchnic and hindlimb muscle vascular beds was measured while recording changes in systemic arterial pressure and heart rate. Activation of groups of neurones in PGL in the cat, by microinjection of D, L-homocysteic acid, showed that the relative contribution from each vascular bed to a given rise in peripheral resistance was not uniform throughout the nucleus (Lovick, 1985a, and unpublished observations; Lovick & Hilton, 1985a, b). Excitation of neurones in the caudal part of PGL caused different degrees of constriction in the splanchnic, renal and hindlimb muscle beds so they would have contributed to a varying extent to the resulting increase in peripheral resistance and hence to the pressor response. In contrast, activation of more rostrally located neurones, superficial to the caudal part of the facial nucleus, usually produced vasodilatation in the hindlimb muscles and constriction of the renal and splanchnic beds, particularly the former. Indeed, at many sites the magnitude of the muscle dilatation was sufficient to counterbalance the increase in vascular resistance in the other beds so that there was little net change in systemic arterial pressure. The dilatation was found to be resistant to atropine, thus excluding an involvement of sympathetic cholinergic dilator fibres. However, it was greatly reduced, although not completely abolished, by intravenous administration of β-blocking agents, and is probably mediated in part by circulating catecholamines released from the adrenal medulla. Indeed, Ross *et al.* (1984b) and McAllen *et al.* (1985) have demonstrated large increases in plasma catecholamine levels following activation of neurones in the pressor area of the ventrolateral medulla in the rat and cat.

Differential effects on heart rate were observed to accompany the pressor response produced by stimulating neurones in PGL. Bradycardia was the predominant response (Fig. 10.2) although an increase in heart rate could be evoked by activating neurones in the rostral part of PGL (Fig. 10.2). The

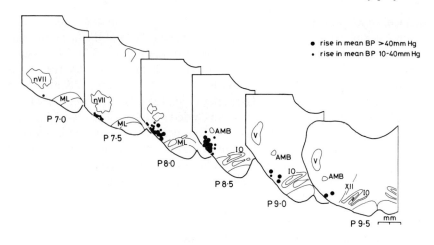

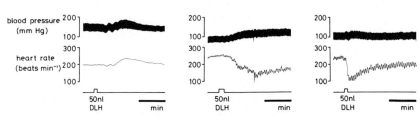

Fig. 10.2. Upper part of the diagram shows the location of sites in the ventrolateral medulla where microinjection of D, L-homocysteic acid (DLH) produced pressor responses. Lower part of the diagram shows examples of changes in blood pressure and heart rate evoked by microinjection of 50 nl 0.2 M DLH at three different sites within the pressor area. Abbreviations: AMB, nucleus ambiguus; IO, inferior olive; ML, medial lemniscus; nVII, facial nucleus; V, spinal trigeminal tract; XII, hypoglossal nerve rootlets.

tachycardia was seen more clearly after cholinergic blockade or vagotomy. Vagal cardiomotor neurones are known to be mainly localised to the region ventrolateral to and within nucleus ambiguus (Sugimoto *et al.*, 1979; Miura and Okada, 1981) and therefore the bradycardia was probably due to direct excitation of these motoneurones (see Fig. 10.2). On the other hand, the tachycardia was likely to result from stimulation of neurones that project to the cardioacceleratory portion of the intermediolateral cell column. Such neurones are known to lie rostrally in PGL at the level of the caudal pole of the facial nucleus (Miura *et al.*, 1983). It is interesting that in the rat, in which there is very little vagal tone, the pressor responses evoked by stimulating neurones in the ventrolateral medulla were usually accompanied by tachycardia (Howe *et al.*, 1983; Ross *et al.*, 1984b; Lovick, 1985b), although bradycardia of vagal origin was sometimes seen.

These studies clearly demonstrate that there are neurones within PGL that can produce cardiac or differentiated vasomotor effects and so may be properly considered as cardiovascular control neurones. The pattern of cardiovascular changes which is evoked by microinjection of excitant amino acids into PGL will thus depend both on the relative numbers and on the degree of activation of the functionally different neurones within the nucleus which have been stimulated.

## 10.4. Descending projections from PGL

Neuroanatomical studies have shown that cells in PGL project almost exclusively to the intermediolateral and intermediomedial cell columns in the spinal cord (Amendt *et al.*, 1979; Loewy *et al.*, 1981; Martin *et al.*, 1981; Miura *et al.*, 1983; Ross *et al.*, 1984a). Most of the descending axons appear to run bilaterally in the dorsolateral funiculus although labelled fibres have also been found in the ventrolateral white matter (Martin *et al.*, 1981; Loewy *et al.*, 1981). Estimations of conduction velocity in the spinally projecting axons, calculated from the latency of antidromic spikes evoked by stimulating the spinal cord at a known distance from the recording site in PGL, suggest that there is a heterogeneous population of neurones in PGL with axonal conduction velocities that range from 0.4 to 61 ms$^{-1}$ (Lebedev *et al.*, 1984a; Brown & Guyenet, 1985; Lovick, 1985a; McAllen, 1985). Only those cells with conduction velocities below 8 ms$^{-1}$ are likely to be involved in sympatho-excitation (Satoh & Schmidt, 1973; Krasiukov *et al.*, 1981; Coote & Macleod, 1984; Lebedev *et al.*, 1984a, b). Nevertheless, this group of ventrolateral medullary neurones appears to provide a major source of descending tonic excitatory drive to sympathetic preganglionic vasomotor neurones, and may also be able to initiate phasic changes in sympathetic activity. There is also the possibility that some of these neurones exert inhibitory actions at the spinal level on preganglionic vasoconstrictor neurones to muscle, either directly or via an interneurone, and produce vasodilatation by reducing tonic vasoconstrictor nerve activity (Fig. 10.3).

## 10.5. Afferent input to PGL

Afferents to PGL arise from a number of structures that are known to play a role in cardiovascular control, viz. the medial division of nucleus tractus solitarius, the parabrachial complex, periaqueductal grey matter and the dorsomedial and lateral parts of the hypothalamus (Andrezik *et al.*, 1981b; Dampney *et al.*, 1982; Li & Lovick, 1985; Lovick, 1985c). Electrophysiological studies have demonstrated that many of the connections from the periaqueductal grey matter and hypothalamus are excitatory and converge on the same neurones in PGL, including those that project to the spinal cord (Hilton & Smith, 1984; Lovick *et al.*, 1984; Brown & Guyenet, 1985; Li &

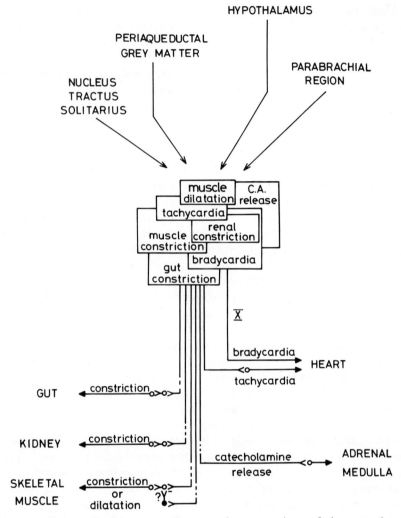

Fig. 10.3  Schematic diagram to illustrate the connections of the ventrolateral medullary sympathoexcitatory cell group. Distinct but overlapping neuronal pools within the area control the level of activity of sympathetic preganglionic neurones which in turn modify the activity of postganglionic fibres supplying the splanchnic, renal and muscle vasculature, the heart and adrenal medulla.

Lovick, 1985). Many neurones in PGL, including those with spinally projecting axons, show rhythmic activity which is time locked to the ECG (Brown & Guyenet, 1985). These cells were also inhibited when blood pressure was raised by intravenous injection of noradrenaline or by aortic occlusion. However, both their pulse-synchronous rhythmicity and their sensitivity to the level of arterial pressure were markedly attenuated after denervation of the baroreceptors (Brown & Guyenet, 1984, 1985). These findings are supported by the observation that the activity of spinally projecting neurones in the ventrolateral medulla could be inhibited during increased baroreceptor input produced by raising the pressure in a carotid sinus 'blind sac' preparation (McAllen, 1985). Baroreceptor afferents are thought to terminate in the medial division of the nucleus tractus solitarius (Berger, 1979), and so increased baroreceptor drive appears to excite an inhibitory projection from the medial solitary nucleus to neurones in PGL.

## 10.6. **PGL and integration of cardiovascular reflexes**

Several groups of workers have shown that the cardiovascular responses to baroreceptor, midbrain and hypothalamic stimulation can be attenuated following inhibition of synaptic activity in PGL by topical application of glycine, GABA or neurotoxic agents to the neuropil superficial to these neurones (McAllen *et al.*, 1982; Hilton *et al.*, 1983; Yamada *et al.*, 1984). At the same time the resting level of arterial pressure fell, showing that an essential tonic drive to the spinal sympathetic outflow had been removed. It seems unlikely that this drive depends to any great extent on the afferent input to PGL from the diencephalon, at least in anaesthetised animals, as resting blood pressure is little changed after complete midpontine transection which would deprive the medulla of all inputs from higher levels (Alexander, 1946; T. A. Lovick, unpublished experiments). On the other hand, removal of any source of input derived from the baroreceptor drive could only serve to increase the activity of the ventrolateral medullary neurones, by removal of an inhibitory input (Brown & Guyenet, 1984, 1985; McAllen, 1985).

It is possible that the ventrolateral medullary sympatho-excitatory neurones display intrinsic ongoing activity which is responsible for maintaining a tonic excitatory drive to the spinal sympathetic outflow. When the neuraxis is intact, their resting discharge rate is undoubtedly biased by inputs originating from a number of sources. Inputs derived from baroreceptor afferents via a relay in nucleus tractus solitarius appear to exert a strong inhibitory infuence, while phasic inputs from the periaqueductal grey matter and the dorsomedial and lateral regions of the hypothalamus provide excitatory drive. The nature of the afferent input that arises from the parabrachial region has yet to be investigated, as have possible direct or indirect influences from other systems involved in generating distinctive patterns of cardiovascular change such as those that occur during exercise, temperature regulation or sleep.

Neurones in nucleus paragigantocellularis lateralis constitute one of the most important sources of sympatho-excitatory drive to originate from the medulla. Fine adjustments to the pattern of efferent discharge in the neuronal pools within this nucleus that control the level of activity in individual sympathetic outflows could be initiated by changes in the level of activity in one or more sources of afferent inputs to the nucleus. Differential changes in heart rate, regional vascular resistance and circulating catecholamine levels would then be produced sufficient to generate patterns of cardiovascular response appropriate to the moment-to-moment needs of the organism.

## References

Alexander, R. S. (1946). Tonic and reflex functions of medullary sympathetic cardiovascular centers. *J. Neurophysiol.* **8**, 205–17.

Amendt, K., Czachurski, J., Dembowsky, K. & Seller, H. (1979). Bulbospinal projections to the intermediolateral cell column: a neuroanatomical study, *J. Auton. Nerv. Syst.* **1**, 103–17.

Andrezik, J. A., Chan-Palay, V. & Palay, S. L. (1981a). The nucleus paragigantocellularis lateralis in the rat. Conformation and cytology. *Anat. Embryol.* **161**, 355–71.

Andrezik, J. A., Chan-Palay, V. & Palay, S. L. (1981b). The nucleus paragigantocellularis lateralis in the rat. Demonstration of afferents by retrograde transport of horseradish peroxidase. *Anat. Embryol.* **161**, 373–90.

Bard, P. (1960). Anatomical organisation of the central nervous system in relation to control of the heart and blood vessels. *Physiol. Rev.* **40**, Suppl. 4, 3–26.

Berger, A. J. (1979). Distribution of carotid sinus nerve afferent fibres to solitary tract nuclei of the cat using transganglionic transport of horseradish peroxidase. *Neurosci. Lett.* **14**, 153–8.

Brown, D. L. & Guyenet, P. (1984). Cardiovascular neurons of brain stem with projections to spinal cord. *Am. J. Physiol.* **247**, R1009–16.

Brown, D. L. & Guyenet, P. (1985). Electrophysiological study of cardiovascular neurons in the rostral ventrolateral medulla in rats. *Circ. Res.* **56**, 359–69.

Coote, J. H. & Macleod, V. H. (1984). Estimation of conduction velocity in bulbospinal excitatory pathways to sympathetic outflows in cat spinal cord. *Brain Res.* **311**, 99–107.

Dampney, R. A. L. & Moon, E. A. (1980). Role of ventrolateral medulla in vasomotor response to cerebral ischemia. *Am. J. Physiol.* **239**, H349–58.

Dampney, R. A. L., Goodchild, A. K., Robertson, L. G. & Montgomery, W. (1982). Role of the ventrolateral medulla vasomotor regulation: a correlative anatomical and physiological study. *Brain Res.* **249**, 223–35.

Dampney, R. A. L., Goodchild, A. K. & Tan, E. (1984). Identification of cardiovascular cell groups in the brainstem. *Clin. Exp. Hypert.* **A6**, 205–20.

Feldberg, W. & Guertzenstein, P. G. (1972). A vasodepressor effect of pentobarbitone sodium. *J. Physiol.* (*Lond.*) **224**, 83–103.

Goodchild, A. K., Dampney, R. A. L. & Bandler, R. (1982). A method for evoking physiological responses by stimulation of cell bodies, but not axons of passage, within localized regions of the central nervous system. *Neurosci. Methods* **6**, 351–64.

Guertzenstein, P. G. & Silver, A. (1974). Fall in blood pressure produced from discrete regions of the ventral surface of the medulla by glycine and lesions. *J. Physiol.* (*Lond.*) **242**, 489–503.

Hilton, S. M. Marshall, J. M. & Timms, R. J. (1983). Ventral medullary relay neurones in the pathway from the defence areas of the cat and their effect on blood pressure. *J. Physiol.* (*Lond.*) **345**, 149–66.

Hilton, S. M. & Smith, P. R. (1984). Ventral medullary neurones excited from hypothalamic and midbrain defence area. *J. Auton. Nerv. Syst.* **11**, 35–42.

Howe, P. R. C., Kuhn, D. M., Minson, J. B., Stead, B. H. & Chalmers, P. (1983). Evidence for a bulbospinal serotonergic pressor pathway in the rat brain. *Brain Res.* **270**, 29–36.

Keeler, J. R., Shults, C. W., Chase, T. N. & Helke, C. J. (1984). The ventral surface of the medulla in the rat: pharmacological and autoradiographic localisation of GABA-induced cardiovascular effects. *Brain Res.* **297**, 217–24.

Krasiukov, A. V., Lebedev, V. P. & Nikitin, S. A. (1981). White rami responses to stimulation of the ventral surface of the medulla. *Fiziol. Zh. USSR* **6**, 1057–66.

Lebedev, V. P., Krasiukov, A. V. & Nikitin, S. A. (1984a). Neuronal organization of the sympathoactivating structures of the bulbar ventrolateral surface. *Fiziol. Zh. USSR* **70**, 761–72.

Lebedev, V. P., Krasiukov, A. V. & Nikitin, S. A. (1984b). The role of sympatho-activating structures of the bulbar ventrolateral surface in vasomotor regulation. *Fiziol. Zh. USSR* **70**, 1221–32.

Li, P. & Lovick, T. A. (1985). Excitatory projections from hypothalamic and midbrain defence areas to nucleus paragigantocellularis lateralis in the rat. *Exp. Neurol.* **89**, 543–53.

Loewy, A. D. & Sawyer, W. B. (1982). Substance P antagonists inhibit vasomotor responses elicited from ventral medulla in rat. *Brain Res.* **245**, 379–83.

Loewy, A. D., Wallach, J. H. & McKellar, S. (1981). Efferent connections of the ventral medulla oblongata in the rat. *Brain Res. Rev.* **3**, 63–80.

Lovick, T. A. (1985a). Descending projections from the ventrolateral medulla and cardiovascular control. *Pflügers Arch.* **404**, 197–202.

Lovick, T. A. (1985b). Cardiovascular and antinociceptive responses to stimulating neurones in the ventrolateral medulla. *Neurosci. Lett. Suppl.* **21**, 558.

Lovick, T. A. (1985c). Projections from the diencephalon and mesencephalon to nucleus paragigantocellularis lateralis in the cat. *Neuroscience* **14**, 853–61.

Lovick, T. A. & Hilton, S. M. (1985). Vasodilator and vasoconstrictor neurones in the ventrolateral medulla in the cat. *Brain Res.* **331**, 353–7.

Lovick, T. A. & Hilton, S. M. (1986). Cardiovascular neurones in the ventrolateral medulla. *J. Auton. Nerv. Syst. Suppl.* 121–4.

Lovick, T. A., Smith, P. R. & Hilton, S. M. (1984). Spinally projecting neurones near the ventral surface of the medulla in the cat. *J. Auton. Nerv. Syst.* **11**, 27–33.

McAllen, R. M. (1985). Bulbospinal neurones of the 'glycine-sensitive' area in the cat. *J. Physiol.* **361**, 48P.

McAllen, R. M., Killpatrick, I. C., Jones, M. W. & Woollard, S. (1985). Adrenal catecholamine release following chemical activation of ventrolateral brainstem neurones in cats. *Neurosci. Lett. Suppl.* **21**, 557.

McAllen, R. M., Neil, J. J. & Loewy, A. D. (1982). Effects of kainic acid applied to the ventral surface of the medulla oblongata on vasomotor tone, the baroreceptor reflex and hypothalamic autonomic responses. *Brain Res.* **238**, 65–76.

Martin, G. F., Cabana, T., Humbertson, A. O., Laxson, L. C. & Panneton, W. M. (1981). Spinal projections from the medullary reticular formation of the North American opossum: evidence for connectional heterogeneity. *J. Comp. Neurol.* **196**, 663–82.

Miura, M. & Okada, J. (1981). Cardiac and non-cardiac preganglionic neurons of the thoracic vagus nerve: an HRP study in the cat. *Jap. J. Physiol.* **31**, 53–66.

Miura, M., Onai, T. & Takayama, K. (1983). Projections of upper structure to the spinal cardioacceleratory center in cats: an HRP study using a new microinjection method. *J. Auton. Nerv. Syst.*, **7**, 119–39.

Ross, C. A., Ruggiero, D. A., Joh, T. H., Park, D. H. & Reis, D. J. (1984a). Rostral ventrolateral medulla: selective projections to the thoracic autonomic cell column from the region containing $C_1$ adrenaline neurons. *J. Comp. Neurol.* **228**, 168–85.

Ross, C. A., Ruggiero, D. A., Park, D., Joh, A., Sved, A. F., Fernandez-Pardal, J., Saavedra, J. M. & Reis, D. J. (1984b). Tonic vasomotor control by the rostral ventrolateral medulla: effect of electrical and chemical stimulation of the area containing $C_1$ adrenaline neurons on arterial pressure, heart rate and plasma catecholamines and vasopressin. *J. Neurosci.* **4**, 474–94.

Satoh, A. & Schmidt, R. F. (1973). Somatosympathetic reflexes: afferent fibers, central pathways, discharge characteristics. *Physiol. Rev.* **53**, 916–47.

Sugimoto, T., Itoh, K., Mizuna, N., Nomura, S. & Konishi, A. (1979). The site of origin of cardiac preganglionic fibers in the vagus nerve: an HRP study in the cat. *Neurosci. Lett.* **12**, 53–8.

Taber, E. (1961). The cytoarchitecture of the brain stem of the cat — I. Brain stem nuclei of cat. *J. Comp. Neurol.* **116**, 27–70.

Yamada, K. A., McAllen, R. M. & Loewy, A. D. (1984). GABA antagonists applied to the ventral surface of the medulla oblongata block the baroreceptor reflex. *Brain Res.* **297**, 175–80.

Yamada, K. A., Norman, W. P., Hamosh, P. & Gillis, R. A. (1982). Medullary ventral surface GABA receptors affect respiratory and cardiovascular function. *Brain. Res.* **248**, 71–8.

# 11

# The function of atrial receptors

**R. J. Linden**

*Department of Cardiovascular Studies, University of Leeds, Leeds LS9 2JT, UK*

## 11.1. Introduction

The left and right atria are small chambers of the heart which act as booster pumps to the ventricles. In the walls of the atria are to be found three groups of receptors, two discharging into afferent nerves in the vagi and one into the sympathetic nerves.

Only the functions of one type, the so-called Paintal-type atrial receptors discharging into myelinated fibres in the vagi, will be described here; the functions of the other two, one discharging into non-myelinated fibres in the vagi and the other into sympathetic nerves, are unknown.

## 11.2. The receptors

The Paintal-type atrial receptors are unencapsulated and have been the subject of histological investigation since last century (Berkley, 1895); a review of this subject and subsequent work including the electron microscopy of Tranum-Jensen (1979) has been published recently (Linden & Kappagoda, 1982). The receptors are to be found in the atrial endocardium which is the most profusely innervated area of the heart.

These complex unencapsulated sensory endings have been found mainly at the junctions of the superior and inferior vena cava and the right atrium and of the pulmonary veins and left atrium, as described by Nonidez (1937). Only one study (Coleridge *et al.*, 1957) has defined the position of the receptors physiologically and then gone on to examine histologically the tissue beneath the surface of the endocardium to which a point stimulus had been applied using a fine glass probe; complex unencapsulated nerve endings were always observed in the stimulated areas.

Coleridge *et al.* (1964), in a careful study in the manner of Coleridge *et al.* (1957), confirmed that the atrial receptors discharging into myelinated fibres, Paintal-type atrial receptors, were mainly situated at the atrio-venous

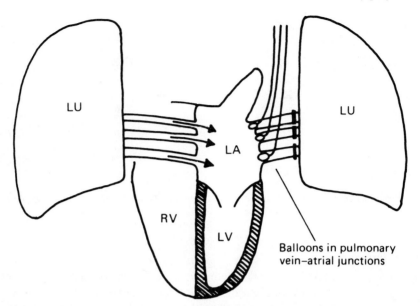

Fig. 11.1.  Diagram of preparation used to stimulate left atrial receptors. LA, left atrium; LU, lung; RV and LV, right and left ventricles. Diagram illustrates left lung root tied off, small balloons at pulmonary vein–atrial junctions and total venous return passing through right lung. Therefore it is possible to distend balloons and stretch junctions without altering flow through the heart or atrial pressure. (From Linden, 1976.)

junctions. All the receptors were within the pericardial sac, and the receptors from the right and left atrium discharged into both vagi. It was also apparent that receptors from the right atrium discharged mainly into the right vagus, and of the receptors in the left atrium there was a preponderance of fibres in the right vagus from those receptors found on the right side of the left atrium.

## 11.3.  Reflex effects

Ledsome & Linden (1964) devised a method of stretching the left pulmonary vein–atrial junctions in a manner which did not interfere with the rest of the circulation (Fig. 11.1). Small latex balloons attached to fine nylon tubing were inserted in the left pulmonary veins and advanced to the pulmonary vein–atrial junctions. The balloons were secured in position and the left lung was ligated. Subsequent distension of the balloons with warm saline (1 ml in each) caused them to attain the shape of a sphere about 0.8 cm in diameter, stretched the vein–atrial junctions, activated the receptors and did not change atrial pressure or interfere with blood flow from the lung through the atrium to the left ventricle.

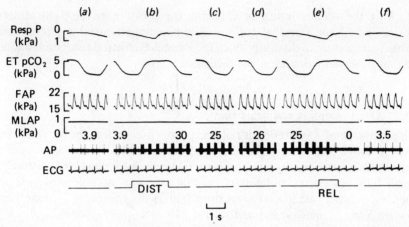

Fig. 11.2. Parts of continuous experimental record showing the effects of distending a small balloon with 1 cm$^3$ saline for 30 min, at the left upper pulmonary vein–atrial junction, on the discharge from a type B atrial receptor. From above downwards, tracheal pressure (Resp P), end-tidal $pCO_2$ (ET $pCO_2$), femoral arterial pressure (FAP), mean left atrial pressure (MLAP), action potentials (AP), electrocardiogram (ECG) and event marker. Changes in event marker signal the distension (DIST) and release of distension (REL) of the balloon. Records were obtained during control (a), and distension (b), 10 (c), 20 (d) and 30 (e) min after distension, final control (f). The numbers above the records of action potentials are mean frequencies (spikes s$^{-1}$). (From Linden & Kappagoda, 1982.)

## 11.4. Atrial receptors and action potentials

Using the technique described briefly above and fully by Ledsome & Linden (1964) it was found that the endings most likely to be stimulated by distension of the small balloons at the pulmonary vein–atrial junctions were the Paintal-type unencapsulated endings (Kidd *et al.*, 1978a); an illustration of the effect of distending the balloons on action potentials in vagal nerves is shown in Fig. 11.2. It can be seen that the distension causes an increase in the number and frequency of the action potentials in each train of impulses which is pulsatile in time with the heart beat and mostly with the 'v' wave of the atrial pressure pulse; it is typical of type B discharge of Paintal-type atrial receptors when subjected to an increased left atrial pressure brought about by infusion. Thus, even though the stimulus is unphysiological, the second-order neurones in the medulla are receiving an increased stimulus in a manner within the physiological range. The increased discharge is observed as long as the stimulus is applied, in this instance for 30 min.

A separate, but similar, technique was used for stimulating the right atrial receptors. A special cannula (Kappagoda *et al.*, 1972a) was created which could be inserted into the external jugular vein of anaesthetised dogs to enable the superior vena caval–right atrial junction to be distended without blocking the venous return or changing the pressure in the right atrium. Distension of the terminal balloon stimulated right atrial receptors and caused an increase in discharge from the Paintal-type atrial receptors, similar to that observed from left atrial receptors.

## 11.5. **Atrial receptors and heart rate**

The methods of stimulating atrial receptors enumerated above were then used to evoke responses in the heart and in the kidney. In the heart a reflex increase in heart rate only was observed. Ledsome & Linden (1964) distended small balloons in the pulmonary vein–atrial junctions and observed an increase in heart rate in every experiment; in 78 distensions in 24 dogs there was an average increase in heart rate of 24 beats $min^{-1}$ (range: 2–89).

Atrial receptors were also discovered in the atrial appendages (Floyd *et al.*, 1972), and another small balloon was placed in the left atrial appendage in addition to the one in the upper pulmonary vein and the one in the middle pulmonary vein; distension of these balloons in order, distending first one, then two, then three, showed increasing responses of an increase in heart rate. Each response was statistically different from the other, demonstrating recruitment of receptor endings from the three areas (Kappagoda *et al.*, 1975).

Stimulating the atrial receptors in the right atrium following the special technique described above, Kappagoda *et al.* (1972a) observed during 65 distensions in 16 dogs that there was an increase in heart rate of 18 beats $min^{-1}$ (mean; range 5–73). There was no relationship between the small changes in arterial pressure and the superior vena caval pressure and the changes in heart rate; also the small changes in right atrial pressure and left atrial pressure were not related to the changes in heart rate (Kappagoda *et al.*, 1972b).

From all our experiments it has been observed that, during 23 investigations reported in 14 publications, 811 distensions of discrete areas of the atria in 251 dogs resulted always in an increase in heart rate, the mean increase being 19 beats $min^{-1}$ (range of means: 10–35) (Linden & Kappagoda, 1982).

## 11.6. **Afferent pathway of the reflex**

Section or cooling of the vagi in the chest and neck has always reduced or abolished the response. Recently, by grading the cooling of the vagi in steps of 2°C, it has been shown that the heart rate responses begin to decrease at about 18°C and are abolished between 12°C and 10°C. It was also shown that the *increase* in discharge from Paintal-type atrial receptors, observed as an increase in frequency and number in trains of impulses in myelinated fibres in the vagi, also followed a similar decremental pattern during this cooling technique. This positive correlation allowed the hypothesis that Paintal-type atrial receptors discharging into myelinated fibres were responsible for the increase in heart rate. Further evidence supporting this hypothesis was obtained by distending the balloons and observing the response in non-myelinated fibres during stepwise cooling of the vagi. In the event, the increase in number and frequency of impulses in non-myelinated fibres did not decrement until the temperature was below 8°C, allowing the conclusion that non-myelinated fibres were not involved in this reflex response. A full account of these results is given by Kappagoda *et al.* (1979).

Coupled with the numerous reports that cutting the vagi or cooling the vagi to 5°C abolishes the response of an increase in heart rate, it may be concluded that 'sympathetic' afferent nerves are also not involved in this reflex response. The afferent limb of the reflex is then solely in the myelinated fibres of the vagi.

### 11.7. Efferent limb of the reflex

Section of the right and left ansae subclavae (which contain all the sympathetic efferent nerves to the heart in the dog) and the use of sympathetic blocking drugs (propranolol; bretylium tosylate) showed that the efferent limb was solely in the efferent sympathetic nerves to the heart (Linden & Kappagoda, 1982). Surprisingly there was no positive inotropic responses accompanying the increase in heart rate. In a further investigation involving the stimulation of left atrial receptors Furnival *et al.* (1971) used a known sensitive index of inotropic responses, i.e. the maximal rate of rise of pressure in the left ventricle ($dP/dt$ max) which had previously been shown to be an adequate index under the circumstances of this investigation (Furnival *et al.*, 1970). Though stimulation of left atrial receptors resulted in an increase in heart rate of up to 90 beats $min^{-1}$, there was no significant concomitant change in $dP/dt$ max. It was concluded that activity in this discrete efferent pathway does not include an inotropic effect on the left ventricle, and therefore the reflex involved only those sympathetic nerves that innervate the sinu-atrial node.

The activity in efferent cardiac nerves to the sinu-atrial node, in response to stimulation of left atrial receptors, was studied by Linden *et al.* (1982). Recording action potentials in single sympathetic efferent fibres, an increased activity was observed in 17 single efferent fibres in 11 dogs during distension of the small balloons. No changes in these fibres were observed during stimulation of arterial baroreceptors over their full range of pressures, or during stimulation of chemoreceptors or peripheral cutaneous nerves. It was concluded that the efferent cardiac sympathetic nerves of the atrial receptor reflex constituted a group of fibres separate from those responding to the stimulation of receptors in other regions.

## 11.8. **Atrial receptors and urine flow**

Karim *et al.* (1972) recorded action potentials in efferent sympathetic nerves and stimulated atrial receptors by distending small balloons at the pulmonary vein–atrial junctions. As well as showing that stimulating atrial receptors caused an increase in trains of impulses in sympathetic nerves to the heart, as was expected, they showed no changes in abdominal or peripheral efferent sympathetic nerves, but, totally unexpectedly, a *decrease* in activity in sympathetic nerves to the kidney. This inhibition of sympathetic activity to the kidney has been shown, by the differential cooling techniques described above, not to be a result of increased activity in non-myelinated fibres in the vagi, but, again, solely to be caused by Paintal-type atrial receptors discharging into myelinated fibres; again 'sympathetic afferent' fibres were not involved (Linden *et al.*, 1980).

The sympathetic efferent fibres to the kidney, in contrast to those to the sinu-atrial node (see above), did not comprise a separate bundle; single efferent fibres responding to stimulation of atrial receptors also responded to stimulation of arterial baroreceptors. However, it was concluded that simple arithmetic summation of effect could explain the phenomena; there was no evidence of interaction between the two systems (Linden *et al.*, 1981).

Distension of the left atrium in the manner of Henry *et al.* (1956) to obstruct the mitral orifice, or distending the pulmonary vein–atrial junctions in the manner of Ledsome & Linden (1964) caused an increase in urine flow (Ledsome & Linden, 1968). Distensions of the two separate balloon systems were carried out in random order in each dog, and in the event all distensions of each of the two balloon systems resulted in an increase in urine flow (Ledsome & Linden, 1968). Results from one of their experiments are shown in Fig. 11.3; there is no evidence to suggest increases in urine flow obtained by the two methods are in any way qualitatively different. It is probable that the large balloons are stimulating more atrial receptors than the smaller ones, resulting in a large increase in urine flow. Evidence that this response involves atrial receptors comes from the blockade of branches of vagal nerves which are known to carry afferent fibres involved in the response of reflex increases in heart rate enumerated above. Vagal section and cooling of the vagi to 5°C abolishes the response, and graded cooling of the vagi at 18°C and 12°C causes a decrementing effect, similar to that observed in the response in myelinated fibres or in the response of an increase in heart rate, when the atrial receptors are discretely stimulated by distending small balloons at the pulmonary vein–atrial junctions. Thus it may be concluded that Paintal-type atrial receptors are responsible for the increase in urine flow following distension of small balloons at the pulmonary vein–atrial junctions (Linden & Kappagoda, 1982).

Kappagoda *et al.* (1973) stimulated right atrial receptors and concluded that this also results in a reflex increase in urine flow in the same manner as stimulating the atrial receptors in the left atrium.

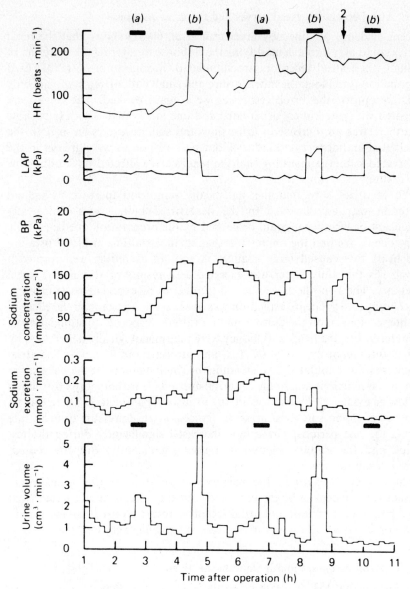

Fig. 11.3. Changes occurring in measured variables during one experiment. During (a) small balloons were distended in the pulmonary vein–atrial junctions. During (b) a balloon was distended in the left atrium to cause mitral obstruction. There is a break in the record at '1', when the atrial balloon was replaced because it leaked. At '2' the right vagal nerve was cut in the neck and the left vagal nerve was cut at the level of the upper border of the aorta. HR, Heart rate; LAP, left atrial pressure. (From Ledsome & Linden, 1968.)

## 11.9. Atrial receptors, renal nerves and the urine response

Recent evidence obtained by Sreeharan *et al.* (1981) shows that the renal nerves could play a role in modifying the response by altering the excretion of sodium when atrial receptors are stimulated. Sreeharan *et al.* (1981) used large balloons to block the mitral orifice and small balloons to stimulate only atrial receptors; the urine responses were again evoked. The dogs were prepared with one kidney denervated and one innervated. The results show that there was an increase in urine flow and sodium excretion in both the innervated and denervated kidneys, but both responses were greater in the innervated kidney, suggesting that the renal nerves affected both urine flow and sodium excretion.

We were not sure that the statistically significant increase in sodium excretion we had observed in the denervated kidney was biologically significant or whether it could be caused by the preparation not being fully 'controlled'. We had the impression that small variations in blood pressure and heart rate caused large changes in sodium excretion, and formed a hypothesis that only water was excreted as a results of stimulating atrial receptors. The hypothesis was tested in a series of experiments (Linden & Sreeharan, 1981). The investigation was made solely to examine the effect of the humoral agent on the diuretic and natriuretic responses to stimulation of atrial receptors; the heart and kidney were pharmacologically denervated by giving, intravenously, bretylium tosylate, atropine and atenolol. The atrial receptors were stimulated by distending the small balloons at the pulmonary vein–atrial junctions and in the left atrial appendage without any obstruction to flow as evidenced by changes in any measured parameters. There was no evidence of changes in atrial pressure, femoral arterial pressure or heart rate during the test periods. Urine flow increased significantly during the test period and the urinary sodium decreased significantly. But the sodium excretion did not change.

Thus, when changes in the haemodynamic state of the animal were prevented as evidenced by the constancy of heart rate, arterial pressure and atrial pressure, stimulation of atrial receptors resulted only in an increase in excretion of water: there was no increase in sodium excretion.

## 11.10. Atrial receptors and a blood-borne agent

It is known that the response of an increase in urine flow to distension of small balloons at the pulmonary vein–atrial junctions, or to distension of a large balloon partially to occlude the mitral orifice, still evokes the response of an increase in urine flow in a denervated kidney (e.g. Ledsome *et al.*, 1961; Kappagoda *et al.*, 1975; Sreeharan *et al.*, 1981). The diuresis was also obtained with the animal and its kidney 'pharmacologically denervated' (Linden & Sreeharan, 1981). These findings suggest that there is a blood-borne agent responsible for a large part of the increase in urine flow.

The identity of this humoral agent is controversial but the popular view has been that the response is mediated solely by a reduction in the concentration of circulating antidiuretic hormone. It is not possible here fully to discuss all the evidence presented for and against this view, but comments are contained in some publications from this laboratory (e.g. Kappagoda *et al.*, 1974, 1975; Linden & Kappagoda, 1982). However, recently we (Bennett *et al.*, 1982, 1983a) have shown conclusively that stimulation of atrial receptors using a large balloon in the lumen of the left atrium in the anaesthetised dog resulted in a decrease in the plasma concentration of vasopressin. Discrete stimulation of the receptors using small balloons in carefully controlled experiments also resulted in a decrease in plasma vasopressin which was independent of secondary haemodynamic changes. Using the technique of graded cooling of the vagi, these responses have been shown to result from the stimulation of Paintal-type atrial receptors and not from receptors discharging into non-myelinated vagal fibres or 'sympathetic afferent' fibres (Bennett *et al.*, 1983b). There is as yet no evidence that these small changes in plasma vasopressin are responsible for the atrial receptor diuresis in the anaesthetised dog. A hypothesis has been proposed which involves a blood-borne agent of an unknown nature, and this hypothetical agent may be a naturally occurring diuretic substance (Linden & Kappagoda, 1982). In Leeds we drew this conclusion because destruction of the posterior pituitary gland and most of the hypothalamus did not abolish the response (Kappagoda *et al.*, 1975). Whether the response was observed in innervated kidneys or denervated kidneys or whether the animal had been injected with bretylium tosylate to abolish the effect of efferent sympathetic nerves following total destruction of the posterior pituitary gland, there was always an increase in urine flow in response to stimulation of atrial receptors. It was shown that there appeared to be no difference between the responses in the two groups, the group with intact posterior pituitary glands and that in which the glands were destroyed.

A technique for the detection of the blood-borne agent, using the Malpighian tubule of the South American blood-sucking bug, *Rhodnius prolixus*, has been evolved (Kappagoda *et al.*, 1979). This preparation does not respond to ADH; incubation of an extract of plasma, obtained during the diuresis, with sodium thioglycollate does not affect the blood-borne agent, which still has an effect on the tubules; such treatment would destroy ADH (Knapp *et al.*, 1981a). All this evidence suggests that the blood-borne agent with which we are dealing is not ADH.

The use of the Malpighian tubules of the *Rhodnius prolixus* as a means of detecting differences in plasma of anaesthetised dogs, obtained during control periods and during periods of stimulation of atrial receptors, has been described by Kappagoda *et al.* (1979). Four Malpighian tubules are obtained from each insect; two are used for control, and two for test purposes. A difference between the results from the two tubules suspended in the butanol extract from control plasma and the tubules suspended in plasma obtained during the diuresis is observed. It was found that this difference could be abolished by cooling or cutting the cervical vagi. The only claim made is that these differences in the plasmas as detected by the behaviour of the Malpighian tubules may reflect the presence of the hypothetical diuretic agent, but it may be a concomitant variable.

Research now involves attempts to identify this hypothetical diuretic agent. Initial purification steps showed the agent to be stabilised in plasma by acidification to pH 3.2, and it was shown to be stable in acidified plasma after heating for up to 20 min (Knapp *et al.*, 1981b). Further purification (Pither *et al.*, 1983) allowed the conclusion that the activity of the humoral agent, as detected by the Malpighian tubule preparation, is associated with a molecule of low molecular weight which may be bound to a larger molecule from which it can be dissociated with acid treatment. It was also shown that cooling the vagal nerves to 9°C abolished the reflex diuresis and abolished the activity of the humoral agent recovered from a Bio-Gel P-2 fraction (mol. wt. range 100–1800). Thus it was suggested that the presence of the substance is dependent on the integrity of the afferent limb of the atrial receptor reflex (Knapp *et al.*, 1983).

It seems that there are changes in two humoral agents in response to stimulation of atrial receptors, one, a decrease in vasopressin and the other an increase in an unknown, possibly diuretic, substance. At the moment it is unkown whether either or both of these events are causatively related to the diuresis of atrial receptor stimulation.

## 11.11. **Blood volume**

Whether or not the proposed 'diuretic' substance or decrease in plasma vasopressin, or both effects, which result from stimulation of atrial receptors, are involved in the control of blood volumes is unknown. Fitzsimons and co-workers (Fitzsimons & Moore-Gillon, 1980; Moore-Gillon & Fitzsimons, 1982) have increased this possibility by suggesting that stimulation of atrial receptors also results in the inhibition of drinking. It is certainly one conclusion which can be drawn from their results, though the possible effects of other cardiovascular receptors were not completely eliminated.

It is possible that atrial receptors are one mechanism involved in the control of blood volume. The first steps in investigating the problem have been taken; Gupta *et al.* (1982) compared the diuretic and natriuretic responses to stimulation of atrial receptors in two groups of anaesthetised dogs, one group with a high blood volume and another group with a low blood volume. The results showed greater diuretic and natriuretic responses in the high blood volume group. These results are not in conflict with the postulate that atrial receptors play a role in the control of heart volumes (Linden, 1976; Gupta *et al.*, 1982).

## 11.12. Conclusion

Thus in summary we conclude that stimulation of Paintal-type atrial receptors results in an increase in heart rate, urine flow and sodium excretion, with the afferent nerves solely in the myelinated nerves in the vagi. The efferent limb of the reflex involved in the heart-rate responses is solely in the sympathetic nerves to the heart, but the efferent limb of the reflex involving the increase in urine flow consists of several components: possibly vasopressin, and another humoral agent, which is possibly diuretic, and these agents only affect water excretion; and efferent sympathetic nerves to the kidney affecting both water and sodium excretion; there is a haemodynamic contribution to the water and sodium excretion secondary to the change in heart rate.

## References

Bennett, K. L., Linden, R. J. & Mary, D. A. S. G. (1982). Left atrial receptors and the antidiuretic hormone. *J. Physiol.* **330**, 23–4P.

Bennett, K. L., Linden, R. J. & Mary, D. A. S. G. (1983). The effect of stimulation of atrial receptors on the plasma concentration of vasopressin. *Quart. J. Exp. Physiol.* **68**, 579–89.

Bennett, K. L., Linden, R. J. & Mary, D. A. S. G. (1984). The nature of atrial receptors responsible for the decrease in plasma vasopressin caused by distension of the left atrium in the dog. *Quart. J. Exp. Physiol.* **69**, 73–81.

Berkley, H. J. (1895). The intrinsic nerve supply of the cardiac ventricles in certain vertebrates. *Johns Hopkins Hosp. Ref.* **4**, 248–74.

Coleridge, H. M., Coleridge, J. C. G. & Kidd, C. (1964). Cardiac receptors in the dog, with particular reference to two types of afferent ending in the ventricular wall. *J. Physiol.* **174**, 323–39.

Coleridge, J. C. G., Hemingway, A., Holmes, R. L. & Linden, R. J. (1957). The location of atrial receptors in the dog: a physiological and histological study. *J. Physiol.* **136**, 174–97.

Fitzsimons, J. T. & Moore-Gillon, M. J. (1980). Pulmo-atrial junctional receptors and the inhibition of drinking. *J. Physiol.* **307**, 74–5P.

Floyd, K., Linden, R. J. & Saunders, D. A. (1972). Presumed receptors in the left atrial appendage of the dog. *J. Physiol.* **227**, 27–8P.

Furnival, C. M., Linden, R. J. & Snow, H. M. (1970). Inotropic changes in the left ventricle: the effect of changes in heart rate, aortic pressure and end-diastolic pressure. *J. Physiol.* **211**, 359–87.

Furnival, C. M., Linden, R. J. & Snow, H. M. (1971). Reflex effects on the heart of stimulating left atrial receptors. *J. Physiol.* **218**, 447–63.

Gupta, B. N., Linden, R. J., Mary, D. A. S. G. & Weatherill, D. (1982). The diuretic and natriuretic responses to stimulation of left atrial receptors in dogs with different blood volumes. *Quart. J. Exp. Physiol.* **67**, 235–58.

Henry, J. P., Gauer, O. H. & Reeves, J. L. (1956). Evidence of the atrial location of receptors influencing urine flow. *Circ. Res.* **4**, 85–90.

Kappagoda, C. T., Knapp, M. F., Linden, R. J., Pearson, M. J. & Whitaker, E. M. (1979). Diuresis from left atrial receptors: effect of plasma on the secretion of the Malpighian tubules of *Rhodnius prolixus*. *J. Physiol.* **291**, 381–91.

Kappagoda, C. T., Linden, R. J. & Mary, D. A. S. G. (1975). Gradation of the reflex response from atrial receptors. *J. Physiol.* **251**, 561–7.

Kappagoda, C. T., Linden, R. J. & Sivananthan, N. (1979). The nature of the atrial receptors responsible for a reflex increase in heart rate in the dog. *J. Physiol.* **291**, 393–412.

Kappagoda, C. T., Linden, R. J. & Snow, H. M. (1972a). The effect of stretching the superior vena caval–right atrial junctions on right atrial receptors in the dog. *J. Physiol.* **227**, 875–87.

Kappagoda, C. T., Linden, R. J. & Snow, H. M. (1972b). A reflex increase in heart rate from distension of the junction between the superior vena cava and the right atrium. *J. Physiol.* **220**, 177–97.

Kappagoda, C. T., Linden, R. J. & Snow, H. M. (1973). Effect of stimulating right atrial receptors on urine flow in the dog. *J. Physiol.* **235**, 493–502.

Kappagoda, C. T., Linden, R. J., Snow, H. M. & Whitaker, E. M. (1974). Left atrial receptors and the antidiuretic hormone. *J. Physiol.* **237**, 663-83.

Kappagoda, C. T., Linden, R. J., Snow, H. M. & Whitaker, E. M. (1975). Effect of destruction of the posterior pituitary on the diuresis from left atrial receptors. *J. Physiol.* **244**, 757–70.

Karim, F., Kidd, C., Malpus, C. M. & Penna, P. E. (1972). The effects of stimulation of the left atrial receptors on sympathetic efferent nerve activity. *J. Physiol.* **227**, 243–60.

Kidd, C., Ledsome, J. R. & Linden, R. J. (1978a). The effect of distension of the pulmonary vein–atrial junction on activity of left atrial receptors. *J. Physiol.* **285**, 445–53.

Knapp, M. F., Linden, R. J. & Pearson, M. J. (1981a). Diuresis from stimulation of left atrial receptors: ADH and the Malpighian tubules of *Rhodnius prolixus*. *Quart. J. Exp. Physiol.* **66**, 333–8.

Knapp, M. F., Linden, R. J. Pearson, M. J., Pither, J. M. & Whitaker, E. M. (1981b). Diuresis from stimulation of left atrial receptors: initial purification steps from plasma of the causative agent. *Quart. J. Exp. Physiol.* **66**, 439–45.

Knapp, M. F., Linden, R. J., Pearson, M. J. & Pither, J. M. (1983). Abolition of atrial receptor diuresis and of release of humoral agent by cooling the vagal nerves *Quart. J. Exp. Physiol.* **68**, 179–88.

Ledsome, J. R. & Linden, R. J. (1964). A reflex increase in heart rate from distension of the pulmonary vein–atrial junctions. *J. Physiol.* **170**, 456–73.

Ledsome, J. R. & Linden, R. J. (1968). The role of the left atrial receptors in the diuretic response to left atrial distension. *J. Physiol.* **198**, 487–503.

Ledsome, J. R., Linden, R. J. & O'Connor, W. J. (1961). The mechanisms by which distension of the left atrium produces diuresis in anaesthetized dogs. *J. Physiol.* **159**, 87–100.

Linden, R. J. (1976). Reflexes from the heart. *Cardiology*, **61**, Suppl. 1, 7–30.

Linden, R. J. & Kappagoda, C. T. (1982). *Atrial Receptors*. Cambridge: Cambridge University Press.

Linden, R. J., Mary, D. A. S. G. & Weatherill, D. (1980). The nature of the atrial receptors responsible for a reflex decrease in activity in renal nerves in the dog. *J. Physiol.* **300**, 31–40.

Linden, R. J., Mary, D. A. S. G. & Weatherill, D. (1981). The responses in renal nerves to stimulation of atrial receptors, carotid sinus baroreceptors and carotid chemoreceptors. *Quart. J. Exp. Physiol.* **66**, 179–91.

Linden, R. J., Mary D. A. S. G. & Weatherill, D. (1982). The response in efferent cardiac sympathetic nerves to stimulation of atrial receptors, carotid sinus baroreceptors and carotid chemoreceptors. *Quart. J. Exp. Physiol.* **67**, 151–63.

Linden, R. J. & Sreeharan, N. (1981). Humoral nature of urine response to stimulation of atrial receptors. *Quart. J. Exp. Physiol.* **66**, 431–8.

Moore-Gillon, M. J. & Fitzsimons, J. T. (1982). Pulmonary vein–atrial junction stretch receptors and the inhibition of drinking. *Am. J. Physiol.* **242**, R452–7.

Nonidez, J. F. (1937). Identification of the receptor areas in the venae cavae and the pulmonary veins which initiate reflex cardiac acceleration (Bainbridge's reflex). *Am. J. Anat.* **61**, 203–31.

Pither, J. M., Knapp, M. F., Linden, R. J. & Pearson, M. J. (1983). Diuresis from stimulation of left atrial receptors in dogs: further purification of the causative agent from plasma. *Quart. J. Exp. Physiol.* **68**, 167–77.

Sreeharan, N., Kappagoda, C. T. & Linden, R. J. (1981). The role of renal nerves in the diuresis and natriuresis caused by stimulation of atrial receptors. *Quart. J. Exp. Physiol.* **66**, 431–8.

Tranum-Jensen, J. (1979). Ultrastructural studies on atrial nerve-end formations in mini-pigs. In *Cardiac Receptors* (eds. R. Hainsworth, C. Kidd & R. J. Linden). Cambridge: Cambridge University Press.

# 12

# Contribution to overall cardiovascular control made by the chemoreceptor-induced alerting/defence response

**J. M. Marshall**

*Department of Physiology, The Medical School, Vincent Drive, University of Birmingham, Birmingham B15 2TJ, UK*

## 12.1. Introduction

It has been recognised since peripheral arterial chemoreceptors were first discovered that stimulation of them can produce striking but complex effects on the cardiovascular system (Heymans & Neil, 1958). The nature of these cardiovascular effects and the mechanisms responsible for them are of physiological and clinical significance, for chemoreceptors have tonic activity at normal levels of arterial $PO_2$ and may be strongly activated in systemic hypoxia at high altitude, in lung disease and during diving, as well as following haemorrhage. In this chapter, emphasis will be placed on recent evidence that carotid chemoreceptor stimulation may activate the defence areas of the brainstem. These are the regions that integrate the behavioural, respiratory and autonomic changes which mammals, including man, show when subjected to a novel or noxious stimulus (see Hilton, 1982). The behaviour observed during activation of the defence areas can range from mild alerting to attack or flight, depending on the strength of the stimulus to the individual concerned. The magnitude of the accompanying respiratory and autonomic changes is correspondingly graded with the stimulus, but the pattern of these visceral changes is constant (Caraffa-Braga *et al.*, 1973; Hilton 1982). This pattern, which will be referred to as the visceral alerting response, includes hyperventilation, tachycardia, renal and mesenteric vasoconstriction, but vasodilatation is skeletal muscle, accompanied by pupillary dilatation, retraction of the nictitating membrane and piloerection. It will be argued not only that stimulation of chemoreceptors may evoke the visceral alerting response, but also that by activating the defence areas they may influence the cardiovascular responses evoked by other incoming stimuli.

In order to set this discussion into its proper context it is necessary to precede it by an account, albeit brief, of the cardiovascular responses which are already well recognised as consequences of chemoreceptor stimulation.

## 12.2. Background

Daly & Scott (1962) showed that carotid chemoreceptor stimulation in dogs anaesthetised with chloralose or urethane and artificially ventilated elicited bradycardia and peripheral vasoconstriction. However, during spontaneous respiration, this primary response was generally overcome by effects that were secondary to the evoked hyperventilation to give tachycardia and vasodilatation, particularly in skeletal muscle. Further experiments revealed that the secondary effects included reflexes initiated by lung stretch receptors whose afferents run in the vagi, and the influence of a fall in $P_aCO_2$ and of increased central inspiratory drive (Daly & Scott, 1963; Daly, 1983).

Results have been obtained in other species, namely the cat, rabbit, seal and primates, which are consistent with these findings, but suggest that in some mammals, notably the cat and rabbit, any effects secondary to hyperventilation are much less striking, probably because the magnitude of the evoked hyperventilation is relatively small (see Korner, 1980; Daly 1983). For example, MacLeod & Scott (1964) found that, in cats anaesthetised with pentobarbitone, chemoreceptor stimulation commonly evoked bradycardia whether or not the animal was allowed to hyperventilate, but the cat showed at most a 100% increase in minute volume in response to chemoreceptor stimulation, whereas the dog showed up to a 500% increase (Daly & Scott, 1962). More recent experiments on the cat suggest that the secondary effects of respiration on the peripheral vasculature may be similarly limited; whereas experimentally induced lung inflation could produce vasodilatation in skeletal muscle, the hyperventilation evoked by chemoreceptor stimulation was never sufficient to reverse the primary reflex vasoconstriction in muscle to vasodilatation (Daly *et al.*, 1983a, b).

Thus the accepted view is that there is a primary bradycardia and generalised peripheral vasoconstriction in response to carotid chemoreceptor stimulation which may be counteracted by effects that are secondary to hyperventilation.

## 12.3. Evidence for activation of defence areas by chemoreceptors

In contrast with this view, Bizzi *et al.* (1961) showed that in unanaesthetised cats, decerebrated at a high level so as to spare the hypothalamus, selective carotid chemoreceptor stimulation or systemic hypoxia evoked the behavioural pattern of 'sham rage' which was indistinguishable from that evoked by known noxious stimuli and was accompanied by a dramatic rise in arterial pressure. Hilton & Joels (1965) confirmed these observations and reported that the sham rage was accompanied by tachycardia and muscle vasodilatation that was not secondary to hyperventilation. Such features would be expected as components of the visceral alerting response, but supporting evidence was not provided since the muscle vasodilatation was not tested for atropine sensitivity — the characteristic of this response in the cat (Abrahams *et al.*, 1960). Nevertheless, the clear implication was that, at least in the high decerebrate preparation, carotid chemoreceptor stimulation can activate the defence areas.

It was pointed out by Hilton (1966) that a reasonable explanation could be provided for the disparity between these observations and those obtained in anaesthetised animals, for conventional laboratory anaesthetics like chloralose and barbiturates depress transmission through the defence areas to the extent that, when employed at full anaesthetic doses, the visceral alerting response cannot be elicited by stimulation of known afferent inputs to the defence areas, i.e. from the amygdala (Hilton & Zbrożyna, 1964), nor by cutaneous nociceptive stimulation (Abrahams *et al.*, 1964). The investigation necessary to test this hypothesis awaited the advent of an anaesthetic which did not have this same central depressant action.

Fortuitously, such a substance arrived in the form of alphaxalone-alphadalone (Althesin, Glaxo). At least, Timms (1976, 1981) demonstrated that Althesin can be given by continuous intravenous infusion in the cat at a dose which produces full anaesthesia and yet still allows the visceral alerting response to be evoked by electrical stimulation in the amygdala. Thus we began a new study of the response evoked by chemoreceptor stimulation in cats anaesthetised with Althesin and more recently in rats so anaesthetised.

### 12.3.1. *The cat*

In cats anaesthetised with Althesin, selective, brief stimulation of carotid chemoreceptors can evoke the pattern of the visceral alerting response (Hilton & Marshall, 1982). There is hyperventilation, usually tachycardia, though sometimes bradycardia, and vasoconstriction in renal and mesenteric vasculature, but pronounced vasodilatation in fore- and hindlimb muscle often preceded by a small constriction and accompanied by synchronisation of the fronto-occipital EEG (Fig. 12.1, C). Concomitantly there is pupillary dilatation, retraction of the nictitating membrane, and sometimes piloerection. The tachycardia and muscle vasodilatation persist virtually unchanged after vagotomy, and under paralysis and artificial ventilation. This is consistent with the evidence that the secondary effects of hyperventilation are not strong in the cat (see above), and indicates that both the tachycardia and muscle vasodilatation are part of a primary response to chemoreceptor stimulation.

Usually, atropine substantially reduced or abolished the chemoreceptor-induced muscle vasodilatation, indicating that it is at least partly mediated by cholinergic fibres. In experiments in which the dilatation was partly atropine resistant and in others in which atropine sensitivity was not tested, guanethidine was given to block the release of transmitter from sympathetic noradrenergic fibres. Thereafter, the increase in muscle vascular conductance evoked by chemoreceptor stimulation was greatly reduced, even under

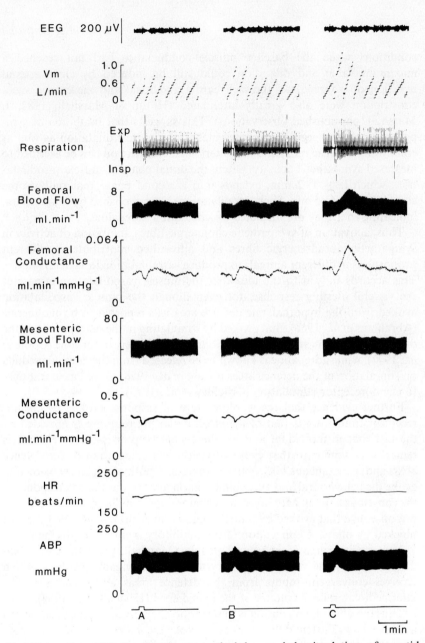

Fig. 12.1. Cat, Althesin. Responses evoked by graded stimulation of carotid chemoreceptors. Traces from above downwards: fronto-occipital electroencephalogram (EEG), respiratory minute volume in litres min$^{-1}$, respiratory air flow, blood flow and vascular conductance in femoral and cranial mesenteric arteries, heart rate and arterial pressure. Stimulus markers show period of injection of 10% (A), 25% (B) and 50% (C) of the 'standard' 0.0245M NaH$_2$PO$_4$ solution described by Hilton *et al.* (1972). Note bradycardia together with constriction in mesenteric and femoral vasculature at (A) but appearance of tachycardia and femoral vasodilatation, graded with stimulus strength, at (B) and (C).

conditions when the baseline muscle conductance had not reached a maximum value and dilatation could still be induced by close arterial injection of isoprenaline; the tachycardia and renal and mesenteric vaso-constriction were also greatly attenuated (Hilton & Marshall, 1982; J. Marshall, unpublished observations). This suggests that inhibition of sympathetic noradrenergic tone contributes to the muscle dilatation as well as confirming that the renal and mesenteric vasoconstriction can be ascribed to increased sympathetic activity. Often, the initial phase of muscle vasodilatation, which lasts 1–2 min, extends into a second phase that outlasts the stimulus by up to 5 min. Such late dilatations were abolished by propranolol, indicating that they are mediated by circulating adrenaline.

Thus, activation of sympathetic cholinergic fibres, inhibition of activity in sympathetic noradrenergic fibres and adrenaline contribute in different proportions in different animals to produce vasodilatation in skeletal muscle. This accords fully with the idea that the muscle vasodilatation is part of the visceral alerting response, for even though the muscle vasodilatation evoked from the hypothalamic defence area was reported to be cholinergic (Abrahams *et al.*, 1960), that evoked by stimulating in the defence area of the dorsal medulla was attributed to inhibition of vasoconstrictor tone (Coote *et al.*, 1973), while adrenaline is known to be released from the adrenal medulla on stimulation of the defence areas (Grant *et al.*, 1958) as well as in response to chemoreceptor stimulation (Critchley *et al.*, 1973).

Further evidence that the whole pattern of response evoked by chemo-receptor stimulation is that of the visceral alerting response is provided by the fact that in individual animals the chemoreceptor-induced response is remarkably similar to that evoked by electrical stimulation in the defence areas and by cutaneous nociceptive stimulation, both of which are known to evoke the behavioural and autonomic components of the alerting response in the conscious animal. Moreover, the chemoreceptor-induced visceral alerting response, like that evoked by central stimulation (Hilton *et al.*, 1983), can be blocked by bilateral application of the inhibitory amino acid glycine to the glycine-sensitive area of the ventral medulla (Marshall, 1986), indicating that it is relayed by the ventral medullary nucleus, paragigantocellularis, which receives convergent inputs from the defence areas and projects to the intermediolateral cell column of the spinal cord (Lovick *et al.*, 1984).

Thus the obvious conclusion is that carotid chemoreceptor stimulation can activate the brainstem defence areas to evoke the visceral alerting response, and that this has been missed in other studies because of the central depressant action of the commonly used anaesthetics. This is not to suggest that the results obtained in animals anaesthetised with more conventional anaesthetics should be regarded just as experimental artefacts. On the contrary, all the evidence we have to date indicates that the primary bradycardia and generalised vasoconstriction (cf. Daly Scott, 1962) are the basic pattern of response upon which the visceral alerting response is superimposed if the stimulus to the chemoreceptors and/or to the defence areas is increased. Thus we have noted (Hilton & Marshall, 1982) that in any given animal, when the level of Althesin anaesthesia is decreased from a surgical level to the lighter level chosen for the experimental period, the response evoked by chemoreceptor stimulation may change from brady-cardia and generalised vasoconstriction, even in skeletal muscle, to that of the visceral alerting response. The response may be converted back to bradycardia and generalised vasoconstriction if the depth of anaesthesia is increased. This presumably means that Althesin, when given at a high dose, does depress transmission through the defence areas just like other anaesthetics; a special property of Althesin would seem to be that such depression can be reduced without forfeiting anaesthesia. Once a stable, light level of Althesin anaesthesia has been attained, the magnitude of the evoked alerting response is graded with the concentration of the solution used to stimulate the chemoreceptors, and if the concentration is substantially reduced, bradycardia and vasoconstriction may be evoked (Marshall, 1986; Fig. 12.1).

Thus in the conscious animal, in the absence of anaesthesia, it would be expected that the response induced by carotid chemoreceptor stimulation would be dependent both on the strength of the stimulus and on the activity already existing in the defence areas as a consequence of other excitatory and inhibitory inputs. As yet, we do not know whether aortic chemoreceptor stimulation can also activate the defence areas.

### 12.3.2. *The rat*

Our observations on the rat are entirely consistent with the evidence discussed above. In spontaneously breathing rats anaesthetised with barbiturate, transmission through the defence areas is presumably blocked, since selective carotid chemoreceptor stimulation consistently evokes hyperventilation, tachycardia and vasoconstriction in skeletal muscle as well as in renal and mesenteric circulation (Marshall, 1984). During paralysis and artificial ventilation, chemoreceptor stimulation evokes bradycardia rather than tachycardia, but the peripheral vasoconstrictor responses are similar in magnitude to those seen during spontaneous respiration. Thus in accord with other species, the rat apparently has the central integrative pathways necessary for chemoreceptor stimulation to elicit bradycardia and generalised vasoconstriction. Effects secondary to chemoreceptor-induced hyperventilation are strong enough to induce tachycardia and overcome the primary bradycardia, as in the dog but, as in the cat, they have little effect on the primary vasoconstriction.

Similar responses to those just described are seen in rats that are *deeply* anaesthetised with Althesin. However, under *light* but adequate Althesin anaesthesia, the block on transmission through the defence areas is lifted and chemoreceptor stimulation evokes the characteristic pattern of the visceral

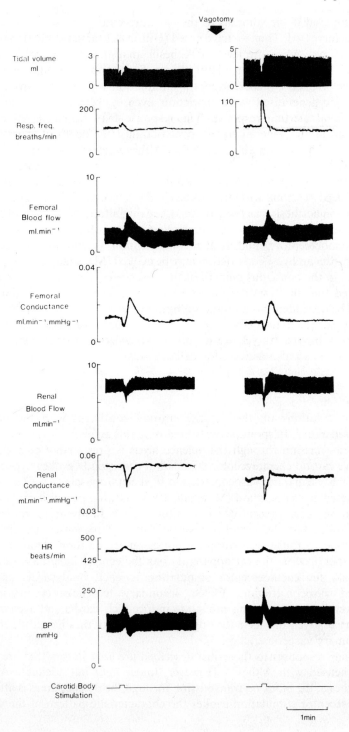

alerting response (Marshall, 1984; Fig. 12.2), comparable with that seen in the cat and with that evoked in the rat on electrical stimulation in the defence areas (Hitlon *et al.*, 1982). Thus, again it may be concluded that when the defence areas are accessible to excitatory inputs, the visceral alerting response may be superimposed upon both the primary bradycardia and peripheral vasoconstrictor response to chemoreceptor stimulation and on effects secondary to hyperventilation.

### 12.4. Systemic hypoxia

The cardiovascular response to systemic hypoxia is generally considered to represent a complex interaction between the direct influence of hypoxia on the central nervous system which elicits tachycardia and peripheral vaso-constriction, the local vasodilating and myocardial depressant action of tissue hypoxia, the reflex effects of peripheral chemoreceptor stimulation and the effects induced by hyperventilation (see Korner, 1959; Daly, 1983). It has been assumed that the reflex effects of chemoreceptor stimulation are bradycardia and peripheral vasoconstriction (cf. Daly & Scott, 1962). But, in view of the results discussed above, it seems likely that activation of the defence areas may be a part of the response to systemic hypoxia which has not yet been recognised.

Observations made in conscious animals suggest that this is the case, though the evidence is not conclusive. It has been reported that hypoxia produces behavioural arousal in rabbits (Korner *et al.*, 1969) and in dogs, and in the latter this was abolished by sino-aortic denervation (Koehler *et al.*, 1980). In the dog, a gradual decrease in $P_aO_2$ from 80 to 25 mmHg induced a progressive increase in arterial pressure, heart rate and cardiac output (Koehler *et al.*, 1980). On the basis of measurements of total peripheral resistance and mesenteric and renal vascular resistances, it was deduced that cardiac output was distributed away from those regional vascular beds. Presumably, the redistribution was towards skeletal muscle, since this is the other major determinant of total peripheral resistance. Such a pattern of change would be comparable with that of the visceral alerting response. However, it must be assumed that the tachycardia and vasodilatation were at least partly secondary to the hyperventilation (see above), as recorded in response to systemic hypoxia in the anaesthetised dog (Kontos *et al.*, 1965)

Fig. 12.2. Rat, Althesin. Pattern of visceral alerting response evoked by stimulation of carotid chemoreceptors before and after vagotomy. Traces from above down-wards: tidal volume, respiratory frequency, blood flow and vascular conductance in femoral and renal arteries, heart rate, arterial pressure and stimulus markers showing period of injection of inorganic phosphate solution. Note that neither the femoral vasodilatation nor the tachycardia were reflex responses mediated by cardiopulmon-ary vagal afferents.

and in the conscious dog in response to brief stimulation of carotid chemoreceptors (Rutherford & Vatner, 1978).

In man, hypoxia has been shown to produce vasodilatation in the skeletal muscle of the forearm, accompanied by an increase in arterial pressure and heart rate (Black & Roddie, 1958). The evidence from those experiments pointed towards circulating adrenaline as the mediator of the dilatation, which as indicated above is part of the alerting response but is not specific to it.

In the rabbit a $P_aO_2$ of 50 mmHg induced tachycardia, but more severe hypoxia ($P_aO_2$ 30 mmHg) induced bradycardia, which may reflect the relatively weak inhibitory influence of increased central inspiratory drive and lung inflation on cardiac vagal motoneurones (see below) in this species and consequent dominance of the primary bradycardia of chemoreceptor stimulation (Korner, 1980). Nevertheless, severe hypoxia did evoke the pattern of splanchnic and renal vasoconstriction and muscle vasodilatation, and the latter was shown to be mediated by circulating adrenaline (Uther *et al.*, 1970).

A firm conclusion as to whether the visceral alerting response is evoked in hypoxia could only be reached by addressing that very question when designing the experimental protocol. We have begun just such a study in the cat and hope to make particular use of the fact that, in this species, muscle vasodilatation mediated by cholinergic fibres is specific to the visceral alerting response.

Results we have already obtained in experiments on the rat are particularly interesting, for not only are they compatible with the idea that activation of the defence areas is an integral part of the response to systemic hypoxia, but also they indicate that in this small mammal the balance between the neurally mediated and local effects of hypoxia is much more easily tipped towards predominance of the latter than in larger mammals like cats, rabbits, dogs and man. Whereas it has been consistently reported that in larger mammals systemic hypoxia elicits a rise in arterial pressure, those who have induced hypoxia in rats anaesthetised with barbiturate or chloralose/urethane have reported a large fall in arterial pressure (Morff *et al.*, 1981; Adams *et al.*, 1982), but have not analysed the underlying mechanisms. Our recent experiments demonstrated that rats which are *deeply* anaesthetised with either barbiturate or Althesin show a fall in arterial pressure when given nitrogen to breathe for 5–10 s (Marshall, 1984). Analysis revealed that the depressor response is due to non-neurally mediated peripheral vasodilatation which is most pronounced in skeletal muscle and is apparently due to vasodilator metabolites released in response to tissue hypoxia. However, in rats which are under *light* barbiturate or Althesin anaesthesia, the locally mediated effects of this short-lasting period of hypoxia are overcome by neurally mediated, generalised vasoconstriction or the pattern of the visceral alerting response, respectively (i.e. responses comparable with those seen on

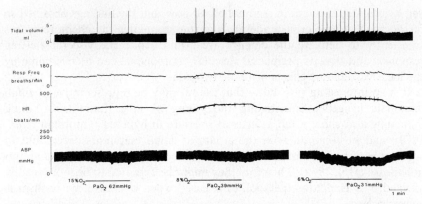

Fig. 12.3. Rat, Althesin. Responses to graded levels of systemic hypoxia. Traces from above downwards: tidal volume, respiratory frequency, heart rate, arterial pressure. Bars indicate periods of breathing 15, 8 or 6% $O_2$ in $N_2$; the figures below indicate arterial $PO_2$ as determined by blood gas analysis of samples taken during final minute of stimulus.

chemoreceptor stimulation alone), and there is a rise in arterial pressure. It is on the basis of these observations that we have begun to interpret the cardiovascular responses evoked in the rat by *graded* levels of hypoxia.

When rats that are lightly anaesthetised with Althesin are exposed to 15, 12, 8 or 6% $O_2$ in $N_2$ for periods of up to 3 min, arterial pressure is maintained for the first minute or so but then falls to an extent which is graded with the level of hypoxia, reaching about 40 mmHg when arterial $PO_2$ is 30 mmHg (Marshall & Paton, 1984; Fig. 12.3). Heart rate increases to reach a peak which is graded with the level of hypoxia, and, particularly when $P_aO_2$ falls below 50–60 mmHg, there is pupillary dilatation, exopthalmus and urination, which are autonomically mediated components of the alerting response in the rat (Barnett, 1975). After vagotomy, or during paralysis and artificial ventilation, the tachycardia at a given $P_aO_2$ is reduced but not abolished, showing that it can only be partly accounted for by effects that are secondary to the hyperventilation; the fall in arterial pressure persists unchanged. Bilateral denervation of the carotid sinus region (the main site of peripheral chemoreceptors in the rat: Sapru & Kreiger, 1977), or administration of guanethidine, greatly accentuates the evoked fall in arterial pressure and abolishes the tachycardia. Since the carotid sinus nerves contain afferents of carotid baroreceptors as well as chemoreceptors, and since guanethidine would have blocked any nerve-mediated release of noradrenaline from sympathetic nerve endings, these results could be explained in part by loss of the baroreceptor reflex. Nevertheless, they are also consistent with the idea that, in the intact animal, reflex changes in sympathetic nerve activity initiated by carotid chemoreceptors attenuate the fall in arterial pressure by offsetting peripheral vasodilatation and increasing heart rate. We have not yet investigated changes in regional blood flow, but the findings obtained so far do suggest that even moderate hypoxia stimulates the chemoreceptors sufficiently to activate the defence areas and evoke the visceral alerting response, and that its peripheral vascular components can be overcome by the local vasodilator effects of tissue hypoxia.

It is an interesting possibility that the rat may be representative of small mammals in general, including the young of large mammals. Young mammals also show a fall in arterial pressure in hypoxia (Gootman et al., 1979), and in common with the adults of small mammal species, but in contrast with large mammals, they show a decrease in oxygen consumption in hypoxia (Hill, 1959). Therefore they might be expected to be more readily affected by vasodilator metabolites released when oxidative metabolism is compromised.

## 12.5. Interaction with the baroreceptor reflex

The fact that chemoreceptor stimulation can raise the level of activity in the defence areas raises the important question of whether that in itself influences the response evoked by other afferent inputs to the central nervous system. An input which is of particular interest is that of the arterial baroreceptors, because electrical stimulation in the defence areas can fully suppress both the cardiac and vascular components of the baroreceptor reflex (Coote et al., 1979). Moreover, in situations in which chemoreceptor activity is increased, there are often accompanying changes in baroreceptor activity, either because the prevailing conditions affect both types of receptor, as in haemorrhage, or because the response to the condition evokes a change in arterial pressure, as in systemic hypoxia.

In cats anaesthetised with Althesin, a chemoreceptor stimulus which evokes the full visceral alerting response can fully suppress both the cardiac and vascular components of the baroreceptor reflex (Marshall, 1981). Thus, when the chemoreceptors were stimulated during the bradycardia and generalised vasodilatation evoked by raising the pressure in one carotid sinus to 210 mmHg for 10s, the characteristic pattern of the visceral alerting response overcame the baroreceptor reflex, and when the baroreceptors were stimulated during a chemoreceptor-induced visceral alerting response, the latter was essentially unchanged. However, when the level of Althesin anaesthesia was relatively deep and the activation of the defence areas by chemoreceptor stimulation was mild, at least as judged by the fact that the muscle vasodilatation was small and there was bradycardia rather than tachycardia, there appeared to be algebraic summation of the chemoreceptor-induced response and the baroreceptor reflex.

It is known that the vagal component of the baroreceptor reflex can be strongly inhibited by increased central inspiratory drive and activation of lung stretch receptor afferents, both of which exert an inhibitory influence on cardiac vagal motoneurones (see Spyer, 1981). An increase in central inspiratory drive also increases the excitability of sympathetic preganglionic neurones, but this has a relatively weak influence on the vascular component of the baroreceptor reflex (see Spyer, 1981). These mechanisms would be expected to contribute to the interaction between baroreceptors and chemoreceptors seen under Althesin, but complete suppression of both the cardiac and vascular components of the baroreceptor reflex is most easily explained by chemoreceptor-induced activation of the defence areas (cf. Coote *et al.*, 1979). The inhibitory influence from the defence areas on the baroreceptor reflex is probably mediated at least in part by mechanisms which are independent of central inspiratory drive, acting early on in the baroreceptor reflex arc (see Spyer, 1981).

That the defence areas can play a role in determining the interaction between chemoreceptors and baroreceptors is reinforced by the fact that the results obtained under Althesin contrast with those obtained under chloralose or barbiturate, when transmission through the defence areas is blocked. Under the latter conditions, carotid chemoreceptor stimulation can completely suppress the vagal component of the baroreceptor reflex, due to the combined inhibitory effects of increased central inspiratory drive and activation of intrapulmonary receptors on cardiac vagal motoneurones (Potter, 1981). However, apart from Trzebski *et al.* (1975), who found that prolonged stimulation of carotid chemoreceptor stimulation could reduce the ability of baroreceptors to inhibit cardiac, renal and lumbar sympathetic activity, the general consensus has been to the contrary that baroreceptor stimulation inhibits peripheral vascular respones produced by carotid chemoreceptor stimulation (Heistad *et al.*, 1974; Mancia, 1975; Wennergren *et al.*, 1976).

It therefore seems that the experiments performed under Althesin have demonstrated a level of interaction between baroreceptors and chemoreceptors that has not been seen in other studies on anaesthetised animals, because of the depressant action of conventional anaesthetics on defence-area function. There is evidence that in conscious cats and man the baroreceptor reflex is progressively suppressed as the level of alertness is increased (Sleight *et al.*, 1978; Schlor *et al.*, 1984). To the extent that chemoreceptor stimulation can cause graded activation of the defence areas this would be expected to be associated with graded suppression of the cardiac and vascular components of the baroreceptor reflex.

## 12.6. Haemorrhage

There is evidence that the activity of peripheral chemoreceptors is increased in haemorrhage, probably as a consequence of reduced tissue $PO_2$ caused by a reduction in glomus blood flow. The latter may be due both to the direct effect of reduced arterial pressure and to local vasoconstriction within the glomus tissue, caused by a reflex increase in the activity of the sympathetic nerve supply and by circulating catecholamines (Lee *et al.*, 1964; Mitchell & McCloskey, 1974). Kenney & Neil (1951) demonstrated that after a severe haemorrhage which reduced arterial pressure to 50–60 mmHg the chemoreceptors were critically important in maintaining that level of arterial pressure. The observation that chemoreceptor stimulation not only induces a rise in arterial pressure but also can suppress the baroreceptor reflex raises the possibility that the chemoreceptors are important in maintaining arterial pressure even after a moderate haemorrhage.

To test this possibility, experiments have been carried out on cats anaesthetised with Althesin in which oxygen was added to the inspired air as a means of unloading the peripheral chemoreceptors. The effect of oxygen on the baroreceptor reflex was tested before and after haemorrhage (J. Marshall, unpublished observations). Before haemorrhage, oxygen administration, which increased $P_aO_2$ to about 250 mmHg, produced only a transient decrease in respiration and arterial pressure and had no effect on the reflex fall in arterial pressure, bradycardia, or peripheral vasodilatation produced by raising the pressure in one carotid sinus to 250 mmHg — a supramaximal stimulus to the baroreceptors. Haemorrhage induced by removing 5–10% of blood volume produced only a slight fall in baseline arterial pressure. There was a significant decrease in mesenteric and hindlimb vascular conductance, but renal vascular conductance and blood flow remained constant, indicating renal autoregulation. After haemorrhage, oxygen produced a sustained fall in baseline arterial pressure of 5–10 mmHg and an increase in the conductances of the regional vascular beds, particularly that of the mesenteric circulation. Moreover, in contrast to the situation before haemorrhage, the reflex evoked by supramaximal baroreceptor stimulation was greater during oxygen breathing than during air breathing; the evoked fall in arterial pressure was greater by approximately 10 mmHg and this reflected larger increases in the regional vascular conductances and usually greater bradycardia. Similar effects of oxygen could be demonstrated after vagotomy, which would have interrupted vagal efferent activity to the heart, as well as afferent activity from aortic chemoreceptors, baroreceptors and cardiopulmonary receptors. However, when the sinus nerve on the side contralateral to the carotid blind sac preparation was cut, so denervating the last peripheral chemoreceptor site which fully experienced the induced rise in arterial $PO_2$, together with the baroreceptors of that side, the effects of oxygen on baseline arterial pressure and on the evoked baroreceptor reflex were abolished.

These observations are entirely consistent with the idea that the effect of oxygen on basline arterial pressure and on the baroreceptor reflex was due to unloading the chemoreceptors rather than to any other effect oxygen may have by acting directly on the central nervous system or on the heart and peripheral vasculature. The corollary of this is that, following even a moderate haemorrhage, raised peripheral chemoreceptor activity plays a significant role in maintaining arterial pressure and partially suppresses the baroreceptor reflex effects on the heart and vasculature. The combined effect of aortic and carotid chemoreceptors may be even greater than could have been demonstrated by the experiments performed, since Lahiri *et al.* (1980) showed that hypotension raises the level of discharge of aortic chemoreceptors far more than that of carotid chemoreceptors, but hyperoxia is more effective in reducing the stimulatory effect of hypotension on carotid chemoreceptors. Notwithstanding this, it is consistent with the evidence already presented to suggest that suppression of the baroreceptor reflex after haemorrhage is mediated at least in part by a central action on the reflex pathway due to the increase in defence area activity caused by carotid chemoreceptor stimulation.

## 12.7. Concluding remarks

Experiments on cats and rats anaesthetised with Althesin have shown that carotid chemoreceptor stimulation is one of the many different types of stimuli that serve as excitatory inputs to the brainstem defence areas. This would not have been apparent in studies carried out under the more commonly used anaesthetics such as chloralose and barbiturates which block transmission through the defence areas. It is already recognised that chemoreceptor stimulation produces behavioural arousal. The evidence presented suggests that the extent to which the characteristic *cardiovascular* changes of the alerting response are apparent during chemoreceptor stimulation depends upon the strength of the stimulus and the level of activity existing in the defence areas. A chemoreceptor stimulus which has low potency to the defence areas may evoke bradycardia and generalised vasoconstriction — the primary cardiovascular response evoked when the functioning of the defence areas is depressed by anaesthesia. A chemoreceptor stimulus which has greater potency to the defence areas will evoke the visceral alerting response whose integral components include tachycardia, and renal and mesenteric vasoconstriction but muscle vasodilatation. These changes are graded in magnitude with stimulus strength, and are superimposed upon and can predominate over the primary response.

Chemoreceptor stimulation also stimulates respiration. The central effects of increased central inspiratory drive and, in an animal that is free to hyperventilate, activation of pulmonary receptors, together induce tachycardia and vasodilatation, particularly in skeletal muscle. These respiratory-dependent effects may overcome the primary bradycardia and vasoconstriction and can probably interfere at least with the components of a mild alerting response. Their potency varies between species, being pronounced in primates and the dog, weak in the cat and rat and virtually absent in the rabbit.

In systemic hypoxia, in addition to the effects of increased peripheral chemoreceptor activity, the influence of hypoxia on the central nervous system tends to induce tachycardia and peripheral vasoconstriction, while the local effect of hypoxia on the heart and peripheral tissues is to cause myocardial depression and vasodilatation, particularly in skeletal muscle, due to accumulation of metabolites. The importance of the local effects is most pronounced in small mammals, e.g. the rat, probably because they have a higher oxygen consumption per body mass which is compromised by a decrease in oxygen supply. Thus the observed pattern of cardiovascular change during systemic hypoxia must depend on the balance of all of the above factors; there are bound to be differences between species.

It is noteworthy that the effects of hyperventilation, the direct effects of tissue hypoxia and the pattern of the alerting response all cause vasodilatation preferentially in skeletal muscle. In species in which the first two mechanisms are inherently weak, or under conditions in which their effect is limited, for example during the apnoea of diving, it may be that activation of the defence areas is of particular importance, not only in inducing behavioural alerting but in generating a pattern of response which redistributes cardiac output from the viscera towards skeletal muscle, perhaps giving a split-second advantage for the muscular exertion necessary to escape from a potentially lethal environment. With this in mind it will be important to establish whether the initiation and maintenance of the alerting response is modified on repeated exposure and during continuing exposure to hypoxic conditions. Is there habituation of the chemoreceptor-induced visceral alerting response as there is of the response evoked by other noxious stimuli (Martin *et al.*, 1976)? Can initiation of the visceral alerting response be suppressed, for example, by the bradycardia and vasoconstriction of the 'diving response' (Butler, 1982; Elsner & Gooden, 1983) if the animal is prevented from surfacing and must conserve oxygen stores?

Whether or not the pattern of cardiovascular response evoked during chemoreceptor stimulation is recognisable as that of the alerting response, excitation of the defence areas may affect the response to other inputs. Thus mild chemoreceptor stimulation may lower the threshold for other noxious stimuli to evoke the behavioural and visceral signs of alerting or aggression. Moreover, chemoreceptor stimulation may fully suppress both the cardiac and vascular components of the baroreceptor reflex. The degree of suppression is likely to be graded with the level of defence area activation and to be achieved in part by a central action early in the baroreceptor reflex arc. This is in addition to the inhibition of the baroreceptor reflex, particularly of its cardiac component, which chemoreceptor stimulation produces via the central and reflex effects of increased central respiratory drive. Such interaction is presumably important in any situation in which chemoreceptor activity is increased. Evidence is presented that, in the particular circumstance of moderate haemorrhage, raised chemoreceptor activity plays a significant role in the maintenance of arterial pressure which is at least associated with, if not due to, partial suppression of both components of the baroreceptor reflex. This finding adds to the general conclusion that peripheral chemoreceptors make an important contribution to the regulation of the cardiovascular system, the full implications of which have yet to be uncovered.

### Achnowledgment

This work was supported by the Medical Research Council, UK.

### Note added in proof

Since this chapter was written we have continued to analyse the cardio-vascular responses evoked in the Saffan-anaesthetised rat by graded hypoxia. The results add further support to the view that activation of the defence areas by peripheral chemoreceptor stimulation and initiation of the visceral alerting response is an integral part of the response to systemic hypoxia (Marshall, J. M. & Metcalfe, J. D., *J. Physiol.* **386**, 77P, 1987; Marshall, J. M. & Metcalfe, J. D., *J. Physiol.* 1987, in press).

### References

Abrahams, V. C., Hilton, S. M. & Zbrożyna, A. W. (1960). Active muscle vasodilatation produced by stimulation in the brain stem. Its significance in the defence reaction. *J. Physiol.* **154**, 491–513.

Abrahams, V. C., Hilton, S. M. & Zbrożyna, A. W. (1964). The role of active muscle vasodilatation in the alerting stage of the defence reaction. *J. Physiol.* **171**, 189–202.

Adams, R. P., Dieleman, L. A. & Cain, S. M. (1982). A critical value for oxygen transport in the rat. *J. Appl. Physiol.* **53**, 660–4.

Barnett, S. A. (1975). *The Rat: a Study in Behaviour.* University of Chicago Press, Chicago, Ill.

Bizzi, E., Libretti, A., Malliani, A. & Zanchetti, A. (1961). Reflex chemoceptive excitation of diencephalic sham rage behaviour. *Am. J. Physiol.* **200**, 923–6.

Black, J. E. & Roddie, I. C. (1958). The mechanism of the changes in forearm vascular resistance during hypoxia. *J. Physiol.* **143**, 226–35.

Butler, P. J. (1982). Respiratory and cardiovascular control during during in birds and mammals. *J. Exp. Biol.* **100**, 195–221.

Caraffa-Braga, E., Granata, L. & Pinotti, O. (1973). Changes in blood-flow distribution during acute emotional stress in dogs. *Pflügers Arch.* **339**, 203–16.

Coote, J. H., Hilton, S. M. & Zbrożyna, A. W. (1973). The ponto-medullary area integrating the defence reaction in the cat and its influence on muscle blood flow. *J. Physiol.* **229**, 257–74.

Coote, J. H., Hilton, S. M. & Perez-Gonzalez, J. F. (1979). Inhibition of the baroreceptor reflex on stimulation in the brain stem defence centre. *J. Physiol.* **288**, 549–60.

Critchley, J. A., Ungar, A. & Welburn, P. J. (1973). The release of adrenaline and noradrenaline by the adrenal glands of cats and dogs in reflexes arising from the carotid chemoreceptors and baroreceptors. *J. Physiol.* **234**, 111P.

Daly, M. de B. (1983). Peripheral arterial chemoreceptors and the cardiovascular system. In *The Physiology of the Peripheral Arterial Chemoreceptors* (pp. 325–93 eds. H. Aker & R. G. O'Regan). Elsevier Science Publishers, Amsterdam.

Daly, M. de B. & Scott, M. J. (1962). An analysis of the primary cardiovascular reflex effects of stimulation of the carotid chemoreceptors in the dog. *J. Physiol.* **162**, 555–73.

Daly, M. de B. & Scott, M. J. (1963). The cardiovascular responses to stimulation of the carotid body chemoreceptors in the dog. *J. Physiol.* **165**, 179–97.

Daly, M. de B., Litherland, A. S. & Wood, L. M. (1983a). The reflex effects of inflation of the lungs on heart rate and hind limb vascular resistance in the cat. *IRCS Med. Sci.* 859–60.

Daly, M. de B., Litherland, A. S. & Wood, L. M. (1983b). The modification of the respiratory, cardiac and vascular responses to stimulation of carotid body chemoreceptors by a laryngeal input in the cat. *IRCS Med. Sci.* 861–2.

Elsner, R. & Gooden, B. (1983). *Diving and Asphyxia.* Cambridge: Cambridge University Press.

Gootman, P. M., Buckley, N. M. & Gootman, N. (1979). Postnatal maturation of neural control on the circulation. *Rev. Perinatal Med.*, **3**, 1–72.

Grant, R., Lindgren, P., Rosen, A. & Uvnas, B. (1958). The release of catecholamines from the adrenal medulla on activation of the sympathetic vasodilator nerves to the skeletal muscles in the cat by hypothalamic stimulation. *Acta Physiol. Scand.* **43**, 135–54.

Heistad, D. D., Abboud, F. M., Mark, A. L. & Schmid, P. G. (1974). Interaction of baroreceptor and chemoreceptor reflexes: modulation of the chemoreceptor reflex by changes in baroreceptor activity. *J. Clin. Investig.* **53**, 1226–36.

Heymans, C. & Neil, E. (1958). *Reflexogenic Areas of the Cardiovascular System.* Churchill, London.

Hill, J. R. (1959). The oxygen consumption of newborns and adult mammals. Its dependence on the oxygen tensions in the inspired air and on the environmental temperature. *J. Physiol.* **149**, 346–73.

Hilton, S. M. (1966). Hypothalamic regulation of the cardiovascular system. *Br. Med. Bull.* **22**, 243–8.

Hilton, S. M. (1982). The defence-arousal system and its relevance for circulatory and respiratory control. *J. Exp. Biol.* **100**, 159–74.

Hilton, S. M. & Joels, N. (1965). Facilitation of chemoreceptor reflexes during the defence reaction. *J. Physiol.* **176**, 20P.

Hilton, S. M. & Marshall, J. M. (1982). The pattern of cardiovascular response to carotid chemoreceptor stimulation in the cat. *J. Physiol.* **326**, 495–513.

Hilton, S. M., Marshall, J. M. & Timms, R. J. (1983). Ventral medullary relay neurones in the pathways from the defence areas of the cat and their effect on blood pressure. *J. Physiol.* **345**, 149–66.

Hilton, S. M., Spyer, K. M. & Timms, R. J. (1972). Stimulating action of inorganic phosphate on chemoreceptor afferent fibres of the carotid body. *J. Physiol.* **226**, 61–2P.

Hilton, S. M. & Zbrożyna, A. W. (1964). Amygdaloid region for defence reactions and its efferent pathway to the brain stem. *J. Physiol.* **165**, 160–73.

Kenney, R. A. & Neil, E. (1951). The contribution of the aortic chemoreceptor mechanisms to the maintenance of arterial blood pressure of cats and dogs after haemorrhage. *J. Physiol.* **112**, 223–8.

Koehler, R. C., McDonald, B. W. & Krasney, J. A. (1980). Influence of $CO_2$ on cardiovascular response to hypoxia in conscious dogs. *Am. J. Physiol.* **239**, H545–58.

Kontos, H. A., Mauck, H. P., Richardson, D. W. & Patterson, J. L. (1965). Mechanisms of circulatory responses to systemic hypoxia in the anaesthetised dog. *Am. J. Physiol.* **209**, 397–403.

Korner, P. I. (1959). Circulatory adaptations in hypoxia. *Physiol. Rev.* **39**, 687–719.

Korner, P. I. (1980). Operation of the central nervous system in reflex circulatory control. *Fed. Proc.* **39**, 2504–12.

Korner, P. I., Uther, M. B. & White, S. W. (1969). Central nervous integration of the circulatory and respiratory responses to arterial hypoxia in the rabbit. *Circ. Res.* **24**, 757–76.

Lahiri, S., Nishino, T., Morashi, A. & Mulligan, E. (1980). Relative responses of aortic body and carotid body chemoreceptors to hypotension. *J. Appl. Physiol.* **48**, 781–8.

Lee, K. D., Mayou, R. A. & Torrance, R. W. (1964). The effect of blood pressure upon chemoreceptor discharge to hypoxia and the modification of this effect by the sympathetic-adrenal system. *Quart. J. Exp. Physiol.* **49**, 171–83.

Lovick, T. A., Smith, P. R. & Hilton, S. M. (1984). Spinally projecting neurones near the ventral surface of the medulla in the cat. *J. Auton. Nerv. Syst.* **11**, 27–33.

MacLeod, R. D. M. & Scott, M. J. (1964). The heart rate responses to carotid body chemoreceptor stimulation in the cat. *J. Physiol.* **175**, 193–202.

Mancia, G. (1975). Influence of carotid baroreceptors on vascular responses to carotid chemoreceptor stimulation in the dog. *Circ. Res.* **36**, 270–6.

Marshall, J. M. (1981). Interaction between the responses to stimulation of peripheral chemoreceptors and baroreceptors: the importance of chemoreceptor activation of the defence areas. *J. Auton. Nerv. Syst.* **3**, 389–400.

Marshall, J. M. (1984). Cardiovascular responses to peripheral chemoreceptor stimulation in the rat. *J. Physiol.* **354**, 64P.

Marshall, J. M. (1986). The role of the glycine-sensitive area of the ventral medulla in cardiovascular responses to carotid chemoreceptor and peripheral nerve stimulation. *Pflügers Archiv.* **406**, 225–31.

Marshall, J. M. & Paton, J. F. R. (1984). The cardiovascular response to systemic hypoxia in a small mammal: the rat. *Arch. Emergency Med.* **1**, 185–6.

Martin, J., Sutherland, C. J. & Zbrożyna, A. W. (1976). Habituation and conditioning of defence reactions and their cardiovascular components in cats and dogs. *Pflügers Arch.* **365**, 37–47.

Mitchell, J. H. & McCloskey, D. I. (1974). Chemoreceptor responses to sympathetic stimulation and changes in arterial pressure. *Resp. Physiol.* **20**, 297–302.

Morff, R. J., Harris, P. D., Weigman, D. L. & Miller, F. N. (1981). Muscle microcirculation: effects of tissue pH, $PCO_2$ and $PO_2$ during systemic hypoxia. *Am. J. Physiol.* **240**, H746–54.

Potter, E. K. (1981). Inspiratory inhibition of vagal responses to baroreceptor and chemoreceptor stimuli in the dog. *J. Physiol.* **316**, 177–91.

Rutherford, J. D. & Vatner, S. F. (1978). Integrated carotid chemoreceptor and pulmonary inflation reflex control of peripheral vasoactivity in conscious dogs. *Circ. Res.* **43**, 200–8.

Sapru, H. N. & Krieger, A. J. (1977). Carotid and aortic chemoreceptor function in the rat. *J. Appl. Physiol.* **42**, 344–8.

Schlor, K.-H., Stumpf, H. & Stock, G. (1984). Baroreceptor reflex during arousal induced by electrical stimulation of the amygdala or by natural stimuli. *J. Auton. Nerv. Syst.* **10**, 157–65.

Sleight, P., Fox, P., Lopez, R. & Brooks, D. E. (1978). The effect of mental arithmetic on blood pressure variability and baroreflex sensitivity in man. *Clin. Sci. Molec. Med.* **55**, 3819–29.

Spyer, K. M. (1981). Neural organisation and control of the baroreceptor reflex. *Rev. Physiol. Biochem. Pharmacol.* **88**, 1–124.

Timms, R. J. (1976). The use of the anaesthetic steroids alphaxalone-alphadalone in studies of the fore-brain in the cat. *J. Physiol.* **256**, 71–2P.

Timms, R. J. (1981). A study of the amygaloid defence reaction showing the value of Althesin anaesthesia in studies of the function of the fore-brain in cats. *Pflügers Archiv.* **391**, 49–56.

Trzebski, A., Lipski, J., Majcherczyk, S., Szulczyk, P. & Chruscielewski, L. (1975). Central organisation and interaction of the carotid baroreceptor and chemoreceptor sympathetic reflex. *Brain Res.* **87**, 227–37.

Uther, J. B., Hunyer, S. N., Shaw, J. & Korner, P. I. (1970). Bulbar and suprabulbar control of the cardiovascular autonomic effects during arterial hypoxia in the rabbit. *Circ. Res.* **26**, 491–506.

Wennergren, G., Little, R. & Oberg, B. (1976). Studies on the central integration of excitatory chemoreceptor influences and inhibitory baroreceptor and cardiac receptor influences. *Acta Physiol. Scand.* **96**, 1–18.

# 13

# Habituation of cardiovascular responses

**A. W. Zbrożyna**

*Department of Physiology, The Medical School, Vincent Drive, University of Birmingham, Birmingham B15 2TJ, UK*

## 13.1. Introduction

Habituation results in diminution and often elimination of a response to a repeated environmental stimulus. It can therefore be considered as the simplest form of learning, and if viewed in this broad sense it is universal in the Animal Kingdom. The first detailed description of habituation was given by Humphrey (1930), who made observations on tentacle withdrawal in snails (*Helix albolabris*), and a large volume of literature has accumulated since that time describing habituation in a great number of species (see review by Thorpe, 1963). In the natural habitat, habituation most often appears to play a prominent role in eliminating flight or attack responses to repeated non-specific stimuli, which are not followed by any significant event in the environment warranting the response. Flight or attack are inborn responses which are dependent to a great extent on the level of arousal, which is usually very high in the natural habitat. It has been suggested that the response to a specific predator is less likely to be habituated than flight induced by generalised and mild warning stimuli (Thorpe, 1963). Once superfluous and useless activities are eliminated, the animal may then proceed with courtship, foraging and fending for its offspring with minimum disruption. On the other hand, stimuli which are followed by food, drink or mating or by an attack by an intruder become conditioned, thus inducing an appropriate response. So gradually by elimination and conditioning the animal builds up a system of meaningful, useful signals.

### 13.1.1. *The neuronal mechanism of habituation*

Habituation is a synaptic process which has been studied extensively in *Aplysia* (Castellucci & Kandel, 1974; Klein *et al.*, 1980). The decline of the gill-withdrawal reflex in *Aplysia* during repeated stimulation is due to reduction in the effectiveness of synaptic connections between the sensory and motor neurones. The reduced synaptic transmission is caused by closing of $Ca^{2+}$ channels in the presynaptic membrane, thus diminishing the output of chemical transmitter. The neuronal basis for habituation has also been studied by Groves & Thompson (1973). They studied habituation of the flexor reflex in a spinal cat. During repeated activation the reflex initially increased (sensitisation) and subsequently decreased (habituation). Analysis of the activity of the spinal interneurones controlling the reflex has shown that during repeated stimulation some interneurones increased their firing rate (sensitising neurones) and some other interneurones decreased their firing rate (habituating neurones). The authors concluded that the sensitising and habituating neurones were responsible for initial facilitation and subsequent suppression of the flexor reflex. These findings are consistent with the observation that repeated activation of a complex behavioural response induces an initial increase followed by decrease in the response (Hinde, 1970). Observations such as these have led to the 'dual-process theory of habituation' (Thompson *et al.*, 1973) and its more recent version, the 'two-factor dual-process theory of habituation and sensitisation' (Petrinovitch, 1984). This proposes that during repeated exposure to a stimulus the two processes, sensitisation and habituation, are activated and develop independently, but through their interaction the magnitude of the response is determined.

Habituation has both short- and long-term effects. A response which is completely suppressed by one train of repeated stimulation will recover after a period of non-exposure to the stimulus. The recovery is not complete, and the next train of repeated stimulation habituates the response more readily. By repeating this procedure the response may be suppressed for a very long period. The rate of habituation and the speed of recovery of a response depend upon the effectiveness of the stimulus (intensity, specificity), frequency of repetition, and the level of excitability (arousal) of the responding organism.

### 13.2. **Habituation of the fight and flight response and its cardiovascular components**

It is now generally accepted that the threatening reaction released in the natural habitat by specific or non-specific stimuli may be habituated (for references see Zbrożyna, 1983). The threatening reaction or as it is often known the defence reaction is a preparatory response for fight or flight and consists not only of postural and vocal threatening components but also of a characteristic pattern of cardiovascular adjustments. Cardiac output, arterial blood pressure and heart rate are increased, the renal, mesenteric and cutaneous vascular beds are constricted, and in the skeletal muscles there is large vasodilatation (Abrahams *et al.*, 1960; Forsyth, 1972; Caraffa-Braga *et al.*, 1973). The same pattern of cardiovascular changes occurs in man in response to noise or trauma, and in turn is comparable with that which

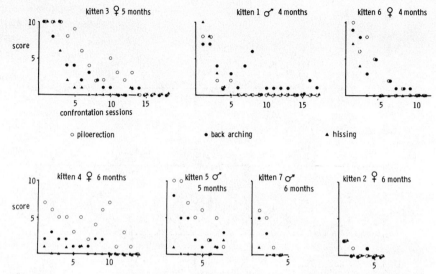

Fig. 13.1. Frequency of occurrence of piloerection, arching of the back and hissing in naive kittens during a series of confrontation sessions. (From Zbrożyna, 1983, reprinted with the permission of the publisher of *Acta Neurobiologiae Experimentalis*, Polish Scientific Publishers.)

occurs in the emotional state of anxiety (Kunkel *et al.*, 1939; Goienhofen and Hildebrandt, 1957; Blair *et al.*, 1959; Barcroft *et al.*, 1960; Dykman and Gantt, 1960; Abrahams *et al.*, 1964; Glaser, 1966; Kelly & Walter, 1968; Mancia *et al.*, 1972; Caraffa-Braga *et al.*, 1973; Breier *et al.*, 1983).

The question that arises is, to what extent can be cardiovascular components of this response undergo habituation? This question is of twofold importance.

(1) Can the behavioural signs of fear or anger be used as indices of the presence of cardiovascular changes?

(2) Can the cardiovascular changes elicited by innate releasers be habituated?

Over the last 15 years we have carried out a number of studies in an attempt to answer these questions. We have established that the threatening posture and vocalisation that occur in cats when confronted by a dog are an innate reaction since it appears in naive kittens (Zbrożyna, 1983). However, even in naive kittens there is great individual variation in the intensity of the individual components of the behavioural response and in the time needed for full habituation of each of the components. Thus the course of habituation was different for each of three components of the threatening reaction — hissing, arching of the back and piloerection — indicating that they were individually suppressed (Fig. 13.1). Since the kittens had not been

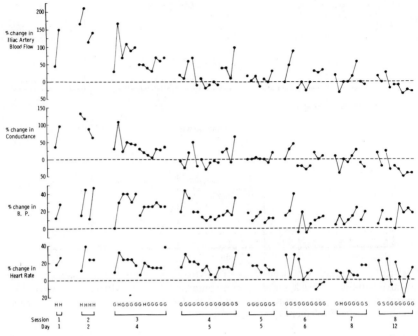

Fig. 13.2.  Habituation of the cardiovascular components of the threatening response elicited in a cat confronted by a dog. Each point corresponds to one bout of rage during confrontation. The points linked by a line refer to one confrontation when a dog was taken into the room and brought close to the cat. On the 5th day there was a morning and afternoon session. H, Hissing; G, growling; S, striking with a front paw in the direction of the dog. (From Martin *et al.*, 1976. Reprinted with the permission of the publisher *Pflügers Archiv*, Springer Verlag.)

confronted by a dog before the experiment began, the individual variation and the selectivity of the suppression of individual components could not have been an effect of previous experience. Of course, in adult cats individual variation in the habituation rate of the individual components of the behavioural response may be partially due to their previous experience.

To answer the question of whether the cardiovascular components of the threatening response can be habituated, we carried out a series of experiments in which the behavioural and cardiovascular aspects of the response were observed simultaneously. In four adult cats, hindlimb blood flow, arterial blood pressure and heart rate were monitored during dailt confrontations by a dog (Martin *et al.*, 1976; Sutherland, 1973). During the first confrontation, the cats displayed the characteristic feline threatening posture and vocalisation. At the same time there was an increase in blood pressure and heart rate and in the conductance of the external iliac artery (Fig. 13.2). This increase in conductance was due to vasodilatation in the skeletal muscles induced by activation of cholinergic sympathetic nerve fibres for it was abolished by atropine. On repeated confrontation there was a gradual change in the pattern of response. The most striking change was a reduction of the magnitude of hindlimb vasodilatation to he extent that, by the 4th session, the vasodilatation was replaced by vasoconstriction in the hindlimb. The muscle vasodilatation would occasionally reappear on subsequent confrontation although it was much reduced.

By contrast the increase of blood pressure and tachycardia persisted, only slightly reduced, in all cats until the end of the experiments, which lasted for up to 12 days. Further the threatening posture and vocalisation also continued unabated in all cats until the end of the series of confrontations. It is therefore obvious that habituation can selectively suppress a single component of the overall response. In particular, since the behavioural components of the response appear to be resistant to habituation, they cannot be used as an indicator of concomitant cardiovascular changes. Moreover, the persistence of the increases in the blood pressure suggests that the vasoconstriction in renal and mesenteric vascular beds which normally occurs during the confrontations (Caraffa-Braga *et al.*, 1973; Seal & Zbrożyna, 1978) is more resistant to habituation than is the vasodilatation in the skeletal muscles.

## 13.3. Renal vasoconstriction

Renal vasoconstriction has been recognised for some time as a particularly important component of naturally elicited fear, of pain and of trauma in animals and man (Smith, 1940; Lauson *et al.*, 1944; Wolff, 1953; Johansson, 1962; Forsyth, 1972; Caraffa-Braga *et al.*, 1973; Mancia *et al.*, 1974). Indeed in repeated confrontation experiments on tree shrews (*Tupaia belangeri*) von Holst (1972) showed that long-lasting renal vasoconstriction occurred in the subordinate animal and this resulted in renal insufficiency eventually leading to uraemia and death. Smith (1940) in his studies on man also observed renal vasoconstriction lasting a few hours in response to fear, and this vasoconstriction persisted even when the patient was calmed and appeared to be relaxed. Wolff (1953) also described renal vasoconstriction in man during mental stress, and showed that it is neurally controlled for it was abolished by thoraco-lumbar sympathectomy. It therefore seemed particularly important to us to investigate whether naturally elicited renal vasoconstriction can be suppressed by habituation. Our experiments were carried out on baboons in which renal blood flow was monitored with electromagnetic flowmeters (Zbrożyna, 1976) during confrontation by a snake. In all four experimental animals the first confrontation evoked a very intense threatening reaction during which arterial blood pressure and heart rate increased while vascular conductance in the renal artery decreased by 80% from the control value (Figs 13.3 and 13.5). However, there was large individual variation between

CARDIOVACSCULAR CHANGES IN THE BABOON 'ARGYL'

DURING A SERIES OF CONFRONTATIONS

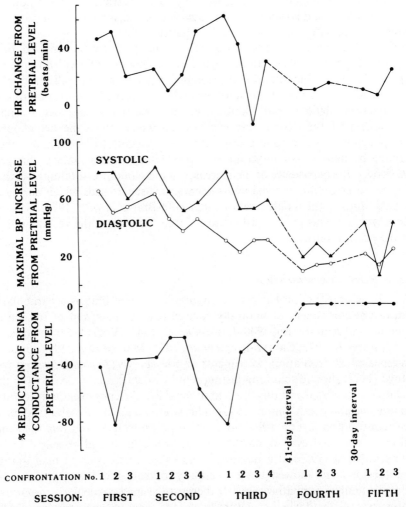

Fig. 13.3. Cardiovascular changes in the baboon 'Argyl' during repeated confrontations by a snake. There is a gradual reduction in blood-pressure increases, transitional decrease in the heart-rate increases and a complete suppression of the renal vasoconstriction response.

### CARDIOVASCULAR CHANGES IN THE BABOON 'ARGYL'

### DURING A SERIES OF CONFRONTATIONS

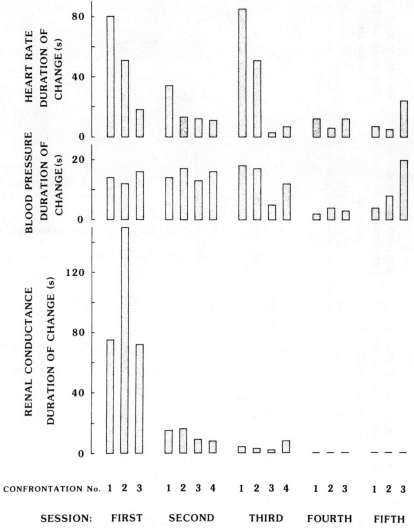

Fig. 13.4. Duration of the cardiovascular changes in the baboon 'Argyl' elicited by confrontation by a snake. There is already a marked reduction in the duration of the renal vasoconstriction starting from the second session and complete absence in sessions 4 and 5. Tachycardia and blood-pressure increase persisted till the end of the experiments although the duration was reduced.

CARDIOVASCULAR CHANGES IN THE  BABOON 'AJAX'

DURING A SERIES OF CONFRONTATIONS

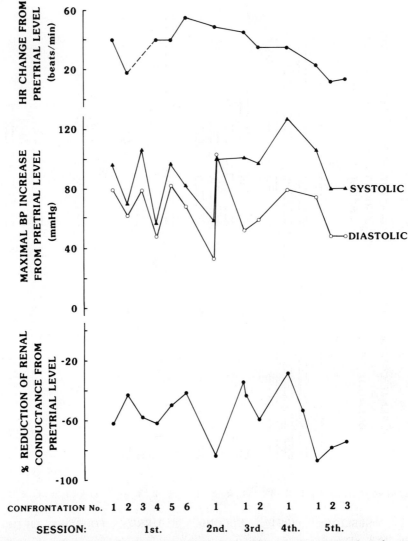

Fig. 13.5.   Cardiovascular changes in the baboon 'Ajax' during repeated confrontations by a snake. There is some reduction in tachycardia after an initial increase. The
blood-pressure increases and the renal vasoconstriction returned to their original level
towards the end of the experiments.

## CARDIOVASCULAR CHANGES IN THE BABOON 'AJAX'

### DURING A SERIES OF CONFRONTATIONS

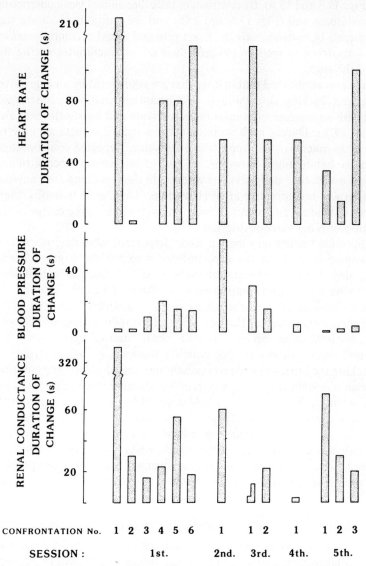

Fig. 13.6. The duration of the cardiovascular changes elicited in the baboon 'Ajax' by confrontation by a snake. There was a marked shortening of the duration of tachycardia and renal vasoconstriction only after the first presentation.

the baboons in the effect habituation had on the renal vasoconstriction; the two extreme cases are shown in the figures. In one animal renal vasoconstriction was habituated completely within three sessions and the effect was lasting (Figs 13.3 and 13.4). By contrast, in the other animal vasoconstriction did not habituate well (Figs 13.5 and 13.6) and the partial habituation was only transient. In both animals the heart rate and blood pressure increases showed a tendency to recover towards their initial magnitudes during the course of the study.

   We have also established that in dogs that are confronted by an aggressive, growling and barking dog there is a substantial renal vasoconstriction together with an increase of arterial blood pressure and heart rate (Seal and Zbrożyna, 1978). During such a confrontation renal conductance may be reduced by as much as 90% from its control value. Repeated confrontation did lead to habituation. However, in two dogs renal vasoconstriction habituated within four daily sessions whereas in the remaining four animals habituation was not complete after 11 sessions. Thus, as in baboons, there were large individual differences between individuals as to the extent of the habituation of renal vasoconstriction.

   An additional finding was that in some dogs renal vasoconstriction was readily conditioned. Thus the experimenter who led the aggressive and growling dog during confrontation very readily became a conditioned stimulus: after a few confrontation sessions, the experimenter entering the cabin alone induced a decrease in reneal vascular conductance (up to 50%). In those instances, however, the dog remained standing quietly. This was particularly interesting because in the confrontation experiments the behavioural aspects of the defence reaction (barking, growling, struggling and attacking the intruder) were completely suppressed within one confrontation session in some dogs, whereas in others the aggressive response to the intruder persisted throughout the whole series of confrontation experiments though at reduced intensity. These observations again confirm that the behavioural and cardiovascular components of the defence reaction may appear independently. On the other hand, when the whole response is habituated, one of the components may recover while the other components remain suppressed (Thon & Pauzie, 1984).

## 13.4. Habituation of the cardiovascular response to physical stimulation

A variety of studies have been carried out that show that the pattern of cardiovascular response associated with fear can also be evoked by physical stimulation, and that the individual components of this response show varying degrees of habituation. However, even very mild stimuli, for example sounds of low intensity, may induce a cardiovascular response. Raskin *et al.* (1969) reported that lower-intensity sounds tend to elicit bradycardia, and high-intensity sounds tachycardia. They showed that whereas bradycardia

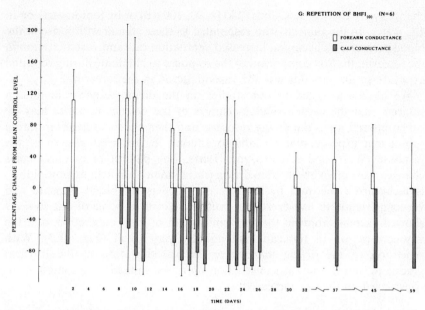

Fig. 13.7. Vascular changes in calf and forearm during diving manoeuvre: facial immersion with 0 mmHg intrathoracic pressure ($BHFI_{(0)}$). Repetition of the manoeuvre leads to reduction of forearm vasodilatation with occasional reversal into vasoconstriction and to gradual increase in vasoconstriction in the calf.

elicited by low-intensity sounds habituated readily, the tachycardia evoked by high-intensity sounds could not be habituated. By contast Sołtysik *et al.* (1961) found that the tachycardia shown by dogs in response to a 65 dB buzzer did habituate. After ten presentations of the buzzer at 2-min intervals, the average increase in the heart rate was reduced from 30 to 15 beats per minute (BPM). Furthermore over the course of six experimental sessions (each with ten repetitions of the sound) the average increase in heart rate was reduced from 25 to 5 BPM. Further repetitions of the sound did not produce any more reduction in response.

The vasoconstriction elicited in the finger by a sound of up to 70 dB has also been shown to habituate readily (Davis *et al.*, 1955; Cohen & Johnson, 1971). However, finger vasoconstriction induced by higher intensity sounds (90–120 dB) could not be habituated and in some instances showed signs of sensitisation. We have since shown in our experiments on dogs that sounds may evoke renal vasoconstriction (Seal & Zbrożyna, 1978). Renal vasoconstriction (a reduction in vascular conductance to 50% of control levels) induced by sounds (2 kHz, 50–110 dB) was habituated after two sessions (37 presentations of the sound). After a further two sessions there was a complete and lasting suppression of the renal vasoconstriction response to the sound.

In our experiments on human subjects (Zbrożyna, 1982) cardiovascular changes were elicited by sounds (2 kHz, 90–100 dB) or by foot immersion in 4°C water. In the subjects who responded to these stimuli with a rise in the blood pressure, tachycardia, increased ventilation rate and vasodilatation in the forearm, the first component of the response to habituate during repeated exposure to the stimulus was the vasodilatation in the forearm.

We have also noted in our studies on the diving response in human subjects that the cardiovascular changes of the defence response may be superimposed upon the diving response and then show habituation during subsequent experimental sessions so altering the manifest pattern of the response (Westwood & Zbrożyna, 1984). The pattern of cardiovascular changes most often observed in diving (facial immersion with breathholding) is tachycardia followed by bradycardia, increase in blood pressure and vasoconstriction in non-exercising muscles. However, some of our subjects showed vasodilatation in the forearm instead of vasoconstriction, and the vasoconstriction in the calf was initially very small (Fig. 13.7). With repetition of the diving manoeuvre the vasodilatation in the forearm gradually waned and vasoconstriction appeared instead; in addition vaso-constriction in the calf increased.

### 13.5. **Habituation in hypertensive patients versus normotensives**

Comparison of habituation of the cardiovascular response to adverse stimuli in young normo- and young hypertensive subjects showed a striking difference between the two groups (Zbrożyna & Krebbel, 1985). The stimulus used was the cold pressor test; the subject was asked to immerse one foot in 4°C water for 1 min. Blood pressure in the brachial artery, blood flow in the calf opposite to the immersed foot, and heart rate were sampled during each immersion and in the intervals between the immersions. In the hypertensive subjects the resting conductance in the calf was approximately 100% higher than in nomotensives (Fig. 13.8). Immersion of the foot in cold water induced tachycardia and an increase in blood pressure in both groups of subjects, and vasodilatation occurred in the calf in some of the hypertensives as well as in normotensive subjects. However, whereas habituation of the vasodilator response to the cold pressor test was very rapid in the normoten-sives (one session), in the hypertensives there was only transient reduction of the conductance increases during the third session. After this the response recovered almost to its original level. Furthermore, whereas the increases in systolic and diastolic blood pressure that occurred habituated almost completely in the normotensive subjects over six sessions, in the hypertensive subjects the increases of systolic blood pressure were only slightly reduced, and the increases in the diastolic pressure remained at the same level until the end of the sixth session. The changes in the heart rate did not differ significantly between the two groups. Thus in the young hypertensive subjects there was little habituation of the muscle vasodilatation evoked by

DILATORS

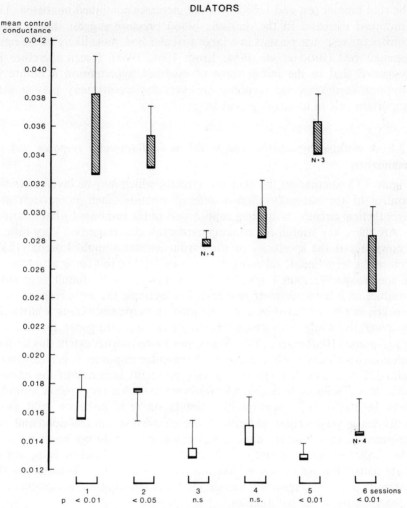

Fig. 13.8. Calf vasodilator responses in hypertensive (hatched columns) and normotensive subjects (open columns) to cold pressor tests. The columns represent the mean areas (across individuals) contained between the regression response line and regression resting line for each session. Calibration is shown on the right-hand side of the graph. The columns are plotted on the resting (control) level of conductance during each session: the heavy line of each column indicates the resting level of conductance. The upward columns indicate increase in conductance, the downward columns decrease in conductance. The bars denote standard deviation. (From Zbrożyna & Krebbel, 1985, reprinted with permission of the publisher of the *European Journal of Applied Physiology and Occupational Physiology*, Springer-Verlag.)

the cold pressor test and blood pressure increases continued unabated. The continued increases in the diastolic blood pressure suggest that a vaso-constrictor response persists in a large vascular bed, most likely in the renal vascular bed (Brod *et al.*, 1954; Brod, 1961, 1963). It can therefore be suggested that in the initial stage of essential hypertension a failure to suppress cardiovascular response to every-day events may play a very important role in its development.

### 13.6. A working hypothesis. The model of cardiovascular response and its habituation

Figure 9.13 summarises the neuronal circuits, which may be involved in the control of the naturally elicited defence reaction, their interaction and hypothetical circuits controlling suppression of the response by habituation.

Are there key stimuli for evoking cardiovascular response? Very little is known about the specificity of the cardiovascular stimuli. Lorenz (1937) coined the term 'innate releasing mechanism' (IRM), this being activated by a species-specific ('key') stimulus, or 'releaser'. Such stimuli invariably produce an inborn adequate response. For example the flight response in a chicken can be activated by a specific moving shape resembling a hawk. If, however, the 'wings' are located close to the tail, as in the goose, then there is no response (Tindbergen, 1951). We do not know to what extent this kind of stimulus specificity applies to the cardiovascular response. It is clear that a stimulus such as a live snake is a very powerful activator of the cardio-vascular response in baboons. The response to such a very specific stimulus may be habituated. Non-specific stimulation (e.g. noise or mild pain) activates a very similar pattern of the cardiovascular reaction; and the response to these stimuli can also be habituated. We do not know whether the cardiovascular response to very intense pain, e.g. visceral pain, can be habituated. But we do know that the rate of habituation depends on the intensity of the non-specific stimulus: the lower the intensity, the quicker and longer lasting is the habituation.

The ability to habituate cardiovascular or galvanic skin response (GSR) depends on the level of *arousal* (Scholander, 1960) or on the level of anxiety (Brierley, 1969); increased arousal or anxiety slows down habituation and may even prevent it altogether. But even the autonomic changes associated with very intense fear occurring during parachuting practice may be habituated (Fenz, 1975). By activation of the reticular formation, habitua-tion is impeded, most likely by increasing the excitatory state on the outgoing pathway to the effectors. Activation of the defence areas (Abrahams *et al.*, 1960; Zbrożyna, 1972) may not only increase the excitatory state of the final pathway but may also influence the 'interpretation' of the incoming sensory information. This might modify the sensory input in such a way that it would

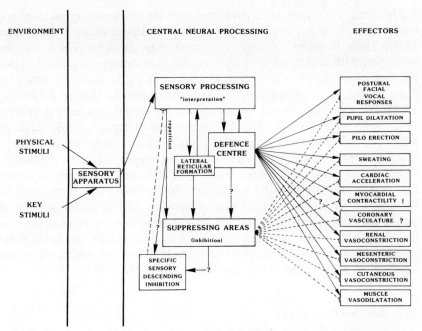

Fig. 13.9. A diagram of the neural circuits controlling the naturally elicited defence reaction and the hypothetical inhibitory neuronal pools which might be activated during habituation.

resemble the specific stimulus pattern eliciting fear or aggression (Sheard & Flynn, 1967; Mark & Ervin, 1970).

The final outcome of the habituation procedure, whether in the laboratory or in a natural habitat, depends upon the algebraic summation of the excitatory state of the final pathway to the cardiovascular effectors induced by the defence areas and by the reticular activating system, and of any inhibition induced by repeated but non-reinforced (non-consequential) presentation of the threatening or disturbing stimulus.

## 13.7. The inhibitory areas responsible for habituation

It is not known which areas of the brain exert the inhibitory influence during habituation. However, there are some areas in the brain known to suppress vasoconstriction. The medial reticular formation in the medulla known as the depressor areas on electrical stimulation induces reduction in the arterial blood pressure and inhibition of the splanchnic nerve activity (Bonvallet & Zbrożyna, 1963). However, it is known that during sleep there is vasodilatation in the mesenteric and renal vascular beds (e.g. Mancia *et al.*, 1971; Seal

& Zbrożyna, 1977) and this is consistent with the observation that there is a suppression of vasoconstrictor fibre activity (Iwamura *et al.*, 1969; Coote, 1982). There is direct evidence to suggest that the areas which may be concerned with repatterning of the vascular tone during sleep (nucl. raphe pallidus, nucl. raphe obscurus and nucl. reticularis paramedialis) also suppress activity of sympathetic vasoconstrictor fibres (Barman & Gebber, 1978). There is also evidence indicating that the lateral amygdala (Fonberg, 1967; Karli *et al.*, 1972) and caudate nucleus (Delgado, 1969) have an inhibitory influence on aggressive behaviour or fear in man and in animals. It is possible that these regions also have a suppressing effect on the cardio-vascular changes accompanying the defence reaction. Furthermore Timms (1977) described in cats the inhibitory effect of electrical stimulation in the anterior or lateral sigmoid gyri or anterior part of the orbital gyrus on the muscle vasodilatation elicited by stimulation in the defence areas of the amygdala. Also, Löfving (1961) showed that in cats the reflex renal vasoconstriction induced by electrical stimulation of the sciatic nerve was inhibited by stimulation in the cingulate gyrus of the cerebral cortex.

### 13.8. Concluding remarks

It is now well established that habituation may suppress cardiovascular responses to alerting or aversive stimuli, but we do not understand why some components are more readily suppressed during habituation than others. The fact that there are large differences between individuals in the cardiovascular sensitivity to extraneous stimulation requires further investigation.

The importance of habituation of the cardiovascular response in anxiety in practical medicine was pointed out for the first time by Celsus (AD 30). In his treatise, Celsus gives this advice on taking the pulse:

> ... the bath and exercise and fear and anger and any other feeling of the mind is often apt to excite the pulse; so that when the practitioner makes his first visit, the solicitude of the patient who is in doubt as to what the practitioner may think of his state, may disturb his pulse. On this account a practitioner of experience does not seize the patient's forearm with his hand as soon as he comes, but first sits down and with a cheerful countenance asks how the patient finds himself; and if the patient has any fear, he calms him with entertaining talk, and only after that moves his hand to touch the patient.

We have made very little progress in this area since the days of Celsus, probably because it has not attracted much interest as a subject worthy of scientific investigation and because it is a very complex and difficult field to work in. Further progress in this field is essential if we are to gain a better understanding of how the individual may maintain cardiovascular homeostasis when facing in his natural environment new challenges and real dangers. Through better understanding of the mechanisms of neural control of the cardiovascular response to sensory stimuli and of its habituation we may come to a better understanding of the success and failure of therapy for essential hypertension by yoga, meditation or sleep.

## Acknowledgements

I would like to express my gratitude to Dr Janice Marshall for reading the manuscript and for her valuable criticism.

## References

Abrahams, V. C., Hilton, S. M. & Zbrożyna, A. W. (1960). Active muscle vasodilatation produced by stimulation of the brain stem: its significance in the defence reaction. *J. Physiol.* **154**, 491–513.

Abrahams, V. C., Hilton, S. M. & Zbrożyna, A. W. (1964). The role of active muscle vasodilatation in the alerting stage of the defence reaction. *J. Physiol.* **171**, 189–202.

Barcroft, H., Brod, J., Heil, Z., Hirsjarvi, E. A. & Kitchin, A. H. (1960). The mechanism of the vasodilatation in the forearm muscle during stress (mental arithmetic). *Clin. Sci.* **19**, 577–86.

Barman, S. M. & Gebber, J. L. (1978). Tonic sympathoinhibition in the baroreceptor denervated cat. *Proc. Soc. Exp. Biol. & Med.* **157**, 648–55.

Blair, D. A., Glover, W. E., Greenfield, A. D. M. & Roddie, J. C. (1959). Excitation of cholinergic vasodilator nerves to human skeletal muscles during emotional stress. *J. Physiol.* **148**, 633–47.

Bonvallet, M. & Zbrożyna, A. (1963). Les commandes reticulaires du systeme autonome et en particulier de l'innervation sympatique et parasympatique de la pupille. *Arch. Ital. Biol.* **101**, 174–207.

Breier, C., Kain, H. & Konzett, H. (1983). The variance of forearm blood flow as an indicator of emotional stress. *Eur. J. Clin. Pharmacol.* **25**, 535–8.

Brierley, H. (1969). The habituation of forearm blood flow in phobic subjects. *J. Neurol. Neurosurg. Psychiat.* **32**, 15.

Brod, J. (1961). Haemodynamic changes in the body during severe muscular exercise and preparation for exercise under physiological and pathological conditions. *Proc. 5th Nat. Cong. Czechoslovak Physiol. Soc.*, Karlovy Vary, 13–16 June 1961. IV. *Regulation of the Circulation*, pp. 217–31.

Brod, J. (1963). Haemodynamic basis of acute reactions and hypertension. *British Heart J.* **25**, 227–45.

Brod, J., Fencl, V., Gerova, M., Hejl, Z., Jirka, J., Kotanova, E., Prat, V., Seidlova, P. & Zajc, F. (1954). Changes of renal haemodynamics and function following a cold stimulus in normal subjects and in subjects with hypertensive disease. In *Hypertensivni Choroba*. Statni Zdravotnicke Nakladelstvi: Prague.

Caraffa-Braga, E., Granata, L. & Pinotti, O. (1973). Changes in blood-flow distribution during acute emotional stress in dogs. *Pflügers Arch.* **339**, 203–16.

Castellucci, V. F. & Kandel, E. R. (1974). A quantal analysis of the synaptic depression underlying habituation of the gill-withdrawal reflex in *Aplysia*. *Proc. Nat. Acad. Sci. US* **71**, 5004–8.

Celsus, Cornelius A. (AD 30). *De Medicina*. Alexandrian School. Quoted after Cule, J.

(1980). *A Doctor to the People. 2000 Years of General Practice in Britain.* London: Update Books.

Cohen, M. J. & Johnson, H. J. (1971). Effects of intensity and the signal value of stimuli on the orienting and defensive responses. *J. Exp. Psychol.* **88**, 286–8.

Coote, J. H. (1982). Respiratory and circulatory control during sleep. *J. Exp. Biol.* **100**, 223–44.

Davis, R. C., Buchwald, A. M. & Frankmann, R. W. (1955). Autonomic and muscular responses and their relation to simple stimuli. *Psychol. Monogr.* **69**, 1–71.

Delgado, J. M. R. (1969). *Physical Control of the Mind.* New York: Harper & Row.

Dykman, R. A. & Gantt, W. H. (1960). Experimental psychogenic hypertension: blood pressure changes conditioned to painful stimuli (schizokinesis). *Bull. Johns Hopkins Hosp.* **107**, 72–84.

Fenz, W. D. (1975). Strategies for coping with stress. In *Stress and Anxiety*, vol. 2, pp. 305–36 (eds. I. G. Saranson & C. D. Spielberger). New York and London: John Wiley.

Fonberg, E. (1967). The role of the amygdaloid nucleus in animal behaviour. *Progr. Brain Res.* **22**, 273–81.

Forsyth, R. P. (1972). Sympathetic nervous system control of distribution of cardiac output in unanaesthetized monkeys. *Fed. Proc.* **31**, 1240–4.

Glaser, E. M. (1966). *The Physiological Basis of Habituation.* London: Oxford University Press.

Golenhofen, K. & Hildebrandt, G. (1957). Psychische Einflusse auf die Muskeldurch-blutung. *Pflügers Arch.* **263**, 637.

Graham, J. (1945). High blood pressure after battle. *Lancet*, **1**, 239–40.

Groves, P. M. & Thompson, R. F. (1973). A dual-process theory of habituation: neural mechanisms. In *Habituation*, vol. 2, pp. 175–203 (eds. H. V. S. Peeke & M. J. Herz). London: Academic Press.

Herd, A. J., Morse, W. H., Kelleher, R. T. & Jones, L. G. (1969). Arterial hypertension in the squirrel monkey during behavioural experiments. *Am. J. Physiol.* **217**, 24–9.

Hinde, R. A. (1970). Behavioural habituation. In *Short-term Changes in Neural Activity and Behaviour*, pp. 3–40 (eds G. Horne & R. A. Hinde). Cambridge University Press, London and New York.

von Holst, D. (1972). Renal failure as the cause of death in *Tupaia belangeri* exposed to persistent social stress. *J. Comp. Physiol.* **78**, 236–73.

Humphrey, G. (1930). Le Chatelier's rule and the problem of habituation and dehabituation in *Helix albolabris*. *Psychol. Forsch.* **13**, 113–27.

Iwamura, Y., Uchino, Y., Ozawa, S. & Torii, S. (1969). Spontaneous and reflex discharge of a sympathetic nerve during 'para-sleep' in decerebrate cat. *Brain Res.* **16**, 359–67.

Johansson, B. (1962). Circulatory responses to stimulation of somatic afferents. *Acta Physiol. Scand.* **57**, Suppl. 198, 1–91.

Karli, P., Vergnes, M., Eclancher, F., Schmitt, P. & Chaurand, J. P. (1972). Role of amygdala in the control of 'mouse-killing' behaviour in the rat. In *The Neurobiology of Amygdala*, pp. 553–80 (ed. B. E. Eleftheriou). New York and London: Plenum Press.

Kelly, D. H. W. & Walter, C. J. S. (1968). The relationships between clinical diagnosis and anxiety, assessed by forearm blood flow and other measurements. *Br. J. Psychiat.* **114**, 611–26.

Klein, M., Shapiro, E. & Kandel, E. R. (1980). Synaptic plasticity and the modulation of the $Ca^{++}$ current. *J. Exp. Biol.* **89**, 117–57.

Kunkel, P., Stead, E. A. Jr & Weiss, S. (1939). Blood flow and vasomotor reactions in the hand, forearm, foot and calf in response to physical and chemical stimuli. *J. Clin. Invest.* **18**, 225–38.

Lauson, H. D., Bradley, S. E., Cournand, A. & Andrews, V. V. (1944). The renal circulation in shock. *J. Clin. Invest.* **23**, 381–402.

Löfving, B. (1961). Cardiovascular adjustments induced from the rostral cingulate gyrus. *Acta Physiol. Scand.* **53**, Suppl. 184, 1–82.

Lorenz, K. Z. (1937). The companion in the birds' world. *Auk* **54**, 245–73.

Mancia, G., Baccelli, G., Adams, D. B. & Zanchetti, A. (1971). Vasomotor regulation during sleep in the cat. *Am. J. Physiol.* **220**, 1086–93.

Mancia, G., Baccelli, G. & Zanchetti, A. (1972). Hemodynamic responses to different emotional stimuli in the cat: patterns and mechanisms. *Am. J. Physiol.* **223**, 925–33.

Mancia, G., Baccelli, G. & Zanchetti, A. (1974). Regulation of renal circulation during behaviour changes in cat. *Am. J. Physiol.* **227**, 536.

Mark, V. & Ervin, F. (1970). *Violence and the Brain*, pp. 97–99, London: Harper & Row.

Martin, J., Sutherland, C. J. & Zbrożyna, A. W. (1976). Habituation and conditioning of the defense reactions and their cardiovascular components in cats and dogs. *Pflügers Arch.* **365**, 37–47.

Petrinovich, L. (1984). A two-factor dual-process theory of habituation and sensitization. In *Habituation, Sensitization and Behaviour*, pp. 17–55 (eds H. V. S. Pecke & C. Petrinovich). New York: Academic Press.

Raskin, D. C., Kotses, H. & Bever, J. (1969). Autonomic indicators of the orienting and defensive reflexes. *J. Exp. Psychol.* **80**, 423–33.

Scholander, T. (1960). Habituation of autonomic response elements under two conditions of alertness. *Acta Physiol. Scand.* **50**, 259–68.

Seal, J. B. & Zbrożyna, A. W. (1977). Cardiovascular changes in various states of alertness in dogs. *Int. Congr. Physiol. Sci. Paris.* **2022**, 680.

Seal, J. B. & Zbrożyna, A. W. (1978). Renal vasoconstriction and its habituation in the course of repeated auditory stimulation and natural elicited defence reactions in dogs. *J. Physiol.* **280**, 56P.

Sheard, M. & Flynn, J. P. (1967). Facilitation of attack behaviour by stimulation of the midbrain of cats. *Brain Res.* **4**, 324–33.

Smith, H. W. (1940). Physiology of the reneal circulation. *Harvey Lectures 1939–40*, **35**, 205–6.

Sołtysik, S., Jaworska, K., Kowalska, M. & Radom, S. (1961). Cardiac responses to simple acoustic stimuli in dogs. *Acta. Biol. Exp.* **21**, 235–52.

Sutherland, C. J. (1973). Cardiovascular participation in unconditioned and conditioned defence reactions. Ph.D. Thesis, University of Birmingham.

Thompson, R. F., Groves, P. M., Teyler, T. J. & Roemer, R. A. (1973). A dual-process theory of habituation: theory and behaviour. In *Habituation*, vol. 1, pp. 239–69 (eds H. V. S. Peek & M. J. Herz). New York: Academic Press.

Thon, B. & Pauzie, A. (1984). Differential sensitization, retention and generalization of habituation in two response systems in the blowfly (*Calliphora vomitoria*). *J. Comp. Psychol.* **98**, 119–30.

Thorpe, W. H. (1963). *Learning and Instinct in Animals*. London: Methuen.

Timms, R. J. (1977). Cortical inhibition and facilitation of the defence reaction. *J. Physiol.* **266**, 98–9P.

Tindbergen, N. (1951). *The Study of Instinct*. London: Oxford University Press.

Westwood, D. M. & Zbrożyna, A. W. (1984). Muscle vasodilatation occurring during diving and its habituation in man. *J. Physiol.* **357**, 85P.

Wolff, H. G. (1953). *Stress and Disease*, pp. 76–8. Springfield, Ill: G. Thomas.

Zbrożyna, A. W. (1982). Habituation of cardiovascular responses to aversive stimulation and its significance for the development of essential hypertension. *Contr. Nephrol.* **30**, 78–81.

Zbrożyna, A. W. (1972). The organization of the defence reaction elicited from amygdala and its connections. In *The Neurobiology of the Amygdala*, pp. 597–606 (ed. B. E. Eleftheriou). New York and London: Plenum Press.

Zbrożyna, A. W. (1976). Renal vasoconstriction in naturally elicited fear and its habituation in baboons. *Cardiovasc. Res.* **10**, 295–300.

Zbrożyna, A. W. (1983). Habituation of the threatening response in cats and kittens. *Acta Neurobiol. Exp.* **43**, 183–92.

Zbrożyna, A. W. & Krebbel, F. (1985). Habituation of the cold pressor response in normo- and hypertensive human subjects. *Eur. J. Appl. Physiol.* **54**, 136–44.

# 14

# Cardiac reactions to psychological challenge: implications for essential hypertension

**D. Carroll, J. R. Turner, J. K. Hewitt and J. Sims**

*Department of Psychology, University of Birmingham, Birmingham B15 2TT, UK*

## 14.1. Introduction

The psychosomatic hypothesis that directed the research reported below is an old and relatively unsophisticated one. In its most basic form, it postulates merely that the manner in which our biology comports itself in the face of environmental challenges has implications for the development of pathology. More recently, a number of researchers have attempted to describe more fully the psychophysiological processes involved. On the whole their deliberations have concentrated on the cardiovascular system and the way in which reactions of that system to psychological challenge might contribute to the development of one particular pathological state: essential hypertension (e.g. Guyton *et al.*, 1970; Light, 1981; Obrist, 1981).

A central proposition is that the orderly linkage between cardiac and metabolic activity, most compellingly displayed in the context of varying physical exercise loads, is far from inviolate, and that certain psychologically challenging situations, namely those that continuously engage the individual mentally, demand constant vigilance, but require little in the way of physical exertion provoke cardiac adjustments that are surplus to metabolic requirement. It is these metabolically excessive reactions and the autoregulatory compensations they precipitate, it is argued, which can contribute to the development of hypertension.

It is appreciated that established hypertension is not in the main associated with increased cardiac activity (e.g. see Brod, 1963) and that high blood pressure is sustained by an increase in peripheral resistance. In such circumstances, it is likely that neurogenic influences are minimal. However, this in no way denies the possibility of substantial neurogenic contributions at early stages in the pathological process. It is here that a role is postulated for autonomically mediated increases in heart rate and cardiac output (e.g. see Lund-Johansen, 1980; Obrist, 1981). In fact, findings in a number of areas of research are very much in accord with the view that the early aetiological stages of hypertension may well be characterised by disturbed cardiac functioning.

First of all, research using animal models lends support. For example, in an early study described by Ledingham & Cohen (1963), rats with experimentally induced renal hypertension showed increases in cardiac output when blood pressure started to rise, although peripheral resistance remained normal. It was only after some time that cardiac output returned to normal as resistance rose, maintaining the elevated pressure.

Secondly, studies of both young and borderline hypertensives provide another line of evidence; the haemodynamics of hypertension would seem to vary markedly with the age of the subjects and the severity of the condition. Several studies have reported increased cardiac output in young hypertensives (e.g. Hejl, 1957; Fejfar & Widimsky, 1961). Relatively high heart rates have also been observed in such juvenile hypertensives (e.g. Dustan & Tarazi, 1977). Similar sorts of results have been reported for borderline hypertensives in a large number of studies (e.g. Julius & Conway, 1968; Frohlich *et al.*, 1969; Julius & Esler, 1975). Cardiac output is elevated relative to that found in normotensives, almost always as a function of increased heart rate, since stroke volume is generally normal.

In the present context, though, it must be conceded that, in borderline hypertension, metabolic rate, as indexed by oxygen consumption, has been observed to be inflated as well (Lund-Johansen, 1967; Julius & Conway, 1968). However, the majority of studies have focused on resting physiology; what is central to the psychosomatic hypothesis, outlined above, is the character of reactions to psychological challenges and not simply resting state. In this regard, evidence is accumulating that borderline hypertensives not only display high baseline activity but also show relatively large-magnitude cardiac reactions to psychological challenges. For example, Schultz & Neus (1983) recently compared the responses of mild and borderline hypertensives with age-matched normotensives during mental arithmetic challenge. Both heart rate and cardiac output increased substantially more in the mild and borderline hypertensive subjects than in the normotensive controls. In another recent study, Steptoe *et al.* (1984) found substantially greater increases in heart rate to a video game in what they dubbed 'transient' hypertensives (individuals who registered high blood pressure on initial screening which subsequently fell to normal levels on re-examination) than in normotensive controls. It is perfectly possible that such relatively high cardiac responding is not paralleled by relatively greater increases in energy expenditure, i.e. that the enhanced cardiac reactions of borderline and labile hypertensives are in fact metabolically unwarranted (see Obrist *et al.*, 1983).

These data, then, are broadly supportive of the psychosomatic hypothesis outlined above. The research described below was undertaken to test further various aspects of the hypothesis.

First of all, we were concerned to demonstrate that certain laboratory challenges did indeed provoke, at least in some individuals, cardiac reactions that were greater than would be expected on the basis of contemporary levels of energy expenditure. Secondly, attention focused on the situational and temporal consistency of laboratory cardiac reactions and their relation to the cardiac adjustments observed with every day psychological stressors. Finally, we sought to explore the origins of individual variation in cardiac reactions using a study of identical and fraternal twins, and, at the same time, to examine the relationship between the magnitude of such reactions and parental blood-pressure status.

## 14.2. Metabolically excessive cardiac reactions

In the first study undertaken, heart rate (HR) plus various ventilatory and metabolic indices (oxygen consumption, carbon dioxide production, and respiratory volume and rate) were monitored while 24 healthy young male subjects played a video game of the 'Space Invaders' *genre*. There were various factors to commend video games in this context. First of all, they are actively engaging while demanding only minimal physical effort. Secondly, they are popular with subjects, and subject recruitment is always an important practical concern in human research. Thirdly, and not unrelatedly, they are non-aversive. Fourthly, they are generally accessible; unlike many psychological tasks, they are suitable for subjects with widely varying intellectual capacities. Finally, recent research had indicated that video games provoke sizeable cardiac reactions (Dembroski *et al.*, 1978, 1981).

Subjects in the present study also participated in a control condition in which analogous but ineffective actions were requested and the game proceeded automatically. Here we were endeavouring to control for the game's physical requirements. Full details of the experimental procedures are available elsewhere (Turner *et al.*, 1983).

Relative to a resting baseline, subjects showed significantly larger increases in HR during 'Space Invaders' than during the control condition. However, oxygen consumption ($VO_2$) and carbon dioxide production ($VCO_2$) also increased more; clearly the control condition offered less than perfect control for physical exertion. While the absolute magnitude of metabolic differences between conditions could be regarded as modest relative to HR differences, given the effective range of variations possible for each parameter, the existence of significant differences in $VO_2$ and $VCO_2$ militates against assertions of overall cardiac–metabolic independence during the video game.

However, an analysis of individual differences in HR reactivity would seem to provide evidence that at least some of our subjects were displaying

Table 14.1.  Average changes in HR, $VO_2$ and $VCO_2$ for high and low HR reactors

|                  | High reactors ($N = 10$) | | Low reactors ($N = 14$) | |
| --- | --- | --- | --- | --- |
|                  | *'Space invaders'* | *Control* | *'Space invaders'* | *Control* |
| HR (bpm)         | 15.7 | 2.6  | 1.9  | 1.0  |
| $VO_2$ (mlpm)    | 95.5 | 33.0 | 87.9 | 23.6 |
| $VCO_2$ (mlpm)   | 73.0 | 24.0 | 61.8 | 12.9 |

metabolically excessive cardiac reactions. On the basis of the HR reactions during 'space invaders', subjects were classified as high and low HR reactors (see Turner *et al.*, 1983). The average HR reactions of these two groups are shown in Table 14.1, as are the average changes in $VO_2$.

Crucially, high HR reactors during 'Space Invaders' did not differ from low reactors in either $VO_2$ or $VCO_2$. In addition, this relatively high HR reactivity was specific to the 'Space Invaders' condition; high and low HR reactors displayed no differences in HR, or any other physiological measure, during the control condition.

The results of this study, then, suggest that our video game elicits, at least in some individuals, metabolically excessive HR reactions. However, more definitive evidence is clearly required before making unequivocal pronouncements of cardiac–metabolic independence during psychological challenge.

Accordingly, a second study was undertaken using a somewhat more sensitive methodology, whereby actual HR during the video-game task was compared with HR predicted from the regression of HR against $VO_2$ during graded isotonic exercise and $VO_2$ during the video game. This approach was considered to afford a more precise test of the status of cardiac activity relative to concurrent levels of energy expenditure. In addition, a second psychological challenge, a pressurised mental arithmetic task, was incorporated. This task consisted of addition and subtraction problems involving two two-digit or three-digit numbers. Subjects were presented aurally with the problem and two seconds later with an answer; half of the given answers were correct, and half were incorrect. Subjects were allowed one second to indicate whether the given answer was correct or not, by raising the index finger of their right hand if correct and the index finger of their left hand if incorrect. Monetary incentives were provided to ensure interest.

On completion of these two tasks subjects exercised on a bicycle ergometer. Following a period of simply resting on the bicycle, they undertook four bouts of increasingly demanding exercise. Full details of the procedure are available elsewhere (Turner & Carroll, 1985a).

HR and $VO_2$ values during this exercise phase of the study were then used to obtain a regression line of HR on $VO_2$ for each subject. Individual correlation coefficients were all greater than 0·97, testifying to the quality of

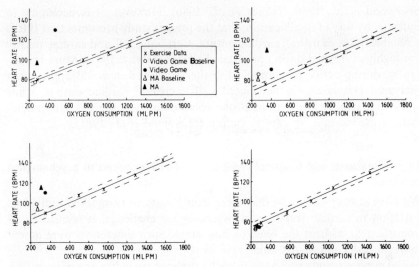

Fig. 14.1.  Heart rate and oxygen consumption for four individual subjects during isotonic exercise and psychological task and baseline conditions. Also shown are regression lines for the exercise data along with 2SEs windows. (Reproduced from Turner & Carroll (1985a) with the permission of *Psychophysiology*.)

the fit in all cases. Examples of the regression lines are presented in Fig. 14.1. Also shown are the data points for the video game and mental arithmetic tasks, as well as the resting baseline periods just prior to each task. These particular examples were chosen to illustrate the range of profiles evident during psychological challenge.

Twenty young healthy male subjects completed this study and the plots for all 20 revealed that the number of data points lying more than two standard errors above the regression lines were 15 and 17 for the video game and mental arithmetic task, respectively. The regression equations calculated for each subject were then used in conjunction with actual $VO_2$ values during the video game and mental arithmetic to predict HR values during the two tasks. These predicted HR values were, as would be expected from our regression plots, considerably less than the HRs actually recorded from subjects ($F(1, 19) = 30.00$, $P < 0.001$). The mean difference between actual and predicted HRs was 9.0 beats per minute (bpm) for the video game and 12.6 bpm for mental arithmetic. These means, though, conceal enormous individual variation; for the video game the differences between actual and predicted HRs ranged from $-4.0$ to $+42.6$ bpm, and for the mental arithmetic from $-3.6$ to $+34.7$ bpm.

These data, then, are much more compelling. HRs for a number of subjects were impressively in excess of what would be expected on the basis of contemporary levels of energy expenditure. As such they are in line with the results of several recent studies (Gliner *et al.*, 1982; Langer *et al.*, 1985;

Sherwood *et al.*, 1986; Turner *et al.*, 1986). However, it is necessary to indicate, by way of qualification, that the present study presumes that HR is a reliable index of overall cardiac output. Certainly, HR and cardiac output are highly correlated during physical challenge (Obrist, 1981). More importantly, during active psychological challenge as well it would appear that increased HR is closely associated with increased cardiac output, while somewhat smaller increases in stroke volume augment the absolute magnitude of the increases in cardiac output (Sherwood *et al.*, 1985).

### 14.3. Situational and temporal consistency of HR reactions to psychological challenge

We have already indicated that there would seem to be marked individual variation in cardiac response to psychological challenge. It seemed to us important to address the issue of how stable such differences were across different tasks and across time.

The previous study provided at least a preliminary indication of inter-task consistency. Additional HR values, computed as the difference between actual and predicted HR levels, were positively, though modestly, correlated across tasks ($r$ (18) = 0·39, $P$ < 0·10). This result contrasts with the extremely high inter-task correlations reported by Light (1981) and Manuck & Proietti (1982). However, these researchers used tasks that were intrinsically more similar than those used in our study. In general, where more diverse tasks have been employed, inter-task consistency has been less striking (e.g. Arena *et al.*, 1983).

In a more recent study in our laboratory (Carroll *et al.*, 1986), using mental arithmetic and another cognitive task, Raven's matrices, we observed much more consistency in HR reaction across tasks ($r$ (22) = 0·66, $P$ < 0·01). In summary, it would seem that while there is a reasonable stability of reaction across tasks, there is also a degree of situational specificity. As intrinsic task demands diverge, so specificity of reaction increases.

Much more impressive is the stability of response over time with the same task. We have recently reported three experiments which all testify to striking temporal consistency of response (Carroll *et al.*, 1984).

In the first of these, the HRs of 42 young healthy males were monitored while they played the 'Space Invaders' video game on two occasions a fortnight apart. HR reactivity, computed as the difference between resting and task HR levels, was highly correlated across occasions of testing ($r$ (40) = 0·80, $P$ < 0·001).

In the second experiment, we selected three extremely high and three extremely low HR reactors from a pool of 23 subjects on the basis of their reactions during an initial session of 'space invaders'. These six subjects then returned to the laboratory a fortnight later and completed four more sessions with the video game; these sessions were scheduled on consecutive days. The

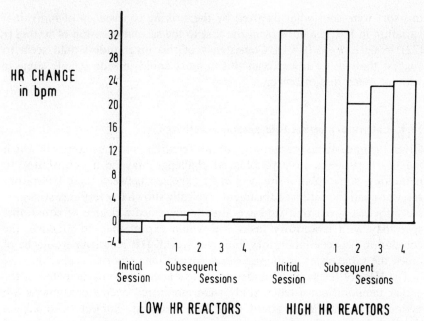

Fig. 14.2. Average heart rate reactivity of high and low reactors. (Reproduced from Carroll *et al.* (1984) with the permission of *Biological Psychology*.)

average HR reactivities for these three high and three low reactors are presented in Fig. 14.2, inspection of which indicates a striking consistency of reaction over time. Although the high reactors showed some attenuation of reaction over sessions, by the final session their average HR reactivity was still around 24 bpm.

In line with the bulk of the research in this field, our studies have employed male subjects only. Given the possibility of intra-menstrual-cycle variation in HR reactivity(Hastrup *et al.*, 1980), most researchers have opted to reduce complexity by including only male subjects. However, as yet few data are available. Accordingly, the third experiment in this series examined the temporal stability of cardiac reactivity in women, and whether temporal consistency was indeed constrained by menstrual-cycle effects.

Twenty-four healthy young women with regular menstrual-cycle lengths and not currently taking oral contraceptives were tested, again using the video game. All subjects were monitored twice. Half were tested first during the preovulatory phase and subsequently postovulatorily, and half were tested first postovulatorily and then preovulatorily. Overall analysis indicated HR reactivity of much the same order as that shown by male subjects, and also that there was a tendency for reactivity to decline from the first to the second occasion of testing. This decline appeared to be somewhat more marked for those whose first test was preovulatory. However, effects of this sort were somewhat dwarfed by the striking consistency of individual variation in HR reactions from the first to the second occasion of testing ($r$ ($\hat{2}2$) $= 0\cdot91$, $P < 0\cdot001$). Consistency of this magnitude would seem to suggest that future research in this context could include female subjects without much loss of power.

## 14.4. Laboratory versus field cardiac reactivity

Given the underlying presumption of this research, that the manner in which the heart responds to psychological challenge may be a contributor to pathology, some relationship would be expected between these laboratory reactions and the cardiac adjustments typically shown to every-day stressors. Nevertheless, given that we have already identified a degree of situational specificity with laboratory tasks, we would expect that, in practice, the correlation between laboratory and 'real world' HR reactivity would be of much the same order as the inter-task correlations reported earlier.

The HRs of the same 42 undergraduate students who participated in the earlier temporal consistency study were monitored over a continuous 8-h period while they went about their daily business. Subjects also kept a detailed diary of their activities, noting time, what they were doing, and whether they were engaged in high or low physical or mental activity. Full details of the procedure are provided by Turner & Carroll (1985b). Minute-by-minute HR records and the subjects' activity records were scrutinised by someone 'blind' to the subjects' laboratory reactions. Attention focused on periods of low physical/low mental activity (invariably periods of 'just relaxing', 'watching TV', 'listening to radio') and periods of low physical/high mental activity. Given the population from which the present sample was drawn, it is perhaps hardly surprising that the vast majority of the latter were periods of study. Other examples were stressful telephone conversations, driving in traffic and, in the case of two subjects, playing 'Astrowars' and 'Tempest' video games. Problems with physiological recording and activity reporting reduced the effective sample size to 31. For each of these subjects, the 'blind' assessor calculated the average HR for low physical/low mental activity periods and for low physical/high mental activity periods. The difference between the two was regarded as an index of 'real world' HR reactivity to stress.

The overall average HR during periods of low physical/low mental activity was 80·3 bpm whereas the average HR during periods of low physical/high mental activity was 84·6 bpm; average 'real world' reactivity, then, was 4·3 bpm. More importantly, HR reactions to the laboratory 'Space Invaders' task were significantly correlated with 'real world' reactivity values: for the first laboratory visit, $r$ (29) $= 0\cdot49$, $P < 0\cdot01$; for the second laboratory visit $r$ (29) $= 0\cdot39$, $P < 0\cdot05$.

## 14.5. The origins and implications of individual variation in cardiac reactivity

Throughout this research programme we have been impressed by the marked individual variation in HR reaction to laboratory challenges. At one extreme we have encountered subjects who display sustained increases in HR of over 30 bpm, and at the other subjects whose HR changes little, if at all, from baseline. The final experiment to be reported uses the standard twin-study methodology to examine the origins of these individual differences. Earlier twin studies of cardiac activity during psychological stress (Shapiro *et al.*, 1968; Theorell *et al.*, 1979), although reporting data broadly suggestive of genetic involvement, have employed either too few subjects or insufficiently sophisticated analytical techniques to afford clear conclusions.

At the same time, we were also keen to start exploring directly the pathological implications of large-magnitude cardiac reactions. Given observed familial aggregation for essential hypertension (Feinleib, 1979), evidence suggestive of a role for high cardiac reactivity in the aetiological process might be obtained by comparing offspring cardiac reactions to psychological challenge with parental blood pressure (BP) status. Three recent studies have attempted such a comparison (Falkner *et al.*, 1979; Hastrup *et al.*, 1982; Manuck & Proietti, 1982) and all reported that the offspring of hypertensive parents displayed greater HR reactions to psychologically challenging tasks than did the offspring of normotensive parents. However, all three studies largely relied on self-report of parental hypertension, with all the attendant uncertainties. It was felt prudent in the present study to monitor parental BP directly.

The HR reactions of 40 monozygotic (MZ) and 40 dizygotic (DZ) pairs of young male twins were monitored at rest and during the 'Space Invaders' video game. In 59 of these 80 families, we were able to interview subjects' parents at home about health, medication, etc., and obtain BP readings, one at the beginning and one at the end of the visit. Full details of the procedures are reported elsewhere (Carroll *et al.*, 1985).

Overall, MZ and DZ twins displayed average HR reactions of the same order. Correlational analysis revealed that whereas HR reactivity, measured again as the difference between rest and task HR levels, was not significantly correlated for DZ twins ($r$ (38) = 0·11, ns), a highly significant correlation was found for the MZ twins ($r$ (38) = 0·56, $p$ < 0·001). This higher correlation for MZ twins certainly suggests the presence of genetic variation for HR reactivity, but correlations alone do not provide the powerful tests of alternative genetic and environmental models afforded by the model fitting technique described below (see Eaves *et al.*, 1978).

The relative contributions of additive genetic variation ($D_R$), shared family environment ($E_2$) and the effects of individual experience ($E_1$) to the variation between and within families of MZ and DZ twins are shown in Table 14.2. Models involving one or more of these parameters can be tested

Table 14.2.   Outome of least squares modelling of within- and between-family variation in HR reactivity

| Source of variation | df | | Mean squares | Full model $E_1 E_2 D_R$ | | |
|---|---|---|---|---|---|---|
| Between MZ families | 39 | | 92.2 | 1 | 2 | 1 |
| Within MZ families | 39 | | 26.2 | 1 | – | – |
| Between DZ families | 39 | | 40.9 | 1 | 2 | 0.75 |
| Within DZ families | 39 | | 32.8 | 1 | – | 0.25 |
| Parameter estimates | $\begin{cases} E_2 \\ D_R \end{cases}$ | 24.4<br>45.8 | | | | |
| Heritability | | | $0{\cdot}48 \pm 0{\cdot}11$ | | | |

by obtaining the 'best' estimates of the parameters in the model by weighted least squares. A chi-square goodness-of-fit test can then be applied to determine whether the parameters fitted are adequate to predict the observed pattern of mean squares. In our case, with four mean squares available from the twin data, we can test simple models involving three effects of fewer. We first test a model involving only the effects of individual experience; this model is $E_1$, which predicts that the four mean squares will be the same. If this model proves inadequate, two further models are tested: an environmental model ($E_1 E_2$) and a simple genetic model ($E_1 D_R$). The first predicts that there are differences between families that are environmentally determined and therefore do not depend on zygosity. The second predicts differences due to genetic variation, and in this case the ratio of between- to within-family mean squares will depend on zygosity. The results of the best models for our data are presented in Table 14.2. Some allowance for familial aggregation is certainly required, as $X^2 (3) = 22{\cdot}91$, $P < 0{\cdot}001$ for the $E_1$ model. However, while the addition of a genetic component (i.e. $E_1 D_R$) gives a fully adequate model, $X^2 (2) = 3{\cdot}98$, ns, the alternative explanation in terms of family environment (i.e. $E_1 E_2$) does not: $X^2 (2) = 6{\cdot}29$, $P < 0{\cdot}05$. Heritability can be estimated as the proportion of total variation which is due to genetic differences between individuals, given by $\frac{1}{2}D_R/(\frac{1}{2}D_R + E_1)$. The present values of $E_1$ and $D_R$ yield a heritability estimate for HR reactivity of $0{\cdot}48 \pm 0{\cdot}11$.

Parental BP readings and general health assessment indicated that in 11 families both parents presented at least marginally high BPs across two readings (had systolic BP $\geqslant 140$ mmHg and/or diastolic BP $\geqslant 90$ mmHg), or were currently receiving antihypertensive medication. The average reactivity of their offspring (11·6 bpm) was significantly higher than that recorded for the rest of the sample (6·2 bpm) ($F (1,57) = 9{\cdot}90$, $P < 0{\cdot}01$).

This study addressed two interrelated issues: first, whether there was a genetic component for variation in HR reactivity to psychological challenge;

secondly, whether HR reactivity in young males would be related to parental BP status. Both received support. In the absence of a longitudinal study, it is impossible to provide an unequivocal test of the underlying hypothesis that excessive cardiac reactivity during psychological challenge represents a heritable predisposition to developing hypertension. However, our present data are certainly in line with such a proposition.

## 14.6. Conclusions

The research reported here provides evidence that psychologically challenging tasks, involving mental but minimal physical effort, provoke, at least in some individuals, cardiac reactions of a magnitude unwarranted in terms of contemporary levels of energy expenditure. The manner in which individuals respond in such circumstances appears to be fairly consistent across different varieties of psychological challenge, although there is clearly a degree of situational specificity, and strikingly consistent over time with the same task. Laboratory reactions, to an extent, reflect the sorts of adjustment observed with every-day stressors. Further, individual variation in HR reactivity to psychological challenge would appear to have a substantial genetic component. Finally, the cardiac reactions of young healthy adults is related to their parents' BP status; reactions are more marked where both parents register relatively high BPs.

Although there remain many unresolved issues, our data are very much in line with the proposition that metabolically excessive cardiac reactions in the face of psychological challenge constitute a heritable risk factor for hypertension.

## Acknowledgements

This chapter includes research presented by JRT for his doctoral thesis while in receipt of a Medical Research Council Studentship. The twin study was also supported by MRC Grant G8207495N.

## References

Arena, J. G., Blanchard, E. B., Andrasik, F., Cotch, P. A. & Myers, P. E. (1983). Reliability of psychophysiological assessment. *Behav. Res. Ther.* 21, 447–60.

Brod, J. (1963). Haemodynamic basis of acute pressor reactions and hypertension. *Br. Heart J.* 25, 227–45.

Carroll, D., Hewitt, J. K., Last, K. A., Turner, J. R. & Sims, J. (1985). A twin study of cardiac reactivity and its relationship to parental blood pressure. *Physiol. Behav.* 34, 103–6.

Carroll, D., Turner, J. R. & Hellawell, J. C. (1986). Heart rate and oxygen consumption during active psychological challenge: the effects of level of difficulty. *Psychophysiol.* 23, 174–81.

Carroll, D., Turner, J. R., Lee, H. J. & Stephenson, J. (1984). Temporal consistency of individual differences in cardiac resonse to a video game. *Biol. Psychol.* **19**, 81–93.

Dembroski, T. M., MacDougall, J. M., Shields, J. L., Petitto, J. & Lushene, R. (1978). Components of the type A coronary-prone behavior pattern and cardiovascular responses to psychomotor performance challenge. *J. Behav. Med.* **1**, 159–76.

Dembroski, T. M., MacDougall, J. M., Slaats, S., Eliot, R. S. & Buell, J. C. (1981). Challenge-induced cardiovascular response as a predictor of minor illnesses. *J. Hum. Stress* **7**, 2–5.

Dustan, H. P. & Tarazi, R. C. (1977). Haemodynamic abnormalities in adolescent hypertension. In *Juvenile Hypertension* (eds M. I. New & L. S. Levine). New York: Raven Press.

Eaves, L. J., Last, K. A., Young, P. A. & Martin, N. G. (1978). Model-fitting approaches to the analysis of human behavior. *Heredity* **41**, 249–320.

Falkner, B., Onesti, G., Angelakos, E. T., Fernandes, M. & Longman, C. (1979). Cardiovascular response to mental stress in normal adolescents with hypertensive parents. *Hypertension* **1**, 23–30.

Feinleib, M. (1979). Genetics and familial aggregation of blood pressure. In *Hypertension: Determinants, Complications and Intervention* (eds G. Onesti & R. Klimt). New York: Grune & Stratton.

Fejfar, Z. & Widimsky, J. K. (1961). Juvenile hypertension. In *The Pathogenesis of Essential Hypertension* (eds J. H. Cort, V. Fencl, Z. Hejl & J. Jirka). Prague: State Medical Publishing House.

Frohlich, E. D., Tarazi, R. C. & Dustan, H. P. (1969). Reexamination of the haemodynamics of hypertension. *Am. J. Med. Sci.* **257**, 9–23.

Gliner, J. A., Bunnell, D. E. & Horvath, S. M. (1982). Hemodynamic and metabolic changes prior to speech performance. *Physiol. Psychol.* **10**, 108–13.

Guyton, A. C., Coleman, T. G., Bower, J. D. & Granger, H. J. (1970). Circulatory control in hypertension. *Circ. Res.* **27**, Suppl. II, 135–48.

Hastrup, J. L., Light, K. C. & Obrist, P. A. (1980). Relationship of cardiovascular stress response to parental history of hypertension and to sex differences. *Psychophysiol.* **17**, 317–18 (abstract).

Hastrup, J. L., Light, K. C. & Obrist, P. A. (1982). Parental hypertension and cardiovascular response to stress in healthy young adults. *Psychophysiol.* **19**, 615–22.

Hejl, Z. (1957). Changes in cardiac output and peripheral resistance during sample stimuli influencing blood pressure. *Cardiologica* **31**, 375–81.

Julius, S. & Conway, J. (1968). Haemodynamic studies in patients with borderline hypertension. *Circulation* **38**, 281–8.

Julius, S. & Esler, M. (1975). Autonomic nervous cardiovascular regulation in borderline hypertension. *Am. J. Card.* **36**, 685–95.

Langer, A. W., McCubbin, J. A., Stoney, C. M., Hutcheson, J. S. Charlton, J. D. & Obrist, P. A. (1985). Cardiopulmonary adjustments during exercise and an aversive reaction time task: effects of beta-adrenoceptor blockade. *Psychophysiol.* **22**, 59–68.

Ledingham, J. M. & Cohen, R. D. (1963). The role of the heart in the pathogenesis of renal hypertension. *Lancet* **ii**, 979–81.

Light, K. C. (1981). Cardiovascular responses to effortful active coping: implications for the role of stress in hypertension development. *Psychophysiol.* **18**, 216–25.

Lund-Johansen, P. (1967). Haemodynamics in early essential hypertension. *Acta. Med. Scand.* Suppl. 482, 1–101.

Lund-Johansen, P. (1980). Haemodynamics in essential hypertension. *Clin. Sci.* **59**, 343s–54s.

Manuck, S. B. & Proietti, J. M. (1982). Parental hypertension and cardiovascular response to cognitive and isometric challenge. *Psychophysiol.* **19**, 481–9.

Obrist, P. A. (1981). *Cardiovascular Psychophysiology: A Perspective.* New York: Plenum Press.

Obrist, P. A., Langer, A. W., Light, K. & Koepke, J. P. (1983). Behavioral–cardiac interactions in hypertension. In *Handbook of Psychology and Health, Vol. 3: Cardiovascular Disorders and Behavior* (eds D. S. Krantz, A. Baum & J. E. Singer) Hillsdale, N J: Erlbaum.

Schultz, W. & Neus, H. (1983) Haemodynamics during emotional stress in borderline and mild hypertension. *Eur. Heart. J.* **4**, 803–9.

Shapiro, A. P., Nicotero, J., Sapira, J. & Scheib, E. T. (1968). Analysis of the variability of blood pressure, pulse rate, and catecholamine responsivity in identical and fraternal twins. *Psychosom. Med.* **30**, 506–20.

Sherwood, A., Allen, M. T., Obrist, P. A. & Langer,' A. W. (1986). Evaluation of beta-adrenergic influences on cardiovascular and metabolic adjustments to physical and psychological stress. *Psychophysiol.* **23**, 89–104.

Steptoe, A., Melville, D. & Ross, A. (1984). Behavioural response demands, cardiovascular reactivity and essential hypertension. *Psychosom. Med.* **46**, 33–48.

Theorell, T., de Faire, U., Schalling, D., Adamson., U. & Askevold, F. (1979). Personality traits and psychophysiological reactions to a stressful interview in twins with varying degrees of coronary heart disease. *J. Psychosom. Res.* **23**, 89–99.

Turner, J. R. & Carroll, D. (1985a). Heart rate and oxygen consumption during mental arithmetic, a video game and graded exercise: further evidence of metabolically exaggerated cardiac adjustments? *Psychophysiol.* **22**, 261–7.

Turner, J. R. & Carroll, D. (1985b). The relationship between laboratory and 'real world' heart rate activity: an exploratory study. In *Psychophysiology of Cardiovascular Control: Methods, Models and Data* (eds J. F. Orlebeke, G. Mulder & L. J. P. van Doornen). New York: Plenum Press.

Turner, J. R., Carroll, D & Courtney, J. (1983). Cardiac and metabolic responses to 'space invaders': an instance of metabolically exaggerated cardiac adjustment? *Psychophysiol.* **20**, 544–9.

Turner, J. R., Hewitt, J. K., Morgan, R. K., Sims, J., Carroll, D. & Kelly, K. A. (1986). Graded mental arithmetic as an active psychological challenge. *Int. J. Psychophysiol.* **3**, 307–9.

# Part III

# Integrative control

# 15

# Cardiovascular–respiratory interactions in fish and crustaceans

**E. W. Taylor**

*Department of Zoology and Comparative Physiology, University of Birmingham, Birmingham B15 2TT, UK*

## 15.1. Introduction

This account concentrates upon the control of external respiration, and more particularly the uptake of oxygen, in fish and decapodan crustaceans. Both groups are active water-breathing animals ventilating and perfusing diffuse gills in order to optimise rates of respiratory gas exchange. The emphasis throughout is on the control of rates of oxygen uptake resulting from integrated changes in the patterns of gill ventilation and perfusion, which, ultimately, together with their detailed morphology, determine the relative effectiveness of the respiratory gas-exchange surfaces. A brief consideration of gill ventilation and perfusion and the reflex changes during hypoxia is followed by a description of the role of receptors monitoring gill function. This leads to an account of the control of respiratory and cardiac rhythms and their temporal relationships, which develops from Chapters 1, 4 and 5 and anticipates Chapters 16 and 17. There have been a number of useful reviews of the control of respiratory gas exchange in water-breathers which represent a suitable background to this account; notably those by Hughes & Shelton (1962), Shelton (1970), Randall (1970, 1982), Johansen (1971), Butler & Metcalfe (1983) and Taylor (1985) on fish; and Wilkens (1981), Taylor (1982) and McMahon & Wilkens (1983) on crustaceans. Dejours (1975) reviewed the principles of comparative respiratory physiology, and the symbols used to represent respiratory variables are largely taken from his account.

Oxygen uptake is by physical diffusion, a process obeying Fick's Law which states that the quantity of oxygen passing over an exchange surface ($\dot{M}O_2$ in moles $O^2$ $min^{-1}$ $kg^{-1}$ tissue) is governed by Krogh's diffusion constant ($K$), for the exchange surface, its surface area ($A$), thickness ($x$), and the gradient for diffusion expressed as partial pressure $PO_2$. This may be expressed as a simple equation:

$$\dot{M}O_2 = \frac{K \cdot A \cdot \triangle PO_2}{x}$$

$\triangle PO_2$ can be controlled by alterations in the relative rates of ventilation of the gills with water and their perfusion with blood; the detailed pattern of ventilation and perfusion of the gills can change their effective diffusive conductance $\dot{M}O_2/\triangle PO_2$.

Water is a relatively dense and viscous medium, and the momentum of the ventilatory stream is typically sustained by unidirectional ventilation. Fish ventilate their gills unidirectionally by means of a double-action pump. Hughes & Shelton (1962) divided ventilation in the trout into four phases with the opercular suction pump (phase 1) and buccal pressure pump (phase 3) separated by periods of transition when differential pressure across the resistance offered by the gill lamellae was much reduced or in some species briefly reversed. A more detailed description of these pumps is given by Ballintijn in Chapter 1. Ventilation in crustaceans is achieved by the rapid oscillations of a pair of specialised appendages, the scaphognathites, which draw water into the branchial chambers, acting as force–suction pumps (Taylor, 1982).

Perfusion of the gill lamellae in fish is direct from the heart, which pumps deoxygenated blood via the ventral aorta and afferent branchial arteries to the afferent filament arteries. Blood flow then separates into a respiratory route which runs via the lamellae where it is oxygenated, then enters the efferent filament arteries which lead to the systemic circulation. This respiratory route interconnects with a non-respiratory blood pathway at various points. Some blood leaves the respiratory, arterio-arterial route to enter a large central canal or venous sinus in the filament which is in turn connected to large sinuses in the interbranchial septum and gill arch. This blood then drains back to the heart along an arterio-venous, non-respiratory route. The complexity of gill perfusion which includes potential shunts has been described in detail for teleosts (Dunel & Laurent, 1980; Laurent & Dunel, 1980) and elasmobranchs (Cooke, 1980; Metcalfe & Butler, 1985) and was summarised by Taylor (1985). In crustaceans the heart pumps oxygenated blood returning from the gills, which receive deoxygenated blood from large venous sinuses (Taylor, 1982).

There is abundant evidence for the existence of counter-current exchange of oxygen between water and blood over the gill lamellae of fish (Hughes & Shelton, 1962). Experimentally this has been demonstrated by examples of measured oxygen tension in arterialised blood ($P_aO_2$) exceeding that in mixed expired water ($P_EO_2$) in both teleosts (e.g. Steen & Kruysse, 1964) and elasmobranchs (Grigg, 1970a). Similar evidence is lacking in crustaceans, though Hughes et al. (1969) described a functional counter-current over the gills of *Carcinus maenas*.

The rates of water flow ($\dot{V}_w$) and blood flow ($\dot{V}_b$) over the counter-current exchanger at the gills are matched according to their relative capacities to carry oxygen (Hughes & Shelton, 1962). Typically in fish the $\dot{V}_w/\dot{V}_b$ ratio is 10–20 (e.g. Piiper & Schumann, 1967) or higher, reflecting the enhanced oxygen capacity of the blood conferred by haemoglobin in the red blood cells (Randall, 1970). In the haemoglobinless ice fish, cardiac output ($\dot{V}_b$) is relatively high and $\dot{V}_w/\dot{V}_b$ is less than 3 (Holeton, 1970), and experimentally induced anaemia reduces the ratio in trout due to a large increase in $\dot{V}_b$ (Cameron & Davis, 1970). Crustaceans have a limited oxygen capacity in the haemolymph conferred by haemocyanin, and consequently have relatively high values of $\dot{V}_b$ when active and low ventilation/perfusion ratios (Taylor & Wheatly, 1980; Taylor, 1982).

## 15.2. Reflex responses to hypoxia

The aquatic environment often varies markedly in oxygen content, and this is reflected immediately as an internal change across the counter-current on the gills. The ability of animals to control the relative diffusive conductance and effectiveness of oxygen transfer over their gills has often been assessed by exposing them to hypoxic water. Some fish and crustaceans show behavioural avoidance reactions to hypoxia (e.g. Jones, 1952; Taylor *et al.*, 1973; Taylor & Wheatly, 1980). The 'typical' hypoxic response in a water-breathing fish or crustacean is an increase in ventilation rate, $\dot{V}_w$, and a reflex bradycardia, which may result in a reduction in cardiac output, $\dot{V}_b$. Consequently, the $\dot{V}_w/\dot{V}_b$ ratio is further increased to compensate for the lower oxygen capacity of the water, and the diffusion time for blood to equilibrate and potentially saturate with oxygen in the gill lamellae is increased.

The increase in ventilation has been described in a number of teleost species (e.g. Randall & Shelton, 1963; Saunders & Sutterlin, 1971) though it has only recently been detected in unrestrained dogfish which show a 50% increase in ventilatory frequency during hypoxic exposure (Metcalfe & Butler, 1984). Ultimately the efficacy of increasing $\dot{V}_w$ may be limited by the decrease in effectiveness at high rates of $\dot{V}_w$ and by the high respiratory cost of ventilation (Hughes, 1964; Jones, 1971). As well as increasing the rate of delivery of oxygen, increased $\dot{V}_w$ may cause turbulent water flow at the exchange surfaces, breaking up stationary water layers close to the lamellae which may present a major obstacle to gas exchange (Piiper & Scheid, 1975). In the crayfish, progressive hypoxia was accompanied by hyperventilation and bradycardia (Wheatly & Taylor, 1981; Taylor, 1981). Despite the increased rate of delivery of water to the gills, effectiveness of removal of oxygen from the water ($E_w$) rose, due to an increase in diffusive conductance which more than doubled during moderate hypoxia. This implies recruitment of a greater area for gas exchange, and/or a change in the flow of water or haemolymph at the exchange surface, which served to increase the effective diffusive conductance or eliminate shunts.

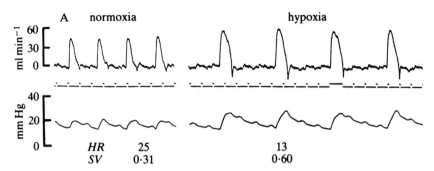

Fig. 15.1.   Blood flow (ml min$^{-1}$), time-base (s) and pressure (mmHg) recorded from the ventral aorta of a dogfish *Scyliorhinus canicula* at 12°C in aerated water ($P_IO_2$ 140 mmHg) and in moderately hypoxic water ($P_IO_2$ 36 mmHg). Values of heart rate (HR in beats min$^{-1}$) and cardiac stroke volume (SV in ml) are given below the traces. A hypoxic bradycardia was accompanied by increases in pulse pressure and stroke volume. Consequently, cardiac output was unchanged from the normoxic value. (Adapted from Butler & Taylor, 1975.)

A reflex hypoxic bradycardia is a well established response to hypoxia in both fish (e.g. Randall & Shelton, 1963; Butler & Taylor, 1971) and crustaceans (Taylor, 1982); though when given time to 'settle' both dogfish (Butler *et al.*, 1979) and lobsters (Butler *et al.*, 1978) showed no cardiac response to moderate hypoxia. The hypoxic bradycardia does not necessarily imply a reduction in blood flow. In dogfish the bradycardia which developed during progressive hypoxia was compensated by a proportional increase in cardiac stroke volume (Fig. 15.1).

The absence of a reduction in $\dot{V}_b$ calls into question the functional significance of the hypoxic bradycardia. Taylor *et al.* (1977) calculated a reduction in apparent power output of the dogfish heart during hypoxia which may reduce overall oxygen demand. More recently, however, Taylor & Barrett (1985) were able to demonstrate a reduction in diffusive capacity and effectiveness of oxygen transfer into the blood of hypoxic dogfish when the reflex bradycardia was abolished by injection of atropine. Apparently the bradycardia subserved a respiratory role which did not involve a reduction in cardiac output but may result from perfusion of previously closed vascular spaces by the increased pulse pressure (Fig. 15.1).

The branchial vasculature in teleosts has neurally and hormonally regulated smooth muscle with a maintained tone (Wood, 1974), and the differential perfusion of gill lamellae reported from intact trout (Booth, 1979) may be actively regulated. In normoxic trout 60% of lamellae were perfused, and during hypoxia or following injection of adrenaline this proportion was reduced in the first gill arch but markedly increased in the last gill arch, with an overall increase in lamellar perfusion approaching 30%. Similar changes in gill perfusion could result in the increases in diffusive conductance during hypoxia reported for fish (Randall, 1970) and crustaceans (e.g. Wheatly & Taylor, 1981).

## 15.3. Receptors in the respiratory and cardiovascular systems

### 15.3.1. *Chemoreceptors*

Studies of the behavioural and physiological responses to hypoxia in both fish and crustaceans have given indirect evidence for the existence of oxygen receptors at various sites in the ventilatory stream or blood system, but as yet no definitive study of an oxygen receptor has been reported for a water-breather. Many studies support the existence of oxygen receptors on or near the gills of fish which monitor environmental $PO_2$ (see Shelton, 1970; Johansen, 1971; Taylor, 1982, 1985). The gill arches in fishes are innervated by cranial nerves IX and X, and it is these nerves which innervate the carotid and aortic bodies of mammals. Bilateral section of IX and X abolished the hypoxic bradycardia in the trout (Smith & Jones, 1978) but in elasmobranchs did not affect the hypoxic response (Satchell, 1959). Butler *et al.* (1977) had to bilaterally section cranial nerves V, VII, IX and X to abolish the hypoxic bradycardia in the dogfish, and concluded that oxygen receptors are distributed diffusely in the orobranchial and parabranchial cavities. Saunders and Sutterlin (1971) were unable to record any change in the level of afferent nervous activity from branchial branches of the vagus nerve during hypoxic exposure of the sea-raven, *Hemitripterus americanus*. In contrast Laurent (1967) recorded oxygen chemoreceptor activity from branches of cranial nerve IX innervating the pseudobranch in the tench. This organ is derived from the spiracle, which is open in elasmobranchs, and as it receives arterialised blood flowing from the gills it is ideally sited to monitor $P_aO_2$ levels. However, bilateral denervation of the pseudobranch in the trout had no effect on the changes in ventilation volume following exposure to hypoxia and hyperoxia (Randall & Jones, 1973). Daxboeck & Holeton (1978) found that irrigation of the anterior region of the respiratory tract of the trout with hypoxic water caused a reflex bradycardia but no change in ventilation, implying that different receptors are involved in the induction of the two overt responses to hypoxic exposure. Saunders & Sutterlin (1971) observed an increase in 'breathing amplitude' in the sea-raven when the dorsal aorta was perfused with hyperoxic blood, and also when perfusing the dorsal aorta with normoxic blood during ambient hypoxia, which they regarded as evidence for both central and peripheral sites of oxygen receptor activity. Eclancher & Dejours (1975) observed a ventilatory and cardiac response to an intravascular injection of cyanide but no response to cyanide in the ventilatory water stream of teleosts, which indicates that the $PO_2$ receptors are located internally. Bamford (1974) concluded that the most important site of oxygen detection in the trout is the brain. Randall (1982) reviewed

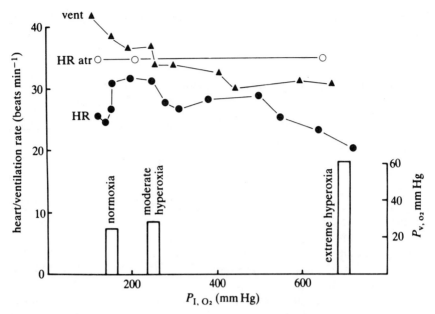

Fig. 15.2. Effect of exposure of the dogfish *Scyliorhinus canicula* to progressive hyperoxia at 15°C on venous oxygen tension ($P_vO_2$) ventilation rate (vent, ▲) and heart rate in both normal (HR, ●) and atropinised (HR atr, ○) fish. An initial tachycardia, towards the atropinised rate, in moderate hyperoxia was followed by a bradycardia in extreme hyperoxia which accompanied an increase in $P_vO_2$. Ventilation rate decreased towards heart rate in moderate hyperoxia.

evidence for the oxygen receptors being sensitive to arterial blood oxygen content or rate of delivery of oxygen to the receptor, which would be singularly appropriate as oxygen supply is thought to be limited by rate of perfusive conductance, $\dot{V}_b\,(C_aO_2 - C_vO_2)$, in fish. Recent evidence suggests the existence of venous $P_vO_2$ receptors in fish. Exposure of the dogfish to progressive hyperoxia caused an initial tachycardia towards the atropinised heart rate, indicating a reduction in vagal tone, followed by a secondary reflex bradycardia at high $PO_2$ levels which corresponded to an increase in $P_vO_2$ (Fig. 15.2). This response was mimicked by injection of hyperoxaemic blood into the venous system (Barrett & Taylor, 1984). Thus, fish may possess receptors monitoring $PO_2$ levels on both the afferent and efferent sides of the counter-current exchanger, potentially enabling them to match the relative flow rates of water and blood over the gill lamellae in order to optimise respiratory gas exchange, saturating the blood with oxygen while minimising the energy cost of ventilation and perfusion.

There is circumstantial evidence for the involvement of oxygen sensitivity at a number of morphological sites in the physiological responses of crustaceans to hypoxia and in particular the initiation of the hypoxic

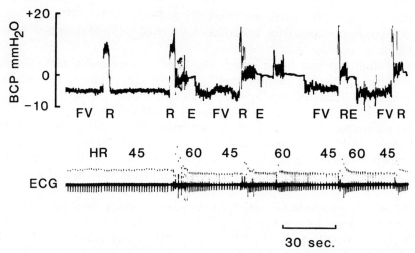

Fig. 15.3. Recordings of hydrostatic pressure from one branchial chamber (BCP) and heart rate (HR beats $min^{-1}$) recorded as the ECG from a shore crab, *Carcinus maenas*. At first the crab was submerged and forward ventilating (FV) in hypoxic water using the scaphognathite to generate an oscillating water pressure below ambient. During this phase it showed a single reversal of ventilation (R). During a second reversal the crab raised its anterior end and emerged into air (E). This resulted in an immediate tachycardia with heart rate rising to a typical normoxic value of 60 beats $min^{-1}$. The crab then commenced alternate bouts of forward ventilation, reversal and emersion, each one accompanied by an immediate switch in heart rate between the hypoxic submerged rate and the normoxic, air-breathing rate. A neurally based link between ventilation and heart rate would account for this rapid response.

bradycardia (Taylor, 1985). The latency of cardiac and ventilatory responses to changes in branchial chamber $PO_2$ (McMahon & Wilkens, 1972) suggests that both the cardiac ganglion and the ventilatory pacemaker neurones in the CNS may respond directly to variations in $PO_2$. Evidence for central receptors does not preclude the existence of peripheral receptors monitoring $PO_2$ levels in the haemocoel or ventilatory stream. Larimer (1964) ascribed initiation of the cardiac and ventilatory responses of the crayfish to hypoxic and hypercapnic water to chemoreceptors located somewhere within the branchial chambers. This suggestion is supported by the instantaneous increase in $f_H$ when air enters the branchial chambers at the onset of the emersion response from hypoxic water in *Carcinus maenas* (Taylor & Butler, 1973; Fig. 15.3). Both this recovery tachycardia following emersion and the similarly high $f_H$ level recorded from *Carcinus* in air (Taylor & Butler, 1978) are associated with internal hypoxia, with $P_aO_2$ values below those normally associated with a bradycardia in submerged, hypoxic animals. The presence of air in the branchial chambers seems to provide a normoxic stimulus to an externally placed oxygen receptor. Direct recordings of oxygen receptor discharge were described from nerves supplying the gills of the chelicerate arthropod *Limulus polyphemus* (Crabtree & Page, 1974), and similar un-published information from a crustacean was cited by McMahon & Wilkens (1983).

The ability to breathe air, which offers the advantage of a continuously high level of $PO_2$ but the problem of carbon dioxide elimination, might be expected to result in development of carbon dioxide sensitivity. This is foreshadowed in aquatic species. Normoxic crayfish show both a ventilatory and associated cardiac response to increases in dissolved carbon dioxide (Larimer, 1964). Land crabs respond to hypercapnia with an increase in ventilation, signifying that they are adapted to function as air-breathers (Cameron, 1975). Injection of buffered $CO_2$-rich saline into the coconut crab *Birgus latro* was without effect, but injection of an acid saline solution caused an immediate increase in ventilation rate, and recovery from post-exercise hyperventilation followed recovery in haemolymph pH values rather than $PCO_2$ (Smatresk & Cameron, 1981). This suggests sensitivity to internal pH (i.e. effectively $[H+]$ or $[HCO_3^-]$, which are components of strong ion difference (Stewart, 1978)) rather than $PCO_2$. A parallel may exist in the responses of the vertebrate medulla to the pH of the cerebrospinal fluid (Loeschcke, 1980) or the intracellular/extracellular pH gradient of chemosensory neurones in the brainstem (Kiwull-Schöne & Kiwull, 1983) which may be anticipated in the ventilatory responses of fishes to carbon dioxide, a sensitivity which may reside in the medulla (Shelton, 1970).

### 15.3.2. *Mechanoreceptors*

The respiratory muscles in fish contain length and tension receptors, in common with other vertebrate muscles (Butler & Metcalfe, 1983) and the gill arches bear a number of mechanoreceptors with various functional characteristics. Satchell & Way (1962) characterised mechanoreceptors on the branchial processes of the dogfish, and Sutterlin & Saunders (1969) described receptors on the gill filaments and gill rakers of the sea-raven. Mechanical stimulation of the gill arches is known to elicite the 'cough' reflex in fish (e.g. Satchell, 1959). These mechanoreceptors will be stimulated by the ventilatory movements of the gill arches and filaments, and afferent information reaching the brain in the IXth and Xth cranial nerves is known to influence the respiratory rhythm with breathing rate slowing in teleosts and increasing in elasmobranchs following transection of the branchial nerves or paralysis of the ventilatory muscles (Johansen, 1971; Barrett & Taylor, 1985a). Stimulation of branchial mechanoreceptors by increasing rates of water- flow may be the trigger for the cessation of active ventilatory movements during ram ventilation in fish (Johansen, 1971; Randall, 1982).

Although there are mechanoreceptors distributed profusely around the inhalent apertures and general surface of the branchial chambers in crustaceans, a leading role in the control of ventilation is played by the oval organ located on the scaphognathite. Imposed movements of the scaphognathite can entrain the central respiratory pacemaker neurones, as is described by Bush *et al.* in Chapter 4.

Historical evidence for the existence of baroreceptor-type responses in elasmobranchs, responsible for regulating blood pressure by reflex alteration of heart rate and peripheral vascular resistance, was reviewed by Johansen (1971). Recent studies on the dogfish, which involved repeated sampling and reinjection of blood, revealed that the resultant changes in blood pressure were largely uncompensated and that the reflex bradycardia induced by injecting 5–10 ml of hyperoxaemic blood did not compensate for the associated increase in blood pressure (Barrett & Taylor, 1984). In contrast, Wood & Shelton (1980) interpreted increases in heart rate during hypoxia in the trout, which paralleled reductions in arterial blood pressure induced by haemorrhage, as interaction between baroreceptor and chemoreceptor drive.

## 15.4. Control of ventilation

As described by Ballintijn in Chapter 1, the respiratory muscles in fish operate around the jaws and gill arches and are innervated by cranial nerves with their motoneurones in the brainstem. This complicates the differentiation between neurones generating the respiratory rhythm and the motoneurones they drive, which supply the respiratory muscles. Neurones which fire rhythmically in phase with ventilation have been located throughout the medulla oblongata of fish, and are adequately described by Ballintijn (1981) and in Chapter 1 of this volume. The neurones in the different motonuclei innervate muscles which generate the complex series of movements involved in ventilation. They all burst rhythmically, with phase relationships dependent upon the muscles they innervate. The phase relationship of activity in the respiratory motoneurones has been monitored as the efferent activity in the nerves supplying the ventilatory muscles (Barrett & Taylor, 1985a). In the dogfish the onset of bursts of activity in the mandibular branch of the Vth cranial nerve supplying muscles in the jaw preceded activity in the glossopharyngeal IXth which innervates the 1st gill arch by a mean of 152 ms. This in turn preceded activity in the four branchial branches of the Xth vagus nerve, which fired simultaneously, by about 30 ms. This independent innervation of the first gill arch may have a functional significance, as Grigg (1970b) found that during experimentally induced hypoxia the Port Jackson shark (*Heterodontus portusjacksoni*) used the first gill slit to admit inhalent water, which was expired from the other gill slits. This ability may enable the fish to continue gill ventilation while its mouth is obstructed during feeding.

The control of ventilation in decapodan crustaceans was reviewed by Taylor (1982), and most recently by Bush *et al.* in Chapter 4. The two scaphognathites supplying the branchial chambers on each side of the animal can beat independently at different intrinsic rates (Batterton & Cameron, 1978). During active forward ventilation of the branchial chambers there is often significant phase coupling between the ventilatory cycles of the two scaphognathites following either drift and lock or absolute phase-locked co-ordination (Wilkens & Young, 1975; Young & Coyer, 1979). Often the scaphognathites beat in synchrony, but other phase relationships also occur. This may imply some advantage from coupling of the rhythms which could result in increased stability and regularity of pumping (Young & Coyer, 1979). Cross-ganglionic motoneuronal processes which could mediate this co-ordination have been described in the lobster (Wilkens & Young, 1975). In settled, inactive animals ventilation may become unilateral for long periods in both water-breathers (McDonald *et al.*, 1977; Butler *et al.*, 1978) and air-breathers (Wood & Randall, 1981). Brief reversals of ventilation may occur simultaneously on both sides or independently (Taylor *et al.*, 1973; Batterton & Cameron, 1978).

### 15.5. Control of the heart and branchial circulation

The fish heart is composed of typical vertebrate cardiac muscle fibres with contraction initiated by a propagated muscle action potential from a myogenic pacemaker and generating a characteristic ECG waveform (Randall, 1968; Satchell, 1971). Heart beat is influenced by intrinsic mechanisms such as the relationship between the force of contraction and stretch applied to the muscle fibres, known as the Frank–Starling relationship. The increase in diastolic filling time, which accompanies cardiac slowing, can, therefore, result in an increase in cardiac stroke volume. Short *et al.* (1977) concluded that the compensatory increases in cardiac stroke volume which maintained cardiac output in the dogfish during a hypoxic bradycardia (see Fig. 15.1) were wholly attributable to the Frank–Starling relationship, and this represents a self-regulating feature of cardiac function.

The heart is supplied with inhibitory parasympathetic innervation via the vagus nerve, which terminates on the heart as a plexus of fibres limited to the sinus venosus in elasmobranchs (Young, 1933) but spreading over the atrium in teleosts (Young, 1936). The inhibitory effect is mediated via muscarinic cholinoreceptors associated with the pacemaker and myocardium (Holmgren, 1977, and see Chapter 5). Recently inhibitory purinoceptors have been detected in the dogfish atrium (Meghji & Burnstock, 1984). The heart typically operates under a degree of inhibitory vagal tone which varies with physiological state and environmental conditions. In the dogfish, cholinergic vagal tone, assessed as the proportional change in heart rate following injection of atropine (which blocks muscarinic receptors), increased with an increasing temperature of acclimation (Taylor *et al.*, 1977). Heart rate in dogfish restrained in a standard set of experimental conditions at 15–17°C varied directly with $PO_2$, so that hypoxia induced a reflex bradycardia and a normoxic vagal tone was released by exposure to moderate hyperoxia (Taylor *et al.*, 1977; Barrett & Taylor, 1984). These data imply that the level of vagal tone of the heart in dogfish is determined peripherally by graded stimulation of $PO_2$ receptors, and variations in this inhibitory tone may result in a reflex bradycardia or tachycardia. There is little morphological or physiological evidence for sympathetic innervation of the elasmobranch heart though it remains possible that some degree of cardioregulation may be exercised by catecholamines, released by activity in sympathetic preganglionic fibres from the chromaffin tissue located in the posterior cardinal sinus, and released directly into the venous drainage to the heart (Johansen, 1971). The levels of circulating catecholamines are extremely high in the dogfish, possibly in some way compensating for the lack of sympathetic innervation of the heart and gills, and the levels increase during hypoxia (Butler *et al.*, 1979). Their major effect on oxygen uptake may be vasodilatation of the branchial vasculature (Capra & Satchell, 1977), and an intrinsic vasoconstriction during deep hypoxia (Satchell, 1962) may be released by a rise in circulating catecholamines (Butler *et al.*, 1979).

In teleosts, the heart receives both a cholinergic vagal supply and an adrenergic sympathetic supply. Goldfish at 25°C had a calculated parasympathetic tone (released by atropine) of 66% of intrinsic heart rate whilst sympathetic tone was 22% and a rapid cardioacceleration induced by enforced swimming was abolished by the sympathetic β-antagonist propranalol (Cameron, 1979). In the trout, vagal tone on the heart, although higher than in the dogfish at all temperatures, decreased at higher temperatures, but the cardioacceleration induced by adrenaline injection into atropinised fish increased with temperature (Wood *et al.*, 1979). A normoxic vagal tone was absent in trout stressed by experimental conditions (Wood & Shelton, 1980). There are sympathetic ganglia associated with cranial nerves IX and X in teleosts, and the branchial nerves are mixed vago-glossopharyngeo–sympathetic trunks (Nilsson, 1983). Stimulation of these nerves may produce a cholinergically mediated constriction. of the respiratory arterio-arterial pathway whereas stimulation of the adrenergic fibres favours blood flow through this respiratory route rather than the parallel, non-respiratory arterio-venous route. Despite the clear demonstration of mixed autonomic innervation of the heart and branchial vasculature in teleosts, it remains probable that much of the functional control of gill perfusion is exercised via circulating catecholamines (Nilsson, 1983, and see Chapter 5), as is the case in elasmobranchs.

The existence of a varying level of inhibitory vagal tone on the heart of the experimentally restrained dogfish prompted our investigation of vagal output to the heart. The heart in the dogfish is supplied with two pairs of cardiac vagi: a branchial cardiac branch leaves the fourth branchial nerve and a visceral cardiac branch is supplied from the visceral branch of the vagus, on either side of the animal (Taylor *et al.*, 1977). Experiments involving transection and electrical stimulation of these nerves revealed that the branchial cardiac branches are more effective in cardioinhibition than the visceral cardiac branches (Short *et al.*, 1977), accounting for the majority of normoxic vagal tone and the reflex bradycardia during hypoxia. Recordings from a branchial cardiac branch contained high levels of spontaneous efferent activity, separable into two types of unit. Some, typically smaller, units fired sporadically and increased their firing rate during hypoxia (Fig. 15.4a). These non-bursting units seem to play the major role in initiating the reflex hypoxic bradycardia, and may also determine the overall level of vagal tone on the heart. Other, larger units fired in rhythmical bursts which were synchronous with ventilatory movements (Taylor & Butler, 1982). These bursts were synchronous with efferent activity in branchial branches of the vagus which innervate respiratory muscles and continued in decerebrate dogfish after treatment with curare which stopped ventilatory movements (Fig. 15.4b).

This evidence suggests that the bursting activity recorded from the cardiac vagus originates in the CNS through some interaction, either direct or indirect, with the respiratory rhythm generator (RRG). The vagal topography of the motor column in the dogfish has been described in detail by Withington-Wray *et al.* in Chapter 16. The majority of vagal motoneurones are located medially, close to the wall of the fourth ventricle, but the branchial cardiac branch supplying the heart is unique in having some of its cardiac vagal motoneurones (CVM) located as a ventro-lateral group which supply axons solely to this branch of the vagus (Barrett & Taylor, 1985b). Extracellular recordings from CVM identified in the hindbrain of decerebrate, paralysed dogfish by antidromic stimulation of a branchial cardiac branch revealed that neurones located in the medial division were spontaneously active, firing in rhythmical bursts which contributed to the bursts recorded from the intact nerve (Fig. 15.5). Neurones located in the ventro-lateral division were either spontaneously active, firing regularly or sporadically but never rhythmically, or were silent (Barrett & Taylor, 1985c). It seems that the two types of efferent activity described in the branchial cardiac branches of the vagus have separate origins in the CNS which may indicate a separation of function. All of the spontaneously active CVM from both divisions and some of the silent CVM fired in response to mechanical stimulation of a gill arch, which infers that they could be entrained to ventilatory movements in the spontaneously breathing fish and that both may be responsible for the reflex bradycardia recorded in response to mechanical stimulation (Taylor & Butler, 1982). Randall (1966) recorded bursting activity from the cardiac vagus of the tench, which he concluded could either originate peripherally from stimulation of receptors on the gills or bloodstream dorsal to the gills (i.e. efferent vessels) or may result from connections between the vagal and respiratory centres in the medulla.

The respiration-related bursting activity recorded from the medial group of CVM is of particular interest because respiratory modulation of CVM has

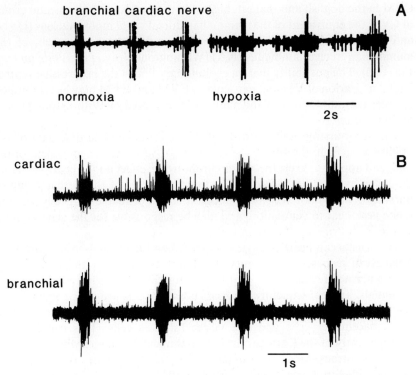

Fig. 15.4. (A) Efferent activity recorded from a cardiac branch of the vagus of a decerebrate dogfish at 15°C in normoxia ($P_IO_2$ 150 mmHg) and hypoxia ($P_IO_2$ 45 mmHg). The smaller, sporadically firing units increased firing rate during hypoxia. The large, bursting units were unaffected by hypoxia. (From Taylor & Butler, 1982.) (B) Simultaneous recordings of activity from the cardiac branch (cardiac) and 3rd branchial branch (branchial) of the vagus on the left side of a decerebrate, curarised dogfish. The animal was continuously ventilated with a stream of hyperoxic water in the absence of normal ventilatory movements. The persistence of rhythmic bursting activity in both nerves indicates that it is generated in the CNS .and not by mechanoreceptors on the gill arches. (From Barrett & Taylor, 1985a.)

been observed in mammals (Spyer, 1982). This modulation, which is the central origin of sinus arrhythmia in the mammal, is thought to arise from direct, inhibitory synaptic contact between collaterals from respiratory vagal motoneurones (RVM) and CVM, and this relationship is described by Jordan & Spyer in Chapter 17. Direct connections between bursting CVM and RVM are possible in the dogfish hindbrain as both are located in the medial division of the vagal motor column with an overlapping rostrocaudal distribution (Barrett *et al.*, 1985). As the bursts are synchronous (Fig. 15.5b) the innervation of CVM is likely to be excitatory rather than inhibitory, and it is equally possible that a direct drive from the RRG operates on the RVM and the CVM. There is a possible parallel between the distribution of

CVM in the dogfish and that established in mammals, with the medial group of CVM the equivalent of the mammalian dorsal vagal motor nucleus (DVN) and the ventro-lateral group the possible evolutionary antecedent of the mammalian nucleus ambiguus (NA) (Withington-Wray *et al.*, 1986; and see Fig. 15.5). The possibility that an evolutionary line in the progressive ventro-lateral migration of VM and particularly CVM and RVM may be established between elasmobranch fish and mammals is explored by Withington-Wray *et al.* in Chapter 16.

The non-bursting units recorded from the branchial cardiac vagi of the dogfish arise from the ventro-lateral group of VM (i.e. the equivalent of the NA) and appear to exert the major chronotropic effect on the heart including the reflex hypoxic bradycardia. The functional role of the medial group of bursting CVM is not yet clear, though it seems probable that they serve to relate heartbeat to ventilation, and may be responsible for the generation of cardiorespiratory synchrony in fish.

The crustacean heart is single-chambered and beats at systole against the elasticity of suspensory ligaments. It responds to stretch by an increase in the force and rate of contraction. Crustacean muscle fibres do not conduct action potentials, and consequently the heart possesses a neurogenic pacemaker in the form of a cardiac ganglion typically consisting of nine neurones, four small pacemaker cells and five larger follower cells. This can function independently of the CNS, producing rhythmical discharges which cause the heart to contract. An account of pacemaker function in the crustacean heart was provided in a recent review (Taylor, 1982).

The crustacean heart receives inhibitor and accelerator nerves from either the suboesophageal or thoracic ganglia which run in separate trunks to the pericardial sinus where some axons supply a pair of neurohaemal, pericardial organs, others supply a plexus on the suspensory ligaments, and one fibre from each trunk is combined into a dorsal nerve which enters the heart to innervate the cardiac ganglion (Maynard, 1960; Taylor, 1982). Peripheral electrical stimulation of the inhibitor nerve trunks causes a marked brady-cardia. The inhibitory transmitter may be aminobutyric acid. Stimulation of the accelerators causes a tachycardia which is mimicked by acetylcholine, though the transmitter is possibly an indolalkylamine (Florey, 1963). Maynard (1960) concluded that the cardioregulatory nerves were probably involved in brief reflex inhibition and acceleration of the heart. They are, however, continuously active in the prepared animal (Taylor, 1970; Field & Larimer, 1975; Young, 1978), and may exert a tonic control over heart rate similar to the vagal tone operating on the fish heart.

The cardioregulatory effects are imposed directly upon the cardiac gan-glion. Intracellular recordings from large follower cells in *Panulirus inter-ruptus* included i.p.s.p. resulting from stimulation of inhibitor nerve trunks which were either hyperpolarising or depolarising depending upon the membrane potential, and showed both facilitation and summation. Stimula-

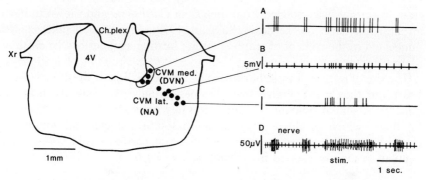

Fig. 15.5. Schematic diagram of the location and properties of cardiac vagal motoneurones (CVM, ●) in the hindbrain of the dogfish. The representative section of the medulla is taken just rostral of obex. All CVM in a medial location (med.) were spontaneously active, firing rhythmically (A) and contributing to the efferent bursting activity recorded from the cardiac branch of the vagus (nerve, D). CVM in the ventrolateral group (lat.) were divided into spontaneously active neurones which fired regularly or sporadically but did not burst (B), or normally silent units (C) which fired in response to mechanical stimulation of the gill septa (stim.), as did all the spontaneously active units. Other silent ventrolateral CVM did not respond to mechanical stimulation and are not represented on the diagram. The medial group of motoneurones (CVM med.) may represent the homologue of the mammalian dorsal vagal motor nucleus (DVN), and the ventrolateral group (CVM lat.) may represent a primitive form of the mammalian nucleus ambiguous (NA). Ch. plex., choroid plexus; 4V, fourth ventricle; Xr, vagal rootlet.

tion of the inhibitor nerves typically caused a drop in the frequency of the trains of impulses from the ganglion plus a reduction in the number and frequency of impulses within each train (Maynard, 1961).

The pericardial organs (PO) located in the pericardial space on either side of the heart, which receive axons from the cardioregulatory nerve trunks, appear to be directly involved in hormonal control of the heart. Extracts of PO increase the frequency and amplitude of heartbeat and may restore steady beating to an arrhythmic preparation (Alexandrowicz & Carlisle, 1953). Cooke (1966) identified the site of action of the extracts as the cardiac ganglion. Electrical stimulation of the PO caused graded cardioacceleration proportional to the number of stimuli given (Cooke, 1964).

The effect of PO extract was mimicked by 5-hydroxytryptamine (5HT) (Carlisle, 1956; Maynard & Welsh, 1959), and the PO produces a range of biogenic amines including HT, octopamine and dopamine. All three amines cause cardioacceleration in the crayfish *Astacus leptodactylus*, with HT the most effective (Florey & Rathmayer, 1978). Berlind & Cooke (1968) concluded that 5HT and dopamine levels in the PO of *Libinia* were too low to be effective in cardioregulation, and attributed this role to peptides released from the PO by electrical stimulation at levels causing cardioacceleration. A substance similar in properties to proctolin, a putative peptide transmitter from insect gut, was isolated from the PO of *Cardisoma* and shown to have an inotropic effect on the heart (Sullivan, 1979). This neuropeptide is also implicated in the control of scaphognathite beating as described by Bush *et al.* in Chapter 4.

The site of release of these hormones by the PO is directly up stream of the heart and they are aspirated from the pericardial space into the heart at diastole. A similar functional location was described above for the chromaffin tissue which produces biogenic amines into the cardinal sinuses of elasmobranch fishes. Tonic control of heart rate, cardiac stroke volume and ventilation may be exerted by hormones released from the PO.

## 15.6. Cardio-respiratory interactions

A link between heartbeat and ventilation in fish was first noted by Schoenlein in 1985 (reported by Satchell, 1960) who described 1 : 1 synchrony in *Torpedo marmorata*. This observation has recently been repeated (Taylor, 1985). Lutz (1930) demonstrated that the cardiac vagus was involved in the maintenance of this link, and a full account of the reflex co-ordination of heartbeat with ventilation in the dogfish was published by Satchell (1960) who concluded that co-ordination was reflexly controlled, with mechanoreceptors on the ventilatory apparatus constituting the afferent limb and the cardiac vagus the efferent limb of a reflex arc. Just as sinus arrhythmia in mammals was previously attributed to stimulation of lung receptors and baroreceptors and is now known to be at least partially centrally generated, cardiorespiratory synchrony in the dogfish could originate centrally with the respiration-related bursting units causing the heart to beat in a particular phase of the ventilatory cycle.

The supposed functional significance of cardiorespiratory synchrony relates to the importance of matching relative flow rates of water and blood over the counter-current at the gill lamellae. Although virtually continuous, both water and blood flow (see Fig. 15.1) over the lamellae are markedly pulsatile. Recordings of differential blood pressure and gill opacity in the dogfish revealed a brief period of rapid blood flow through the lamellae early in each cardiac cycle (Satchell, 1960), and as the ECG tended to occur at or near the mouth-opening phase of the ventilatory cycle, this could result in coincidence of the periods of maximum flow rate of blood and water during each cardiac cycle (Shelton, 1970). The improvement in gill perfusion and consequent oxygen transfer resulting from changes in transmural pressure and intralamellar blood flow, described by Farrell *et al.* (1980), may be further improved by synchronisation of the pressure pulses associated with ventilation and perfusion. Cardiorespiratory synchrony may by a combination of these effects increase the relative efficiency of respiratory gas exchange (i.e. maximum exchange for minimum work).

One problem with this proposal is that ventilation rate is often faster than

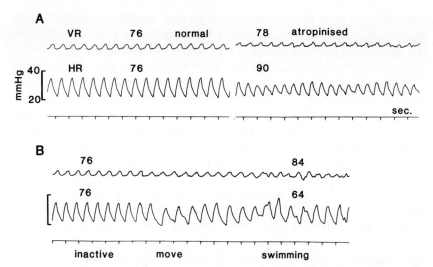

Fig. 15.6. (A) Ventilation rate (VR) measured as water pressure in the orobranchial chamber, and heart rate (HR) measured as ventral aortic blood pressure, recorded from an unrestrained dogfish enclosed in a large tank of running sea water at 23°C. When the animal was stationary, resting on the bottom of the tank (normal), the two rates (beats min$^{-1}$) were identical and synchronous. Atropinisation caused an increase in heart rate and loss of synchrony. (B) When the normal, inactive animal moved (move), then spontaneously commenced gently swimming around the tank (swimming), it showed a bradycardia and an increase in ventilation rate. Consequently, ventilation became faster than heart beat, a condition characteristic of disturbed or experimentally restrained animals. (From Taylor, 1985.)

heart rate. In the restrained dogfish, ventilation rate was approximately twice heart rate, and they showed a drifting relationship (Taylor & Butler, 1971). The absence of synchrony, or even consistent close coupling, as opposed to a drifting phase relationship, was most often attributable to changes in heart rate, which was more variable than ventilation rate (Taylor & Butler, 1971; Hughes, 1972). This may be reliably interpreted in the dogfish as variations in cardiac vagal tone possibly exerted by changes in the rate of firing of the non-bursting units recorded from the branchial cardiac nerves. Activity in these units is high in the restrained dogfish when cardiorespiratory synchrony is absent (Taylor & Butler, 1971, 1982). A decrease in vagal tone on the heart, such as that recorded during exposure to moderately hyperoxic water (Fig. 15.2), causes heart rate to rise towards ventilation rate, suggesting that in the undisturbed fish a 1:1 synchrony may occur. This proves to be the case. When dogfish were allowed to settle in large tanks of running, aerated sea water at 23°C, they showed 1:1 synchrony between heartbeat and ventilation for long periods (Taylor & Barrett, 1985). This relationship was abolished by atropine (Fig. 15.6a), confirming the role of the vagus in the maintenance of synchrony and providing a hypothetical role for the bursting units recorded from the cardiac vagi. Whenever the fish was spontaneously active or disturbed, the relationship broke down due to a reflex bradycardia and acceleration of ventilation (Fig. 15.6b). In disturbed fish the 2:1 relationship between ventilation and heart rate characteristic of the experimentally restrained animal was re-established (Fig. 15.7) and it is possible that the elusiveness of data supporting the proposed existence of cardiorespiratory synchrony is due to experimental procedures which increase vagal tone on the heart exerted by the non-bursting units, and mask the more subtle control exerted by the bursting units recorded from the cardiac vagi. Short periods of 1:1 synchrony were observed in unrestrained cod (Jones *et al.*, 1974). If this hypothesis can be validated, then synchrony may serve to maximise the efficiency of respiratory gas exchange in the 'resting' animal. In the dogfish at least, this probably represents a large proportion of their lifespan because they are observably rather inactive animals, spending a lot of time resting on the substratum, both in aquaria and on the sea bed. Synchrony may yet be observed in cruising fish, as gentle swimming movements, due to contraction of lateral bands of aerobic red muscle, may often entrain to the ventilatory rhythm (Satchell, 1968), but the relationship breaks down in 'disturbed' animals using the large blocks of anaerobic white muscle for sprint swimming. In the trout, synchrony between heart and breathing cycles was induced by hypoxia and abolished by atropine (Randall & Smith, 1967).

This whole discussion is of course hypothetical because we need to know much more in detail about the beat-by-beat control of ventilation and blood flow over the surfaces of the gill lamellae and the resultant instantaneous effects on respiratory gas exchange before the significance of cardiorespiratory synchrony can be properly understood. What emerges from current work is that a potent mechanism for the generation of cardiorespiratory synchrony in fish may exist in the form of the bursting units present in recordings of efferent activity in the cardiac vagi. Stimulation of the vagus nerves of the dog with brief bursts of stimuli, similar to those recorded from efferent vagal fibres to the heart, caused heartbeat to synchronise with the stimulus, beating once for each vagal stimulus burst over a wide frequency range (Levy & Martin, 1984). Similar entrainment with the bursts of activity recorded from the cardiac vagi could explain the 1:1 synchrony observed in 'settled' dogfish. The apparent loose coupling observed in 'disturbed' animals may arise from interactions between the effects of the bursting and non-bursting units when vagal tone is relatively high and the non-bursting units are active.

The control and co-ordination of bilateral ventilation in crustaceans and its relation to perfusion of the gills with haemolymph delivered by the heart has been the subject of a number of studies. Hypoxic or hypercapnic water and solutions of glucose, L-glutamic acid or NaCl applied externally to one side or into the ventilatory stream of the crayfish *Procambarus simulans*

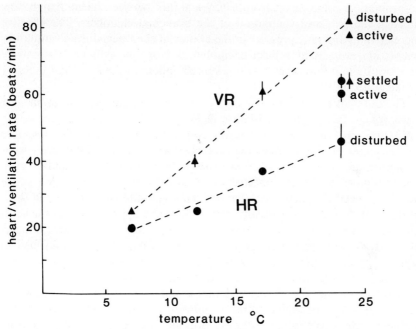

Fig. 15.7.   Heart rate (HR, ●) and ventilation rate (VR, ▲) in the dogfish at a range of acclimation temperatures. At 7°C, 12°C and 17°C, ventilation rate was higher than heart rate in restrained animals. At 23°C, unrestrained animals allowed to settle in large tanks of running sea water (settled) had identical mean rates of VR and HR (64 ± 2 beats min$^{-1}$). Spontaneous bouts of slow swimming (active) were accompanied by an increase in ventilation rate and a slight bradycardia. Disturbed fish (disturbed) showed a further small increase in VR and a marked bradycardia. These disturbed fish had a VR which was approximately twice HR, as reported in restrained fish. The divided lines extrapolate the mean values for VR and HR in restrained animals through the values for disturbed animals at 23°C. Clearly, cardiorespiratory synchrony is characteristic of resting, unrestrained fish. (From Taylor, 1985.)

produced inhibition of the homolateral scaphognathite accompanied by a simultaneous bradycardia or brief cardiac arrest (Larimer, 1964; Ashby & Larimer, 1965). This demonstrates that the scaphognathites can function separately and that changes in their activity are often reflected in responses of the heart. Settling after a period of disturbance is often accompanied by a progressive reduction in ventilation and heart rates culminating in long periods of unilateral ventilation, respiratory pauses and an irregular heartbeat (e.g. McDonald *et al.*, 1977; Butler *et al.*, 1978). Exposure to diluted seawater caused a cardioacceleration, typically accompanied by a slowing in scaphognathite beating in *Carcinus maenas* (Hume & Berlind, 1976) whereas hypoxia typically results in a bradycardia and hyperventilation, as described above. Ventilatory pauses and reversals are often accompanied by changes in heart rate (e.g. McMahon & Wilkens, 1972; Taylor *et al.*, 1973). Part of this co-ordination could result from a physical link between haemolymph flow through the gills and ventilation of the branchial chambers. The effective increase in hydrostatic pressure in the branchial chambers during ventilatory pauses or reversals may flush haemolymph from the gills or alternatively temporarily halt flow when noxious stimuli appear at the gills (McMahon & Wilkens, 1977).

The onset of a respiratory pause is often accompanied by an immediate reduction in heart rate (McMahon & Wilkens, 1972, 1977; Taylor *et al.*, 1973, and see Fig. 15.8). The closely co-ordinated nature of this response suggests a neural link between the ventilatory oscillators and the cardioregulatory centres in the CNS. Wilkens *et al.* (1974) identified command fibres in the circumoesophageal connectives of *Cancer magister* which were active during induced changes in cardiac or scaphognathite rhythms. When these fibres were stimulated electrically, 69% produced responses in both the heart and scaphognathites, 28% in scaphognathites alone, and 3% in the heart alone. By varying the frequency of electrical stimulation, they established an order of response thresholds for both the heart and scaphognathites in the sequences: bradycardia < cardiac arrest and decreased rate and amplitude of forward ventilation < reversed ventilation < ventilatory pause, which resembled observed behavioural responses to increasing levels of disturbance. Reversals often followed stimulation of one command fibre whereas pauses required high-frequency stimulation of several fibres, inferring the involvement of both spatial and temporal summation. The sequence of responses and their co-ordination implied an endogenous programme as suggested by McMahon & Wilkens (1977).

Presumably the command fibres stimulated by Wilkens *et al.* (1974) are the same as those separately identified as affecting the cardioregulatory centres (Wiersma & Novitski, 1942) and the central ventilatory oscillator (Mendelson, 1971). The majority of them are bivalent, innervating two anatomically distinct but functionally correlated systems. Very few command fibres affected the heart alone, and 90% of them caused cardioinhibition which is a common response to sudden disturbance in crustaceans (McMahon & Wilkens, 1972; Wilkens *et al.*, 1974).

A prolonged burst of activity in the cardioinhibitory nerve of the lobster, *Nephrops norvegicus*, caused initial cardiac arrest, followed by adaptation and a postinhibitory rebound, plus persistent cessation of ventilation (Young, 1978). Continuous recordings revealed an inverse relationship between ventilation and activity in the cardioinhibitory nerves, indicating that the cardioregulatory centre interacts with the ventilatory pacemaker. In *Portunus* bursts of activity in the cardioinhibitor nerve may be associated with ventilatory reversals rather than pauses, which agrees with the observations that reversals in *Carcinus* are often accompanied by cardiac arrest (Taylor *et al.*, 1973). Spiking activity in cardioregulator nerves often occurs in preferred phases of the ventilatory cycle (Young, 1978), which is a possible

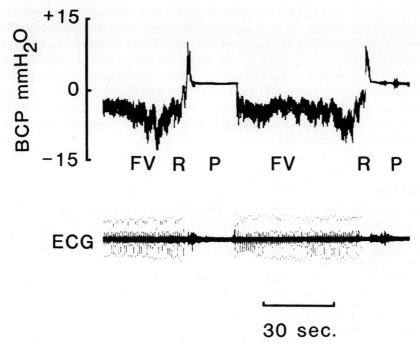

Fig. 15.8. *Carcinus maenas*, the shore crab. Recordings of pressure changes from the left branchial chamber (BCP) and heart rate as ECG. The inactive crab was submerged in normoxic sea water and ventilating the gills in the normal, forwardly directed mode (FV). After a brief reversal of ventilation pressure (R) it exhibited a short pause (P) when the scaphognathite stopped beating, branchial pressure became identical to ambient pressure and ventilation ceased. The pause was accompanied by an immediate cardiac arrest indicating a neural link between the ventilatory oscillator in the CNS and central control of heart rate.

basis for the bimodal and trimodal phase coupling between the heart and scaphognathites described by Young & Coyer (1979).

## 15.7. Conclusion

Both fish and crustaceans can sustain relatively high levels of aerobic activity in their aquatic habitat by virtue of the highly effective transfer of oxygen over the counter-current of water and blood at their gills. Because the counter-current can establish an intimate relationship between oxygen levels in water and blood ($P_aO_2 \simeq P_1O_2$), there is a further significant adaptive advantage to maximising the effectiveness of oxygen transfer by careful control of relative flow rates of water and blood, according to their relative capacities for oxygen. Except for periodic pauses or reversals (coughs), both water flow and blood flow are unidirectional and continuous but pulsatile.

Evidence of beat-by-beat co-ordination between ventilatory and cardiac rhythms is available for both groups of animals. Cardiorespiratory synchrony, with concurrence of periods of maximum blood flow and water flow at the exchange surfaces, may be an important mechanism increasing the efficiency of oxygen transfer in resting fishes (i.e. maximum exchange for minimum effort). The neural mechanisms establishing this relationship are beginning to be described and understood, though more work is needed before we can compare them with those described in greater detail for mammals.

## References

Alexandrowicz, J. S. & Carlisle, D. B. (1953). some experiments on the function of the pericardial organs in Crustacea. *J. Mar. Biol. Assn UK* **32**, 175–92.

Ashby, E. A. & Larimer, J. L. (1965). Modification of cardiac and respiratory rhythms in crayfish following carbohydrate chemoreception. *J. Cell. Comp. Physiol.* **65**, 373–80.

Ballintijn, C. M. (1981). Neural control of respiration in fish and mammals. In *Exogenous and Endogenous Influences on Metabolic and Neural Control* (eds A. D. F. Addink & N. Spronk). Oxford: Pergamon Press.

Bamford, O. S. (1974). Oxygen reception in the rainbow trout *Salmo gairdneri*. *Comp. Biochem. Physiol.* **48A**, 69–76.

Barrett, D. J. & Taylor, E. W. (1984). Changes in heart rate during progressive hyperoxia in the dogfish *Scyliorhinus canicula* L.: evidence for a venous oxygen receptor. *Comp. Biochem. Physiol.* **78A**, 697–703.

Barrett, D. J. & Taylor, E. W. (1985a). Spontaneous efferent activity in branches of the vagus nerve controlling heart rate and ventilation in the dogfish. *J. Exp. Biol.* **117**, 433–48.

Barrett, D. J. & Taylor, E. W. (1985b). The location of cardiac vagal preganglionic neurones in the brainstem of the dogfish. *J. Exp. Biol.* **117**, 449–58.

Barrett, D. J. & Taylor, E. W. (1985c). The characteristics of cardiac vagal preganglionic motoneurones in the dogfish. *J. Exp. Biol.* **117**, 459–70.

Batterton, C. V. & Cameron, J. N. (1978). Characteristics of resting ventilation and response to hypoxia, hypercapnia and emersion in the blue crab *Callinectes sapidus* (Rathbun). *J. Exp. Zool.* **203**, 403–18.

Berlind, A. & Cooke, I. M. (1968). Effect of calcium omission on neurosecretion and electrical activity of crab pericardial organs. *Gen. Comp. Endocrinol.* **11**, 458–63.

Booth, J. H. (1979). The effects of oxygen supply, epinephrine and acetylcholine on the distribution of blood flow in trout gills. *J. Exp. Biol.* **83**, 31–9.

Butler, P. J. & Metcalfe, J. D. (1983). Control of respiration and circulation. In *Control Processes in Fish Physiology* (eds J. C. Rankin, T. J. Pitcher & R. J. Duggan). London: Croom Helm.

Butler, P. J. & Taylor, E. W. (1971). Response of the dogfish (*Scyliorhinus canicula* L.) to slowly induced and rapidly induced hypoxia. *Comp. Biochem. Physiol.* **39A**, 307–23.

Butler, P. J. & Taylor, E. W. (1975). The effect of progressive hypoxia on respiration in the dogfish (*Scyliorhinus canicula*) at different seasonal temperatures. *J. Exp. Biol.* **63**, 117–30.

Butler, P. J. Taylor, E. W. & Davison, W. (1979). The effect of long-term moderate hypoxia on acid–base balance, plasma catecholamines and possible anaerobic end products in the unrestrained dogfish, *Scyliorhinus canicula*. *J. Comp. Physiol. B* **132**, 297–303.

Butler, P. J., Taylor, E. W. & McMahon, B. R. (1978). Respiratory and circulatory changes in the lobster (*Homarus vulgaris*) during long-term exposure to moderate hypoxia. *J. Exp. Biol.* **73**, 131–46.

Butler, P. J., Taylor, E. W. & Short, S. (1977). The effect of sectioning cranial nerves ,V, VII, IX and X on the cardiac response of the dogfish *Scyliorhinus canicula* to environmental hypoxia. *J. Exp. Biol.* **69**, 233–45.

Cameron, J. N. (1975). Aerial gas exchange in the terrestrial Brachyura *Gecarcinus lateralis* and *Cardisoma guanhumi*. *Comp. Biochem. Physiol.* **52A**, 1290–34.

Cameron, J. S. (1979). Autonomic nervous tone and regulation of heart rate in the goldfish, *Carassius auratus*. *Comp. Biochem. Physiol.* **63C**, 341–9.

Cameron, J. N. & Davis, J. C. (1970). Gas exchange in rainbow trout with varying blood oxygen capacity. *J. Fish. Res. Bd Can.* **27**, 1069–85.

Capra, M. F. & Satchell, G. H. (1977). The adrenergic responses of isolated saline-perfused prebranchial arteries and gills of the elasmobranch *Squalus acanthias*. *Gen. Pharmacol.* **8**, 67–71.

Carlisle, D. B. (1956). An indole alkylamine regulating heart beat in Crustacea. *Biochem. J.* **63**, 32–3P.

Cooke, I. C. R. (1980). Functional aspects of the morphology and vascular anatomy of the gills of the Endeavour dogfish *Centrophorus scalpratus* (McCulloch) (Elasmobranchii: Squalidae). *Zoomorphologie* **94**, 167–83.

Cooke, I. M. (1964). Electrical activity and release of neurosecretory material in crab pericardial organs. *Comp. Biochem. Physiol.* **13**, 353–66.

Cooke, I. M. (1966). The sites of action of pericardial organ extract and 5-hydroxytryptamine in the decapod crustacean heart. *Am. Zool.* **6**, 107–21.

Crabtree, R. L. & Page, C. H. (1974). Oxygen sensitive elements in the bookgills of *Limulus polyphemus*. *J. Exp. Biol.* **60**, 631–41.

Daxboeck, C. & Holeton, G. F. (1978). Oxygen receptors in the rainbow trout, *Salmo gairdneri*. *Can. J. Zool.* **56**, 1254–9.

Dejours, P. (1975). *Principles of Comparative Respiratory Physiology*. New York: American Elsevier Publishing Co.

Dunel, S. & Laurent, P. (1980). Functional organisation of the gill vasculature in different classes of fish. In *Epithelial Transport in the Lower Vertebrates* (ed. B. Lahlou). Cambridge: Cambridge University Press.

Eclancher, B. & Dejours, P. (1975). Control de la respiration chez les poissons teleosteens: existence de chemorecepteurs physiologiquement analogues aux chemorecepteurs des vertebres superieurs. *C. r. Acad. Sci. Paris*, Ser. D **280**, 451–3.

Farrell, A. P., Sobin, S. S., Randall, D. J. & Crosby, S. (1980). Interlamellar blood flow patterns in fish gills. *Am. J. Physiol.* **239**, R428–36.

Field, L. H. & Larimer, J. L. (1975). The cardioregulatory system of crayfish: neuroanatomy and physiology. *J. Exp. Biol.* **62**, 519–30.

Florey, E. (1963). Pharmacology of the crayfish heart. In *Problems in Biology* (ed. G. A. Kerkut). Oxford: Pergamon Press.

Florey, E. & Rathmayer, M. (1978). The effects of octopamine and other amines on heart and on neuromuscular transmission in decapod crustaceans: further evidence for role as neurohormone. *Comp. Biochem. Physiol.* **61C**, 229–37.

Grigg, G. C. (1970a). Water flow through the gills of Port Jackson sharks. *J. Exp. Biol.* **52**, 565–8.

Grigg, G. C. (1970b). Use of the first gill slits for water intake in a shark. *J. Exp. Biol.* **52**, 569–74.

Holeton, G. F. (1970). Oxygen uptake and circulation by a haemoglobinless Antarctic fish (*Chaenocephalus aceratus* Lomberg) compared with three red-blooded Antarctic fish. *Comp. Biochem. Physiol.* **34**, 457–71.

Holmgren, S. (1977). Regulation of the heart of a teleost, *Gadus morhua*, by autonomic nerves and circulating catecholamines. *Acta Physiol. Scand.* **99**, 62–74.

Hughes, G. M. (1964). Fish respiratory homeostasis. *Symp. Soc. Exp. Biol.* **18**, 81–107.

Hughes, G. M. (1972). The relationship between cardiac and respiratory rhythms in the dogfish, *Scyliorhinus canicula. J. Exp. Biol.* **57**, 415–34.

Hughes, G. M. & Shelton, G. (1962). Respiratory mechanisms and their nervous control in fish. *Adv. Comp. Physiol. Biochem.* **1**, 275–364.

Hughes, G. M., Knights, B. & Scammell, C. A. (1969). The distribution of $P_{O_2}$ and hydrostatic pressure changes within the branchial chambers in relation to gill ventilation of the shore crab *Carcinus maenas* L. *J. Exp. Biol.* **51**, 203–20.

Hume, R. I. & Berlind, A. (1976). Heart and scaphognathite rate changes in a euryhaline crab, *Carcinus maenas*, exposed to dilute environmental medium. *Biol. Bull. Mar. Biol. Lab., Woods Hole* **150**, 241–54.

Johansen, K. (1971). Comparative physiology: gas exchange and circulation in fishes. *Ann. Rev. Physiol.* **33**, 569–612.

Jones, J. R. E. (1952). The reactions of fish to water of low oxygen concentration. *J. Exp. Biol.* **29**, 403–15.

Jones, D. R. (1971). Theoretical analysis of factors which may limit the maximum oxygen uptake of fish: the oxygen cost of the cardiac and branchial pumps. *J. Theor. Biol.* **32**, 341–9.

Jones, D. R., Langille, B. L., Randall, D. J. & Shelton, G. (1974). Blood flow in dorsal and ventral aortas of the cod, *Gadus morhua. Am. J. Physiol.* **226**, 90–5.

Kiwull-Schöne, H. & Kiwull, P. (1983). Hypoxic modulation of central chemosensitivity. In *Central Neurone Environment* (eds M. E. Schlafke, H. P. Koepchen & W. R. See). Berlin: Springer-Verlag.

Larimer, J. L. (1964). Sensory-induced modifications of ventilation and heart rate in crayfish. *Comp. Biochem. Physiol.* **12**, 25–36.

Laurent, P. (1967). La pseudobranchie des teleostéens: preuves electrophysiologique de ses fonctions chemoreceptrice et baroreceptrice. *C. r. Acad. Sci. Paris*, Ser. D **264**, 1879–82.

Laurent, P. & Dunel, S. (1980). Morphology of gill epithelia in fish. *Am. J. Physiol.* **238**, R147–59.

Levy, M. N. & Martin, P. (1984). Parasympathetic control of the heart. In *Nervous Control of Cardiovascular Function* (ed. W. C. Randall). Oxford: Oxford University Press.

Loeschcke, H. H. (1980). Chemical alterations of cerebrospinal fluid acting on respiratory and circulatory control systems. In *Neurobiology of Cerebrospinal Fluid* (ed. J. H. Wood). New York: Plenum Press.

Lutz, B. R. (1930). Reflex cardiac and respiratory inhibition in the elasmobranch *Scyllium canicula. Biol. Bull., Woods Hole* 59, 170–8.

McDonald, D. G., McMahon, B. R. & Wood, C. M. (1977). An analysis of acid–base disturbances in the haemolymph following strenuous activity in the Dungeness crab *Cancer magister. J. Exp. Biol.* **79**, 47–58.

McMahon, B. R. & Wilkens, J. L. (1972). Simultaneous apnoea and bradycardia in the lobster *Homarus americanus. Can. J. Zool.* **50**, 165–70.

McMahon, B. R. & Wilkens, J. L. (1977). Periodic respiratory and circulatory performance in the red rock crab *Cancer products. J. Exp. Zool.* **202**, 363–74.

McMahon, B. R. & Wilkens, J. L. (1983). Ventilation, perfusion and oxygen uptake.

In *Biology of Crustacea* vol. 5 (eds L. H. Mantel & D. E. Bliss). New York: Academic Press.

Maynard, D. M. (1960). Circulation and heart function. In *The Physiology of Crustacea* (ed. T. H. Waterman). New York: Academic Press.

Maynard, D. M. (1961). Cardiac inhibition in decapod crustacea. In *Nervous Inhibitions*. Oxford: Pergamon.

Maynard, D. M. & Welsh, J. H. (1959). Neurohormones of the pericardial organs of brachyuran crustacea. *J. Physiol.* **149**, 215–27.

Meghji, P. & Burnstock, G. (1984). The effect of adenyl compounds on the heart of the dogfish, *Scyliorhinus canicula*. *Comp. Biochem. Physiol.* **77C**, 295–300.

Mendelson, J. (1971). Oscillator neurons in crustacean ganglia. *Science, N. Y.* **171**, 1170–3.

Metcalfe, J. D. & Butler, P. J. (1984). Changes in activity and ventilation in response to hypoxia in unrestrained, unoperated dogfish (*Scyliorhinus canicula*). *J. Exp. Biol.* **108**, 411–18.

Metcalfe, J. D. & Butler, P. J. (1985). The functional anatomy of the gills of the dogfish (*Scyliorhinus canicula*). *J. Zool. Lond.* **208**, 519–30.

Nilsson, S. (1983). *Autonomic Nerve Function in the Vertebrates*. Berlin: Springer-Verlag.

Piiper, J. & Scheid, P. (1975). Gas transport efficacy of gills, lungs and skin: theory and experimental data. *Resp. Physiol.* **23**, 209–21.

Piiper, J. & Schumann, D. (1967). Efficiency of $O_2$ exchange in the gills of the dogfish, *Scyliorhinus stellaris*. *Resp. Physiol.* **2**, 135–48.

Randall, D. J. (1966). The nervous control of cardiac activity in the tench (*Tinca tinca*) and the goldfish (*Carassius auratus*). *Physiol. Zool.* **39**, 185–92.

Randall, D. J. (1968). Functional morphology of the heart in fishes. *Am. Zool.* **8**, 179–89.

Randall, D. J. (1970). Gas exchange in fish. In *Fish Physiology* (eds W. S. Hoar & D. J. Randall). New York: Academic Press.

Randall, D. J. (1982). The control of respiration and circulation in fish during exercise and hypoxia. *J. Exp. Biol.* **100**, 275–88.

Randall, D. J. & Jones, D. R. (1973). The effect of deafferentation of the pseudobranch on the respiratory response to hypoxia of the trout (*Salmo gairdneri*). *Resp. Physiol.* **17**, 291–301.

Randall, D. J. & Shelton, G. (1963). The effects of changes in environmental gas concentrations on the breathing and heart rate of a teleost fish. *Comp. Biochem. Physiol.* **9**, 229–39.

Randall, D. J. & Smith, J. C. (1967). The regulation of cardiac activity in fish in a hypoxic environment. *Physiol. Zool.* **40**, 104–13.

Satchell, G. H. (1959). Respiratory reflexes in the dogfish. *J. Exp. Biol.* **36**, 62–71.

Satchell, G. H. (1960). The reflex co-ordination of the heart beat with respiration in the dogfish. *J. Exp. Biol.* **37**, 719–31.

Satchell, G. H. (1962). Intrinsic vasomotion in the dogfish gill. *J. Exp. Biol.* **39**, 503–12.

Satchell, G. H. (1968). A neurological basis for the co-ordination of swimming with respiration in fish. *Comp. Biochem. Physiol.* **27**, 835–41.

Satchell, G. H. (1971). *Circulation in Fishes*. Cambridge: Cambridge University Press.

Satchell, G. H. & Way, H. K. (1962). Pharyngeal proprioceptors in the dogfish *Squalus acanthias* L. *J. Exp. Biol.* **39**, 243–50.

Saunders, S. R. L. & Sutterlin, A. M. (1971). Cardiac and respiratory responses to hypoxia in the sea raven, *Hemitripterus americanus*, and an investigation of possible control mechanisms. *J. Fish. Res. Bd Can.* **28**, 491–503.

Shelton, G. (1970). The regulation of breathing. In *Fish Physiology*, vol. IV (eds W. S. Hoar & D. J. Randall). New York: Academic Press.

Short, S., Butler, P. J. & Taylor, E. W. (1977). The relative importance of nervous, humoral and intrinsic mechanisms in the regulation of heart rate and stroke volume in the dogfish *Scyliorhinus canicula*. *J. Exp. Biol.* **70**, 77–92.

Smatresk, N. J. & Cameron, J. N. (1981). Post-exercise acid–base balance and ventilatory control in *Birgus latro*, the coconut crab. *J. Exp. Zool.* **218**, 75–82.

Smith, F. M. & Jones, D. R. (1978). Localisation of receptors causing hypoxic bradycardia in trout (*Salmo gairdneri*) *Can. J. Zool.* **56**, 1260–5.

Spyer, K. M. (1982). Central nervous integration of cardiovascular control. *J. Exp. Biol.* **100**, 109–28.

Steen, J. B. & Kruysse, A. (1964). The respiratory function of teleostean gills. *Comp. Biochem. Physiol.* **12**, 127–42.

Stewart, P. A. (1978). Independent and dependent variables of acid–base control. *Resp. Physiol.* **33**, 9–26.

Sullivan, R. E. (1979). A proctolin-like peptide in crab pericardial organs. *J. Exp. Zool.* **210**, 543–52.

Sutterlin, A. M. & Saunders, R. L. (1969). Proprioceptors in the gills of teleosts. *Can. J. Zool.* **47**, 1209–12.

Taylor, E. W. (1970). Spntaneous activity in the cardioaccelerator nerves of the crayfish *Astacus pallipes* Lereboullet. *Comp. Biochem. Physiol.* **33**, 859–69.

Taylor, E. W. (1982). Control and co-ordination of ventilation and circulation in crustaceans: responses to hypoxia and exercise. *J. Exp. Biol.* **100**, 289–319.

Taylor, E. W. (1985). Control and co-ordination of gill ventilation and perfusion. *Symp. Soc. Exp. Biol.* **39**, 123–61.

Taylor, E. W. & Barrett, D. J. (1985). Evidence of a respiratory role for the hypoxic bradycardia in the dogfish *Scyliorhinus canicula* L. *Comp. Biochem. Physiol.* **80A**, 99–102.

Taylor, E. W. & Butler, P. J. (1971). Some observations on the relationship between heart beat and respiratory movements in the dogfish *Scyliorhinus canicula* L. *Comp. Biochem. Physiol.* **39A**, 297–305.

Taylor, E. W. & Butler, P. J. (1973). The behaviour and physiological responses of the shore crab *Carcinus maenas* during changes in environmental oxygen tension. *Neth. J. Sea Res.* **7**, 496–505.

Taylor, E. W. & Butler, P. J. (1978). Aquatic and aerial respiration in the shore crab *Carcinus maenas* (L.), acclimated to 15°C. *J. Comp. Physiol.* **127**, 315–23.

Taylor, E. W. & Butler, P. J. (1982). Nervous control of heart rate: activity in the cardiac vagus of the dogfish. *J. Appl. Physiol.* **53**, 1330–5.

Taylor, E. W., Butler, P. H. & Sherlock, P. J. (1973). The respiratory and cardiovascular changes associated with the emersion response of *Carcinus maenas* (L.) during environmental hypoxia, at three different temperatures. *J. Comp. Physiol.* **86**, 95–115.

Taylor, E. W., Short, S. & Butler, P. J. (1977). The role of the cardiac vagus in the response of the dogfish *Scyliorhinus canicula* to hypoxia. *J. Exp. Biol.* **70**, 57–75.

Taylor, E. W. & Wheatly, M. G. (1980). Ventilation, heart rate and respiratory gas exchange in the crayfish *Austropotamobius pallipes* (Lereboullet) submerged in normoxic water and following 3 h exposure in air at 15°C. *J. Comp. Physiol.* **138**, 67–78.

Wheatly, M. G. & Taylor, E. W. (1981). The effect of progressive hypoxia on heart rate, ventilation, respiratory gas exchange and acid–base status in the crayfish *Austropotamobius pallipes*. *J. Exp. Biol.* **92**, 125–41.

Wiersma, C. A. G. & Novitski, E. (1942). The mechanism of the nervous regulation of the crayfish heart. *J. Exp. Biol.* **19**, 255–65.

Wilkens, J. L. (1981). Respiratory and circulatory coordination in decapod crustaceans. In *Locomotion and Energetics in Arthropods* (eds C. F. Herreid & C. R. Fourtner). New York: Plenum Press.

Wilkens, J. L. & Young, R. E. (1975). Patterns and bilateral co-ordination of scaphognathite rhythms in the lobster *Homarus americanus. J. Exp. Biol.* **63**, 219–35.

Wilkens, J. L., Wilkens. L. A. & McMahon, B. R. (1974). Central control of cardiac and scaphognathite pacemakers in the crab, *Cancer magister. J. Comp. Physiol.* **90**, 89–104.

Withington-Wray, D. J., Roberts, B. L. & Taylor, E. W. (1986). The topographical organisation of the vagal motor column in the elasmobranch fish, *Scyliorhinus canicula* L. *J. Comp. Neurol.* **248**, 95–104.

Wood, C. M. (1974). A critical examination of the physical and adrenergic factors affecting blood flow through the gills of the rainbow trout. *J. Exp. Biol.* **60**, 241–65.

Wood, C. M., Pieprzak, P. & Trott, J. N. (1979). The influence of temperature and anaemia on the adrenergic and cholinergic mechanisms controlling heart rate in the rainbow trout. *Can. J. Zool.* **57**, 2440–7.

Wood, C. M. & Randall, D. J. (1981). Oxygen and carbon dioxide exchange during exercise in the land crab (*Cardisoma carnifex*). *J. Exp. Zool.* **218**, 7–22.

Wood, C. M. & Shelton, G. (1980). The reflex control of heart rate and cardiac output in the rainbow trout: interactive influences of hypoxia, haemorrhage, and systemic vasomotor tone. *J. Exp. Biol.* **87**, 271–84.

Young, R. E. (1978). Correlated activities in the cardiovascular nerves and ventilatory system in the Norwegian lobster, *Nephrops norvegicus* (L). Comp. Biochem. Physiol. **61A**, 387–94.

Young, R. E. & Coyer, P. E. (1979). Phase co-ordination in the cardiac and ventilatory rhythms of the lobster *Homarus americanus. J. Exp. Biol.* **82**, 53–74.

Young, J. Z. (1933). The autonomic nervous system of selachians. *Quart. J. Microsc. Sci.* **75**, 571–624.

Young, J. Z. (1936). The innervation and reactions to drugs of the viscera of teleostean fish. *Proc. R. Soc. Lond. B.* **120**, 303–18.

# 16

# The location and distribution of vagal preganglionic neurones in the hindbrain of lower vertebrates

**D. J. Withington-Wray\*, E. W. Taylor and J. D. Metcalfe[†]**

*Department of Zoology and Comparative Physiology, University of Birmingham, Birmingham B15 2TT, UK*

## 16.1. Introduction

In this chapter we will review the literature concerning the location of vagal preganglionic motoneurones in the brainstem of lower vertebrates. When we first examined the literature we were surprised by the paucity of information on this subject. This prompted us to fill in some of the gaps ourselves. The 'lower vertebrates' used in this study are an elasmobranch fish, the lesser spotted dogfish *Scyliorhinus canicula*; two species of teleost fish, the cod *Gadus morhua* and trout *Salmo gairdneri*; and two species of anuran amphibians, the South African clawed 'toad' *Xenopus laevis* and the marine toad *Bufo marinus*. Since embarking on this study a number of laboratories have provided new information which we have incorporated into the review. Much of the emphasis in our discussion will be placed on the distribution of vagal motoneurones in the elasmobranch fish, since it is in this area that the majority of our work has concentrated. Additionally, a brief discussion of the vagal motor column in mammals will be included, but a long description is not warranted since this topic has been covered extensively elsewhere (e.g. Kalia & Mesulam, 1980a, b).

In some vertebrate groups such as the amphibians, as represented by the frog, the peripheral course of the vagus and its role in the control of the heart have been known for over 100 years (e.g. Harris *et al.*, 1951). Only recently, however, has the central origin of cell bodies, with axons contributing to the various branches of the vagus, been elucidated. A great advance has been made in this field since the introduction of horseradish peroxidase (HRP) as a neural tracer. The information on the location of vagal preganglionic

Present addresses: \*Department of Neurophysiology and Neuropharmacology, National Institute of Medical Research, The Ridgeway, Mill Hill, London NW7 1AA, UK; [†]Department of Physiology, The Medical School, University of Birmingham, Birmingham B15 2TT, UK.

motoneurones which we present in this chapter was obtained from the use of the retrograde intra-axonal transport of HRP into the cell bodies of vagal motoneurones in the brainstem, after its application to selected branches of the vagus nerve. It is appropriate here to give a brief outline of the methodology used. Animals were anaesthetised prior to surgery. HRP (Sigma, Type VI) was inserted into the exposed vagus nerve (or selected branches of the vagus) on one side of the animal, as a dried concentrated solution on the tip of a fine insect pin (Barrett & Taylor, 1985b). The wound was then sutured and the animal was returned to a holding tank for an appropriate period of time, depending on the transport distance for the HRP and the temperature at which the animal was maintained. Each animal was then reanaesthetised and perfused with fixative. Serial transverse sections of the hindbrain, cut on a freezing microtome at 60 μm, were reacted using a slightly modified version (Barrett, 1984) of the tetramethyl benzidine procedure (Mesulam, 1978).

## 16.2. Cyclostomes

This group of vertebrates is composed of the myxinoids (e.g. *Myxine*, the hagfish) and the petromyzonts (e.g. *Lampetra*, the lamprey). According to Ariens Kappers (1929, 1947) the central nervous system of the cyclostomes represents the prototype of the vertebrate brain. The hindbrain is identical in superficial appearance to that of the rest of the vertebrates, with vagal rootlets leaving on either side to innervate the viscera. The heart of myxinoids is aneural, that is, it is not innervated by the vagus or the sympathetic nervous system (Green, 1902; Carlson, 1904); whereas the heart of the lamprey (although similarly devoid of a sympathetic supply) is innervated by the vagus (Augustinsson *et al.*, 1956). However, these animals are unique among vertebrates in that the acetylcholine released by the vagus has an excitatory action on the heart (Falck *et al.*, 1966).

No study has been made of the topographical representation of vagally innervated structures within the vagal motor column of cyclostomes. In *Lampetra* two separate divisions of the vagal motor column have been identified using normal staining techniques: a rostral and a caudal motor nucleus of X (Niewenhuys, 1972). The caudal motor nucleus of X, which cannot be delineated from the spinal visceromotor cells, is thought to represent a splanchnic centre, and the rostral nucleus is considered to be branchiomotor in nature (i.e. to innervate the branchial pouches) (Addens, 1933). The location of the caudal motor nucleus in cyclostomes, which centres around the obex, is similar to the region of the dorsal vagal motor nucleus (dmnX) in the cat (Bennett *et al.*, 1981) and to the nucleus motorius nervi vagi medialis (Xmm) in the dogfish (Barrett & Taylor, 1985b) in which the cell bodies contributing axons to the cardiac vagi are found.

### 16.3. **Elasmobranchs**

In the elasmobranch fish *Scyliorhinus canicula* the vagus nerve divides to form, at its proximal end, branchial branches 1, 2 3 and 4 which contain skeletomotor fibres innervating the intrinsic respiratory muscles of gill arches 2, 3, 4 and 5 respectively. The first gill arch is innervated by the glosso-pharyngeal (IXth cranial) nerve. The vagus also sends, on each side of the fish, two branches to the heart; the branchial cardiac branch, which arises from the 4th branchial branch (Norris & Hughes, 1920), and the visceral cardiac branch, which arises close to the visceral branch of the vagus (Marshall & Hurst, 1905). The remainder of the vagus is termed the visceral branch, and this innervates the anterior part of the gut down to the pylorus and the anterior part of the spiral intestine (Young, 1933). More recent descriptions of the route of the vagus nerve in *Scyliorhinus* were provided by Taylor *et al.* (1977) and Withington-Wray *et al.* (1986).

The gross location of the vagal motor column in the hindbrain has been described in a number of elasmobranchs (e.g. Black, 1917; Ariens Kappers, 1920; Addens, 1933, Smeets & Niewenhuys, 1976; Smeets *et al.*, 1983); although until recently almost nothing was known of the topographical origin of vagal preganglionic fibres in elasmobranchs (Smeets *et al.*, 1983). The vagal motor nucleus was shown to consist of a continuous column of large, bipolar, tripolar and (less frequently) quadripolar cells in conjunction with the motor nuclei of the IXth and VIIth cranial nerves in a number of elasmobranchs, namely *Selache maxima* (Black, 1917), *Squalus acanthias* and *Scyliorhinus canicula* (Smeets & Niewenhuys, 1976) and *Hydrolagus collei* and *Raja clavata* (Smeets *et al.*, 1983).

In the shark *Cetorhinus* and in the Holocephali, Addens (1933) divided the vagal motor nucleus into separate rostral and caudal parts and suggested that the rostral portion is specialised to subserve either a visceromotor or branchiomotor function, whereas the caudal portion represents a general visceromotor or splanchnic centre. Smeets *et al.* (1983) observed that in *Hydrolagus* the vagal nucleus can readily be divided into a caudodorsal nucleus and a rostroventral nucleus, the latter being continuous with the nuclei of IX and VII. A similar subdivision into a dorsal and a ventral nucleus could be recognised at some levels in *Raja*, and the authors noted that the dorsal portion appeared to contain somewhat smaller neurones than the ventral portion.

In *Squalus* an area lateral to the caudal part of the visceromotor column contains a distinct aggregation of large bipolar and triangular cells (Smeets & Niewenhuys, 1976). These authors considered this aggregation of cells represented a part of the motor nucleus of X and named it accordingly the nucleus motorius nervi vagi lateralis (Xml). The Xml extended from 2·0 mm rostral to approximately 4·0 mm caudal to the obex. The vagal part of the visceromotor column was designated the nucleus motorius nervi vagi medialis (Xmm). The Xmm and Xml may, by virtue of their locations, be the homologues of the mammalian dorsal vagal motor nucleus and the nucleus ambiguus, respectively (Smeets & Niewenhuys, 1976; Barrett *et al.*, 1983). In *Squalus* the cells in the Xmm are somewhat larger than those in the lateral nucleus. In *Scyliorhinus* a medial vagal motor nucleus has been described (Smeets & Niewenhuys, 1976), but no lateral nucleus was identified. The Xmm of *Scyliorhinus* extended from approximately 2·7 mm rostral to 2·25 mm caudal to the obex (on the basis of sections of the hindbrain illustrated in the atlas of Smeets & Niewenhuys, 1976).

Our studies using the retrograde intra-axonal transport of HRP for the identification of vagal preganglionic neurones showed that the vagal motor column of *Scyliorhinus* extends over 5 mm in the hindbrain (2.1 mm caudal to 2·9 mm rostral to obex), which agrees well with the extent described by Smeets and Niewenhuys (1976) for fish of similar size. Further, the use of HRP histochemistry has shown that the vagal motor column is more complex than had previously been thought (Fig. 16.1). Caudal to obex there appeared to be two distinct groups of vagal motoneurones, the majority found dorsomedially, and a smaller ventromedial group, both close to the lateral edge of the 4th ventricle. The ventromedial group were continuous with cells in the spino-occipital motor nucleus (Black, 1917) and may constitute a forward extension of this nucleus, contributing axons to the hypobranchial nerve which innervates the ventral muscles of the gill region (J. J. Levings, unpublished observations). The majority of vagal moto-neurones caudal to obex contribute axons to the visceral branch of the vagus. The other branch of the vagus whose motoneurones were found caudal to obex was the visceral cardiac branch. Visceral cardiac motoneurones were found in the dorsomedial division of the vagal motor column. Rostral to obex the medial motoneurones were no longer distinguishable into dorsal and ventral divisions: for the remainder of the rostral part of the vagal motor column the medial cells were found clustered close to the ventrolateral edge of the 4th ventricle. Most of the vagal motoneurones were found in this rostromedial division of the vagal motor column. This division contributed axons to the branchial cardiac branch and to the visceral branch in its most caudal one-third, and contributed axons to the branchial branches of the vagus in its rostral two-thirds (Fig. 16.1). A clearly distinguishable lateral group of cells was identified which had a rostrocaudal extent of approxi-mately 1 mm, rostrally from obex. This population of motoneurones contributed axons solely to the branchial cardiac branch of the vagus (Barrett *et al.*, 1983; Barrett & Taylor, 1985b) and comprised 8% of the total population of vagal motoneurones. The cells in the lateral division supply 60% of the efferent axons running in the branchial cardiac nerve, with the other 40% supplied by cells in the rostromedial division. When the medial cells contributing efferent axons to the heart via the visceral cardiac branches are taken into account, then the lateral cells are found to supply 45% of vagal efferent output to the heart.

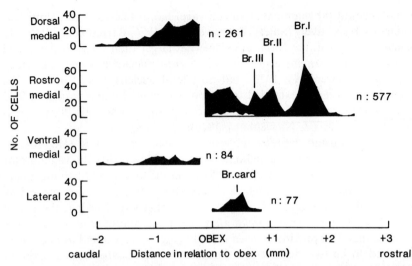

Fig. 16.1. *Scyliorhinus canicula*, the dogfish. The rostrocaudal distribution either side of obex of the divisions of the vagal motor column determined from the application of HRP to the whole vagus nerve. *n* is the number of cells identified in each division. The peaks on the distribution of cells in the rostromedial division coincide with the peripheral insertion of the first, second and third branchial branches of the vagus (Br I–III). The clear area in this division indicates the distribution of medial cells supplying the branchial cardiac nerve (Br. card.) which has the rest of its cells in the lateral division.

The four divisions of the vagal motor column described in *Scyliorhinus* (Barrett *et al.*, 1984) do not seem to be directly comparable to divisions of the vagal motor nucleus previously described for any one species of selachian. Indeed, even the similarity between the lateral vagal motor division in *Scyliorhinus* and the Xml described in *Squalus* is perhaps questionable. In *Scyliorhinus* the lateral division is composed of cells of a similar size to those in rostro- and dorsomedial divisions. It extends over a short distance (1 mm) within the hindbrain, rostral to obex, and the cells have a scattered mediolateral distribution (Fig. 16.2A). In contrast, the cells comprising the Xml of *Squalus* are smaller than those of the Xmm; the nucleus extends over a longer distance both rostral and caudal to obex and is composed of a discrete aggregation of cells (Smeets & Niewenhuys, 1976). The division of the caudal portion of the vagal motor nucleus of *Raja* into dorsal and ventral populations, with the ventral cells being larger than the dorsal population, is similar to the situation described in *Scyliorhinus* (Smeets *et al.*, 1983).

In *Hydrolagus* the dorsal and ventral populations are not restricted to the caudal part of the vagal nucleus, and are found together approximately 3.2 mm rostral to obex (determined from the atlas provided by Smeets *et al.*, 1983). In neither *Raja* nor *Hydrolagus* was a lateral division of the vagal motor column identified. These differences in the distribution of vagal motoneurones between species of selachians may be real since in mammals there are species differences in the cytoarchitectural divisions of the dorsal vagal motor nucleus (e.g. Kimmel, 1940 (rabbit), Contreras *et al.*, 1980 (cat)), or they may, at least in part, result from the use of Nissl-stained material in these earlier studies in contrast to the current use of HRP for the identification of vagal motoneurones. This applies particularly to the lateral division of the vagal motor nucleus identified in *Scyliorhinus* (Barrett *et al.*, 1983) which had not previously been described, presumably through the paucity of cells and their scattered distribution.

The branchial cardiac and visceral branches of the vagus are supplied by neurones of two topographically distinct origins in the hindbrain in *Scyliorhinus*. Motoneurones supplying axons to the visceral branch of the vagus may be found dorsomedially and ventromedially in the caudal part of the vagal motor column. The cells in the two locations are very different in size; the ventromedial cells are approximately twice the size of the dorsomedial cells and there are fewer of them (Withington-Wray *et al.*, 1986). The innervation of the gastrointestinal tract of elasmobranchs includes both a submucosal and a myenteric plexus (Kirtisinghe, 1940; Nicol, 1952). We originally suggested that the ventromedial cells in *Scyliorhinus* may give rise to the innervation of the gut musculature, and that the dorsomedial cells may supply fibres which are secretomotor in function. This attractive hypothesis is, however, currently being questioned by further detailed neuranatomical studies in our laboratory, which have revealed that the ventromedial cells are similar in location and size to the occipital and anterior spinal motoneurones supplying the hypobranchial nerve (J. J. Levings, unpublished observation), so that the visceral vagus may have all its motoneurones in the dorsomedial division described by Barrett *et al.* (1984).

The branch of the vagus which certainly receives axons from two different locations in the hindbrain is the branchial cardiac vagus (Fig. 16.2A). Branchial cardiac motoneurones are found rostromedially, and solely comprise the lateral division of the vagal motor column. It is thought that these two locations of cardiac vagal preganglionic neurones give rise to the two different types of efferent activity recorded from the cardiac vagi of this animal (Taylor & Butler, 1982; Barrett & Taylor, 1985a, c). This functional separation is described by Taylor in Chapter 15.

In summary, the vagal motor column of *Scyliorhinus* consists of distinct divisions. Caudal to obex it contains dorsomedial and possibly ventromedial divisions, and rostral to obex there is a single rostrosmedial division and a short lateral division which contains 8% of the vagal preganglionic neurones. There is a sequential topographic representation of the vagus nerve in the vagal motor column with neurones supplying the structures distal to the hindbrain (gastrointestinal tract) located caudally, those supplying the cardiac nerves located in the mid-portion of the column and those supplying the proximal structures (gill arches) located most rostrally. There is a small

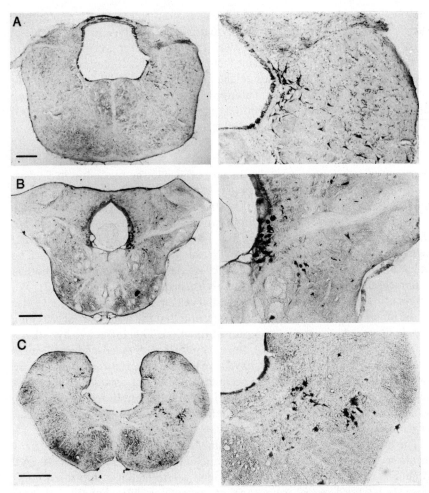

Fig. 16.2.   Transverse sections (60 μm) of the hindbrain to show vagal motoneurones labelled with HRP. Scale bars indicate 500 μm, the plates to the right of the figure are in each case 2.2 × enlargements of the same or a neighbouring section; to show details of the distribution of motoneurones. (A) *Scyliorhinus canicula*, the dogfish. Section cut at obex showing some cells grouped in a medial division close to the wall of the fourth ventricle and a more scattered ventrolateral division of cells which extends to the outer edge of the medulla (section supplied by Jennifer J. Levings). (B) *Gadus morhua*, the cod. Section taken 0.1 mm caudal of obex to show medial and lateral groups of vagal motoneurones. (C) *Xenopus laevis*, the African clawed 'toad'. Section taken 0.1 mm rostral of obex to show two groups of vagal motoneurones at different mediolateral locations with respect to the fourth ventricle.

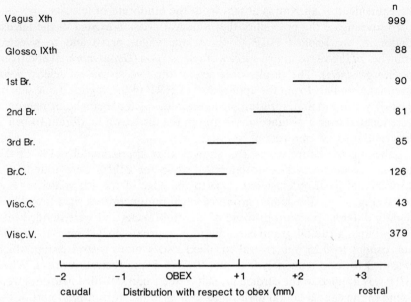

Fig. 16.3. *Scyliorhinus canicula*, the dogfish. Topographical organisation of the vagal motor column. The rostrocaudal distribution either side of obex of the pools of motoneurones that supply the vagus and its constituent branches and the glosso-pharyngeal nerve (Glosso IXth). The extent of the motoneurones supplying each vagal branch is represented by a solid line; *n* = the number of labelled cell bodies identified from the best backfill of each branch. 1st–3rd Br., 1st 2nd and 3rd branchial branches; Br. C., branchial cardiac; Visc.C., visceral cardiac; Visc.V., visceral vagus.

degree of overlap between these pools of neurones supplying adjacent branches of the vagus (Barrett *et al.*, 1984, Withington-Wray *et al.*, 1986) (Fig. 16.3).

## 16.4. Teleosts

In teleost fish the vagus innervates the gills, the heart and the viscera (pharynx, oesophagus, stomach and swimbladder). In contrast to elasmobranchs where the branchial branches are solely skeletomotor (Metcalfe & Butler, 1984), the branchial branches of the vagus (going to the gills) have both a vasomotor and skeletomotor function (Pettersson & Nilsson, 1979) described by Nilsson and Axelsson in Chapter 5.

Previous topological studies of the brain of teleosts have concentrated on the rather 'atypical' teleosts, e.g. the reedfish *Erpetoichthys* (Niewenhuys & Oey, 1983), the Crossopterygian fish *Latimeria* (Kremers & Niewenhuys, 1979), and *Gnathonemus* (Szabo & Liboubans, 1979). In all these studies a single vagal motor nucleus was described. It seemed from these studies that the equivalent of an Xml is absent from the hindbrain of teleosts.

To investigate the possibility that a lateral division existed in the teleost hindbrain, we applied HRP to the whole vagus nerve and to selected branches of the vagus in two species of teleost, cod (*Gadus morhua*) and trout (*Salmo gardneri*). The results obtained in the two species of teleost were essentially similar. From the application of HRP to the vagus on one side of the fish, we found that, for example in the cod, vagal preganglionic neurones were located over a distance of 2·8 mm in the ipsilateral hindbrain from 1·2 mm caudal to 1·6 mm rostral to obex.

Labelling the entire vagus also showed that approximately 11% of the neurones were located ventrolaterally, while the others were found in a dorsomedial location clustered close to the edge of the 4th ventricle (Fig. 16.2B, Fig. 16.4). The lateral group of vagal motoneurones were found in a slightly different position to those of elasmobranchs and were divided into two groups: a caudal group extending for approximately 1 mm (from 0·75 mm caudal to 0·25 mm rostral to obex) and a more rostral group which extended for approximately 0·75 mm (0·75–1·5 mm rostral to obex). When HRP was applied to the cardiac branch of the vagus, labelled neurones were found in the caudal lateral division as well as in the dorsomedial part of the vagal motor column. The application of HRP to one of the branchial branches of the vagus also labelled both lateral and dorsomedial cells, this time with the lateral cells located more rostrally than the cardiac neurones.

The identification of lateral cardiac vagal preganglionic neurones is similar to our findings in elasmobranchs. In contrast, however, some branchial motoneurones are located in the lateral division in teleosts, whereas they are confined to a medial location in elasmobranchs. This may reflect the observation that the branchial branches of the vagus serve both a vasomotor and skeletomotor function in teleosts but only a skeletomotor function in elasmobranchs (see earlier). We suggest that the dual function of the branchial branches in teleosts may be reflected in the dual origin of the branchial fibres in the brain, and that the medial neurones may give rise to the skeletomotor fibres whereas the lateral neurones may give rise to the vasomotor fibres. A larger percentage of vagal preganglionic neurones is located in a lateral division in teleosts (11%) when compared to elasmobranchs (8%), and the lateral neurones in teleosts send axons along the branchial and cardiac branches of the vagus.

In teleosts there is also a sequential topographic representation of the vagus within the vagal motor column. The most rostral neurones give rise to fibres supplying the most proximal organs (gills), and the caudal neurones give rise to fibres innervating the viscera. The cardiac neurones are located in the middle of the vagal motor column. So in both classes of fish in which the topographical layout of the vagus has been studied there is a sequential representation of the vagus.

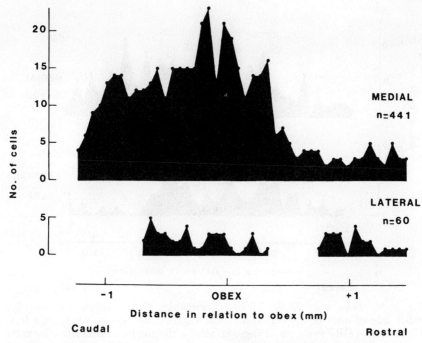

Fig. 16.4. *Gadus morthua*, the cod. The rostrocaudal distribution either side of obex of the divisions of the vagal motor column determined from application of HRP to the whole vagus nerve. *n* is the number of cells identified in the medial and lateral divisions.

## 16.5. **Amphibians**

In amphibians the vagus innervates the viscera, the heart and, in the air-breathing adults, the lungs. It also innervates the hyoid apparatus and the larynx. In the last decade the topological analysis of the hindbrain performed on various species of amphibian had identified only one vagal motor nucleus (e.g. *Rana esculenta, Rana catesbeiana*, Opdam *et al.*, 1976; and *Ambystoma*, the axolotl, Opdam & Niewenhuys, 1976). A more recent study (Struesse *et al.*, 1984), which utilised HRP histochemistry, found labelled vagal neurones only in a 'ventrolateral' location in the medulla. The position of these cells was, however, in an intermediate location between the mammalian dorsal vagal motor nucleus and the nucleus ambiguus. The authors concluded that there was only a single column of vagal motoneurones in the hindbrain of the two ranid species *R. pipiens* and *R. catesbeiana*. The topographical representation of the vagus was also examined by Struesse *et al.* (1984). They found that visceral vagal neurones were located throughout the rostrocaudal extent of the vagal motor column. Cardiac neurones tended to be more rostral than

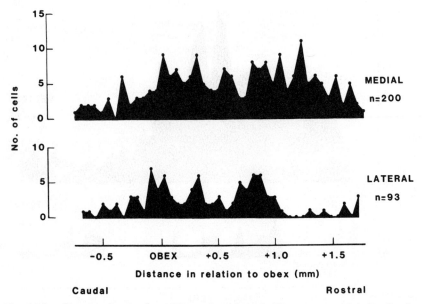

Fig. 16.5. *Xenopus laevis*, the African clawed toad. The rostrocaudal distribution either side of obex of the divisions of the vagal motor column determined from application of HRP to the whole vagus nerve. *n*. is the number of cells identified in the medial and lateral divisions.

pulmonary neurones, and both groups were located in the middle of the column with laryngeal neurones located more caudally in the nucleus.

A somewhat dissimilar story seems to be the case for the African clawed 'toad' *Xenopus laevis* (family Pipidae). In a topological analysis of the brainstem of this animal, Nikundiwe & Niewenhuys (1983) observed two cell groups which constituted the motor nuclei of the vagus and the glosso-pharyngeal nerves, one group in the most superficial zone of the central grey and a second group more laterally in the white matter overlying this central gray. Recently, we administered HRP into the vagus nerve on one side of *Xenopus* and our findings were essentially the same as those of Nikundiwe & Niewenhuys (1983). Neurones were located ipsilaterally in the hindbrain over a distance of 2·5 mm (from 0·7 mm caudal to 1·8 mm rostral to obex). In this amphibian the mediolateral distribution of vagal preganglionic neurones differed markedly from that of the fishes. Approximately 32% of the neurones were identified in a ventrolateral location, with the remainder located slightly more dorsally and medially (Figs 16.2C and 16.5). We attributed the increase in the number of lateral preganglionic neurones to the additional 'respiratory' structures innervated by the vagus in these animals and perhaps particularly to the change from gill to lung breathing. A similar distribution of vagal motoneurones was revealed when we applied HRP to the vagus of the marine toad *Bufo marinus* (family Bufonidae). The vagal motonucleus extended over a distance of 2·5 mm around obex with 20% of motoneurones in a ventrolateral and more caudal group (Innes *et al.*, 1986).

It is surprising that there seems to be this major difference in the distribution of vagal preganglionic neurones between the ranid and pipid and bufonid amphibians, with the latter two groups falling neatly into an interamediate position between the fishes and the reptiles.


## 16.6. Reptiles

In reptiles the vagus nerve sends branches for the innervation of the heart, lungs, trachea and viscera. Few studies have concentrated on the topology of the cell masses in the brainstem of reptiles, and nothing is known of the possible functional subdivisions of the vagal motor column (Schwab, 1979). An early study by Black (1920) described two divisions (medial and ventrolateral) of the vagal motor column. Black studied a variety of species (turtles, *Damonia* and *Chelone*, lizard, *Varanus*, alligator, *Alligator*, and snake, *Boa*), he noted that the lateral division, although present in *Damonia* and *Chelone*, was more prominent in *Varanus* and *Alligator*, whereas it was absent from *Boa*. More recently Cruce & Niewenhuys (1974) identified a 'nucleus ambiguus' adjacent to the dorsal motor nucleus of X in the tortoise *Testudo*. Cruce & Niewenhuys did not discuss the function of the nA apart from including it with the branchiomotor nuclei. However, vocal control neurones have been located in the nA of the gekko (Kennedy, 1981), and comparable motoneurones are present in the nA of mammals (Getz & Sirnes, 1949; Szabo & Dussardier, 1964). A study by Barbas-Henry & Lohman (1984) using HRP histochemistry has clearly shown the two divisions of the vagal motor column in *Varanus*. One group was found as a compact mass dorsally in the brainstem which consisted of medium-sized round and polygonal cells and extended rostrocaudally from a level just rostral to the hypoglossal nuclear complex to the upper cervical spinal cord. Rostrally the group was located immediately ventral to the solitary tract, and in the cervical cord its position was dorsolateral to the central canal. A second group of more lateral cells divided into two populations, a rostral portion which contained smaller cells than the caudal portion. The number of cells in the medial location exceeded that in the lateral location (H. A. Barbas-Henry, pers. comm.). Recently, Leong *et al.*(1984), using HRP to localise vagal neurones in the terrapin, reported that between 36 and 50% of vagal preganglionic neurones are located in the reptilian nucleus ambiguus, a greater proportion than is found in fishes and amphibians.

A detailed study of the somatotopic representation of the vagus in reptiles should yield interesting and important new data contributing to our knowledge of the evolution of vagal control of visceral function, including cardiorespiratory regulation.

## 16.7. **Birds**

The vagally innervated structures in birds are the pharynx, larynx, trachea, heart, lungs and viscera. The central origin of vagal efferent fibres in birds has been the subject of a number of studies. Black (1922), Sanders (1929) and Ariens Kappers *et al.* (1960) identified cells in the ventrolateral medulla of birds that they felt were the avian homologue of the nucleus ambiguus in mammals. A recent study on the pigeon by Katz & Karten (1983) demonstrated, using HRP, that vagal motoneurones are localised to the dorsal motor nucleus of the vagus complex, the region of the nA and the region of the reticular formation extending between the dmnX and the nA. Wild (1981) working on the cockatoo found vagal motoneurones both in the dmnX and the nA. The nA was composed of both glossopharyngeal and vagal motoneurones intermixed to form a single nucleus with a considerable mediolateral and rostrocaudal extension. The subnuclear architectonic divisions of the dmnX in birds have been described by Sanders (1929) for the duck, chicken, dove and sparrow and for the pigeon by Cohen *et al.* (1970). These studies largely concur in the identification of three distinct cell groups: a large-celled dorsal group, a group of medium-sized cells at an intermediate dorsoventral position, and a group of small cells ventrally. A more comprehensive study by Katz & Karten (1983) on the pigeon has demonstrated at least 11 cytoarchitecturally distinct subnuclei of the dmnX.

The peripheral representation of the vagus nerve in birds was described by Cohen *et al.* (1970) as having a partially inverted topographic representation in the dorsal motor nucleus. The visceral representation was located in the rostral two-thirds of the nucleus; the pulmonary representation (although small) straddled the obex; and the recurrent laryngeal representation was confined to the caudal one-third of the nucleus. This interpretation has been found to be an oversimplification. Katz & Karten (1985) found that individual vagal target organs in the pigeon have discrete and topographic representations which may be within more than one cytoarchitecturally distinct subnucleus of the dmnX complex. For example the thoracic oesophagus was supplied by groups of neurones up to 1 mm caudal of obex and up to 1·7 mm rostral of obex in the posterior and anterior mediocellular subnuclei. The description of a partially inverted representation only holds in that some neurones supplying the viscera are located rostral to obex, whereas others are located in a typically sequential position caudal to obex. The cardiac representation in birds is also inconsistent with a strictly inverted somatotopy, since cardiac neurones are located rostral to obex. There are no figures available for the proportions in birds of vagal neurones located in the medial (dmnX) or lateral (nA) division of the vagal motor column.

## 16.8. **Mammals**

In mammals the vagus innervates the larynx, trachea, extrathoracic trachea, bronchi, lungs, heart and viscera. Until recently it has been generally accepted that these visceromotor fibres in the vagus nerve originated from two distinct nuclear subgroups in the medulla: the dorsal motor nucleus of the vagus (dmnX) and the nucleus ambiguus (nA). This concept was based upon the observations of Marinesco (1897, quoted in Kalia, 1981). The most recent evidence suggests, however, that vagal motor fibres in the cat originate not only in the dmnX and the nA, but also from the nucleus retroambigualis (nRA), the nucleus dorsomedialis (ndm), the spinal nucleus of the accessory (nspA), and the reticular formation between the dmnX and the nA (Kalia & Mesulam, 1980a, b; Kalia, 1981). In the rat similar nuclei in the brainstem, the dmnX, nA, nRA and the nspA, contribute fibres to the vagus, but no contribution to the rat vagus was found to originate in the ndm (Kalia & Sullivan, 1982). In the pig *Sus scrofa* (Hopkins *et al.*, 1984) vagal motoneurones are found in the dmnX, nucleus of the solitary tract, nA, ventrolateral nA (VLnA) and in an intermediate zone between the dmnX and the nA. Recently (Gwyn *et al.*, 1985), vagal efferent fibres of the squirrel monkey, *Saimuri sciureus*, have been shown to originate in the dmnX, nA and the region between these two nuclei.

Neurones giving rise to fibres supplying all of the vagally innervated structures (except the extrathoracic trachea) arise from the dmnX, and there is no element of somatotopy within this nucleus (Kalia & Mesulam, 1980b). The nA also contributes efferents to all of the vagally innervated structures, and again there is no discernible topographic representation of the thoracic and abdominal organs (Kalia & Mesulam, 1980b). Kalia (1981) does, however, note that there is a preferential innervation of a given organ from a particular nucleus, e.g. dmnX or nA.

In mammals there is little published data available for the proportions of vagal motoneurones located in the various divisions of the vagal motor complex. In one study on the pig (Hopkins *et al.*, 1984) the majority of vagal motoneurones were found in a lateral location in the brainstem (nA and VLnA), whereas recent work on the rat revealed that approximately 30% are located in a lateral location with reference to the dmnX (D. J. Withington-Wray, unpublished observation). There are, however, published figures for some of the branches of the vagus. For example, in the cat (Bennett *et al.*, 1981; Jordan *et al.*, 1985), both pulmonary and cardiac vagal motoneurones are found predominantly in the nA, with up to 78% of cardiac and 68% of pulmonary neurones found in this location. This compares with 45% of cardiac vagal motoneurones located ventrolaterally in the dogfish, and indicates that in mammals, compared with lower vertebrates, a greater proportion of cardiac and pulmonary vagal motoneurones originate in this division.

In mammals during embryological development, neurones which form the nA migrate from a dorsomedial position to a final ventrolateral position within the brainstem (Windle, 1933). In birds the ventral motor nucleus (nA) also arises from a ventral migration of ventrolateral dmnX cells (Katz & Karten, 1983). No data exist on the embryological development of the vagal motor column in lower vertebrates. Determination of the criteria involved in the migration of vagal motoneurones during development in lower vertebrates may serve as a key to our understanding of the differentiation of function between the dmnX and the nA. It is interesting that both cardiac and pulmonary vagal motoneurones are located in ventrolateral subdivisions of the motor column in the majority of vertebrates. In mammals their juxtaposition has functional correlates in the direct neuronal interaction described by Jordan and Spyer in Chapter 17.

## 16.8. Summary

Although this chapter includes in its title the words 'lower vertebrates', the reader will have observed that we have included sections on all the major vertebrate groups. It is clear that the sequential topographical representation in the hindbrain of vagally enervated structures which is so apparent in fishes, and possibly in amphibians, has been lost during the evolution of other vertebrate groups. One of our interests is in mediolateral location of vagal preganglionic neurones and how this differs between the groups. In the vertebrate groups where the number of neurones located in each division has been calculated (elasmobranchs, teleosts, amphibians and reptiles), we find an increase in the number of cells located in the lateral division of the vagal motor column as one moves from fishes up to mammals. In elasmobranchs, where only 8% of the cells are located laterally, these neurones supply axons to the cardiac branch of the vagus only. In teleosts (11%), both branchial and cardiac neurones are located laterally. In amphibians this proportion rises to between 20 and 32%, and this increase may be associated with the acquisition of air-breathing structures. This trend is supported by the work of Leong *et al.* (1984), who found between 36 and 50% of vagal motoneurones in the reptilian nucleus ambiguus. We propose that the increase in the number of preganglionic vagal motoneurones found in a ventrolateral position as one ascends through the lower vertebrates towards mammals may reflect a shift in the importance of the lateral location of the vagal motor column, particularly with respect to the vagal control of the cardiorespiratory system and its interactions.

## References

Addens, J. L. (1933). The motor nuclei and roots of the cranial and first spinal nerves of vertebrates. I. Introduction and cyclostomes. *Z. Anat. Entwicklungesch.* **101**, 307–410.

Ariens Kappers, C. U. (1920). *Die vergleichende Anatomie des Nervensystems des Wirbettier und des Menschen.* Haarlem: Bohn.

Ariens Kappers, C. U. (1929). *The Evolution of the Nervous System.* Haarlem: Bohn.

Ariens Kappers, C. U. (1947). *Anatomie comparée du système nerveux.* Haarlem: Bohn.

Ariens Kappers, C. U., Huber, G. C. & Crosby, E. C. (1960). *The Comparative Anatomy of the Nervous System of Vertebrates, Including Man.* V. L. New York: Haffner.

Augustinsson, A., Fange, R., Johnels, A. & Ostlund, E. (1956). Histological, physiological and biochemical studies on the heart of two cyclostomes, hagfish (*Myxine*) and lamprey (*Lampetra*). *J. Physiol. Lond.* **13**, 257–76.

Barbas-Henry, H. A. & Lohman, A. H. M. (1984). The motor nuclei and primary projections of the IXth, Xth, XIth and XIIth cranial nerves in the monitor lizard *Varanus exanthematicus. J. Comp. Neurol.* **226**, 565–79.

Barrett, D. J. (1984). The Xth cranial nerve (the vagus) in the elasmobranch fish *Scyliorhinus canicula*, and its role in the control of the heart. Ph.D. Thesis, University of Birmingham.

Barrett, D. J., Roberts, B. L. & E. W. Taylor (1983). The identification of the cell bodies of cardiac vagal efferent fibres in the dogfish *Scyliorhinus canicula. J. Physiol. Lond.* **338**, 9P.

Barrett, D. J., Roberts, B. L. & E. W. Taylor (1984). The topographical organisation of vagal motoneurones in the dogfish *Scyliorhinus canicula. J. Physiol. Lond.* **350**, 32P.

Barrett, D. J. & Taylor, E. W. (1985a). Spontaneous efferent activity in branches of the vagus nerve controlling heart rate and ventilation in the dogfish. *J. Exp. Biol.* **117**, 433–48.

Barrett, D. J. & Taylor, E. W. (1985b). The location of cardiac vagal preganglionic neurones in the brainstem of the dogfish. *J. Exp. Biol.* **117**, 449–58.

Barrett, D. J. & Taylor, E. W. (1985c). The characteristics of cardiac vagal preganglionic motoneurones in the dogfish. *J. Exp. Biol.* **117**, 459–70.

Bennett, J. A., Kidd, C., Latif, A. B. & McWilliam, P. N. (1981). A horseradish peroxidase study of vagal motoneurones with axons in cardiac and pulmonary branches of the cat and dog. *Quart. J. Exp. Physiol.* **66**, 145–54.

Black, D. (1917). The motor nuclei of the cerebral nerves in phylogeny I. Cyclostomi and Pisces. *J. Comp. Neurol.* **27**, 467–564.

Black, D. (1920). The motor nuclei of the cerebral nerves in phylogeny III. Reptilia. *J. Comp. Neurol.* **32**, 61–98.

Black, D. (1922). The motor nuclei of the cerebral nerves in phylogeny IV. Aves. *J. Comp. Neurol.* **34**, 233–75.

Carlson, A. J. (1904). Contributions to the physiology of the heart of the California hagfish (*Bolellostoma dombeyi*). *Z. Allg. Physiol.* **4**, 259–88.

Cohen, D. H., Schnall, A. M., MacDonald, R. L. & Pitts, L. H. (1970). Medullary cells of origin of vagal cardioinhibitory fibres in the pigeon. I. Anatomical structure of peripheral vagus nerves and the dorsal vagal motor nucleus. *J. Comp. Neurol.* **140**, 299–320.

Contreras, R. J., Gomez, M. M. & Norgren, R. (1980). Central origins of cranial nerve parasympathetic neurons in the cat. *J. Comp. Neurol.* **190**, 373–94.

Cruce, W. L. R. & Niewenhuys, R. (1974). The cell masses in the brain stem of the turtle (*Testudo hermanni*): a topographical and topoligical analysis. *J. Comp. Neurol.* **156**, 277–306.

Falck, B., Mecklenburg, C., Myhrberg, H. & Persson, H. (1966). Studies on adrenergic and cholinergic receptors in the isolated hearts of *Lampetra fluviatilis* (Cyclostomata) and *Pleuronectes platessa* (Teleostei). *Acta. Physiol. Scand.* **68**, 64–71.

Getz, B. & Sirnes, T. (1949). The localization within the dorsal motor vagal nucleus. *J. Comp. Neurol.* **90**, 95–110.

Green, C. W. (1902). Contributions to the physiology of the California hagfish

*Polistrotremas stoutii* II. The absence of regulative nerves for the systemic heart. *Am. J. Physiol.* **6**, 318–24.

Gwyn, D. G., Leslie, R. A. & Hopkins, D. A. (1985). Observations on the afferent and efferent organization of the vagus nerve and the innervation of the stomach in the squirrel monkey. *J. Comp. Neurol.* **239**, 163–75.

Harris, D. T., Gilding, H. P. & Smart, W. A. M. (1951). *Experimental Physiology for Medical Students* (5th edn). London: J. & A. Churchill.

Hopkins, D. A., Gootman, P. M., Gootman, N., Di Russo, S. M. & Zeballos, M. E. (1984). Brainstem cells of origin of the cervical vagus and cardiopulmonary nerves in the neonatal pig (*Sus scrofa*). *Brain Res.* **306**, 63–72.

Innes, A. J., Levings, J. J., Taylor, E. W. & Withington-Wray, D. J. (1986).The distribution of vagal preganglionic motoneurones in two species of Amphibia. *J. Physiol.* **376**, 55P.

Jordan, D., Spyer, K. M., Withington-Wray, D. J. & Wood, L. M. (1985). Histochemical and electrophysiological identification of cardiac and pulmonary vagal preganglionic neurones in the cat. *J. Physiol.* **372**, 87P.

Kalia, M. (1981). Brain stem localization of vagal preganglionic neurons. *J. Auton. Nerv. Syst.* **3**, 451–81.

Kalia, M. & Mesulam, M-M. (1980a). Brain stem projections of afferent and efferent fibres of the vagus nerve in the cat. I. The cervical vagus and nodose ganglion. *J. Comp. Neurol.* **193**, 435–65.

Kalia, M. & Mesulam, M-M. (1980b). Brain stem projections of afferent and efferent fibres of the vagus nerve in the cat. II. Laryngeal, tracheobranchial, pulmonary, cardiac and gastrointestinal branches. *J. Comp. Neurol.* **193**, 467–508.

Kalia, M. & Sullivan, J. M. (1982). Brain stem projections of sensory and motor components of the vagus nerve in the rat. *J. Comp. Neurol.* **211**, 248–64.

Katz, D. M. & Karten, H. J. (1983). Subnuclear organization of the dorsal motor nucleus of the vagus nerve in the pigeon *Columbia livia*. *J. Comp. Neurol.* **217**, 31–46.

Katz, D. M. & Karten, H. J. (1985). Topographic representation of visceral target organs within the dorsal motor nucleus of the vagus nerve of the pigeon *Columbia livia*. *J. Comp. Neurol.* **242**, 397–414.

Kennedy, M. C. (1981). Motoneurons that control vocalization in a reptile: an HRP histochemical study. *Brain Res.* **218**, 337–44.

Kimmel, D. L. (1940). Differentiation of the bulbar nuclei and the coincident development of associated root fibres in the rabbit. *J. Comp. Neurol.* **72**, 183–248.

Kirtisinghe, P. (1940). The myenteric nerve-plexus in some lower chordates. *Quart. J. Microsc. Sci.* **81**, 521–39.

Kremers, J. W. P. M. & Niewenhuys, R. (1979). Topological analysis of the brain stem of the crossopterygian fish *Latimeria chalumnae*. *J. Comp. Neurol.* **187**, 613–38.

Leong, S. K., Tay, S. W. & Wong, W. C. (1984). The localization of vagal neurons of the terrapin (*Trionyx sinensis*) as revealed by the retrograde horseradish peroxidase method. *J. Auton. Nerv. Syst.* **11**, 373–82.

Marshall, A. H. & Hurst, C. H. (1905). *Practical Zoology*. London: John Murray.

Mesulam, M. M. (1978). Tetramethyl benzidine for horseradish peroxidase neurohistochemistry: a non-carcinogenic blue reaction product with superior sensitivity for visualizing neural afferents and efferents. *J. Histochem. Cytochem.* **2612**, 106–17.

Metcalfe, J. D. & Butler, P. J. (1984). On the nervous regulation of gill blood flow in the dogfish *Scyliorhinus canicula*. *J. Exp. Biol.* **113**, 253–67.

Nicol. J. A. C. (1952). Autonomic nervous systems in lower chordates. *Biol. Rev. Cambridge Phil. Soc.* **27**, 1–49.

Niewenhuys, R. (1972). Topological analysis of the brain stem of the lamprey *Lampetra fluviatilis*. *J. Comp. Neurol.* **145**, 165–77.

Niewenhuys, R. & Oey, P. L. (1983). Topological analysis of the brainstem of the reedfish, *Erpetoichthys calabaricus*. *J. Comp. Neurol.* **213**, 220–32.

Nikundiwe, A. M. & Niewenhuys, R. (1983). The cell masses in the brainstem of the South African clawed frog *Xenopus laevis*: a topographical analysis. *J. Comp. Neurol.* **213**, 199–219.

Norris, H. W. & Hughes, S. P. (1920). The cranial occipital and anterior spinal nerves of the dogfish *Squalus acanthias*. *J. Comp. Neurol.* **31**, 293–400.

Opdam, P. & Niewenhuys, R. (1976). Topological analysis of the brainstem of the axolotl *Ambystoma mexicanum*. *J. Comp. Neurol.* **165**, 285–306.

Opdam, P., Kemali, M. & Niewenhuys, R. (1976). Topological analysis of the brainstem of the frogs *Rana esculenta* and *Rana catesbeiana*. *J. Comp. Neurol.* **165**, 307–32.

Pettersson, K. & Nilsson, S. (1979). Nervous control of the branchial vascular resistance of the Atlantic cod *Gadus morhua*. *J. Comp. Physiol.* **129**, 179–83.

Sanders, E. B. (1929). A consideration of certain bulbar, midbrain and cerebellar centres and fibre tracts in birds. *J. Comp. Neurol.* **49**, 155–22.

Schwab, M. E. (1979). Variation in the rhombencephalon. In *Biology of the Reptilia*, vol. 10 (eds C. Gans, R. G. Northcutt & P. S. Ulinski). San Francisco: Academic Press.

Smeets, W. J. A. J. & Niewenhuys, R. (1976). Topological analysis of the brainstem of the sharks *Squalus acanthias* and *Scyliorhinus canicula*. *J. Comp. Neurol.* **165**, 333–68.

Smeets, W. J. A. J., Niewenhuys, R. & Roberts, B. L. (1983). *The Central Nervous System of Cartilaginous Fishes*. Berlin: Springer-Verlag.

Struesse, S. L., Cruce, W. L. R. & Powell, K. S. (1984). Organization within the Cranial IX–X complex in ranid frogs: a horseradish peroxidase transport study. *J. Comp. Neurol.* **222**, 358–65.

Szabo, T. & Dussardier, M. (1964). Les noyaux d'origine du nerf vague chez le mouton. *Z. Zellforsch.* **63**, 247–76.

Szabo, T. & Liboubans, S. (1979). On the course and origin of cranial nerves in the teleost fish *Gnathonemus* determined by antero- and retrograde horseradish peroxidase axonal transport. *Neurosci. Lett.* **11**, 265–70.

Taylor, E. W. & Butler, P. J. (1982). Nervous control of heart rate: activity in the cardiac vagus of the dogfish. *J. Appl. Physiol.* **53**, 1330–5.

Taylor, E. W., Short, S. & Butler, P. J. (1977). The role of the cardiac vagus in the response of the dogfish *Scyliorhinus canicula* to hypoxia. *J. Exp. Biol.* **70**, 57–75.

Wild, J. N. (1981). Identification and localization of the motor nuclei and sensory projections of the glossopharyngeal, vagus and hypoglossal nerves of the cockatoo (*Cacatuo roseicapilla*). Cacatuidae. *J. Comp. Neurol.* **203**, 351–77.

Windle, W. F. (1933). Neurofibrillar development in the central nervous system of cat embryos between 8 and 12 mm long. *J. Comp. Neurol.* **58**, 643–723.

Withington-Wray, D. J., Roberts, B. L. & Taylor, E. W. (1986). The topographical organisation of the vagal motor column in the elasmobranch fish, *Scyliorhinus canicula* L. *J. Comp. Neurol.* **248**, 95–104.

Young, J. Z. (1933). The autonomic nervous system of Selachians. *Quart. J. Microsc. Sci.* **15**, 571–624.

# 17

# Central neural mechanisms mediating respiratory–cardiovascular interactions

**D. Jordan and K. M. Spyer**

*Department of Physiology, Royal Free Hospital School of Medicine, Rowland Hill Street, London NW3 2PF, UK*

## 17.1. Introduction

The importance of links between the cardiovascular and respiratory control systems has been noted for many years. In particular, cardiopulmonary coupling, which occurs during exercise, has been widely investigated (Whipp & Ward, 1982) since it is of importance in maintaining both adequate ventilation and perfusion of the lungs. However, even at rest respiratory–cardiovascular interactions can be observed. Rhythmical changes in arterial blood pressure (Traube–Hering waves) are due in part to the mechanical effects of the respiratory muscles affecting venous return to the heart, and also to a central action on vasomotor activity. There are also the variations in heart rate related to respiration known as sinus arrhythmia. In addition to these variations in resting heart rate and blood pressure, respiratory-related activity is also known to modify profoundly the effectiveness of many cardiovascular reflexes. The modification of the chemoreceptor reflex has been investigated in a variety of species since simultaneous alterations in both respiratory activity and chemoreceptor drive occur during breath-hold diving in most animals studied. These responses have been thoroughly reviewed recently (Butler & Jones, 1982; Daly, 1983, 1984) and will not be dealt with further here. This review will restrict itself to the phenomenon of sinus arrhythmia and the central nervous mechanisms underlying it, and the respiratory variations in the effectiveness of the baroreceptor reflex. It will become apparent that these two topics are in fact closely allied.

The inspiratory-related tachycardia of sinus arrhythmia was first thoroughly investigated by Anrep *et al.* (1936a, b) who showed it to be effected by two distinct mechanisms. One was the result of an inhibitory sensory input related to lung inflation, and the other a centrally generated input related to respiratory drive. Indeed, little further was elucidated until the work of Koepchen and his colleagues (Koepchen *et al.*, 1961a, b). In their study of baroreceptor control of heart period these authors showed that a stimulus to the carotid sinus nerve (CSN) evoked a fall in heart rate only if timed to coincide with expiration, a similar stimulus given in inspiration producing a severely attenuated response. Indeed, this marked respiratory variation in the baroreceptor control of heart rate has been confirmed in dogs, cats and human volunteers (Katona *et al.*, 1970; Haymet & McCloskey, 1975; Neil & Palmer, 1975; Davidson *et al.*, 1976; Eckberg & Orshan, 1980; Trzebski *et al.*, 1980).

## 17.2. Central respiratory drive and vagal efferent activity

Since both sinus arrhythmia and the baroreceptor-evoked cardiac slowing are primarily effected by the vagal innervation of the heart, though not entirely (Davis, *et al.*, 1977), it is not surprising that the respiratory variations in basal and evoked changes in heart rate are mirrored in recordings from cardiac vagal efferent (CVE) fibres in either the cervical vagus or its cardiac branches (Iriuchijima & Kumada, 1963, 1965; Jewett, 1964; Katona *et al.*, 1970; Kunze, 1972; Neil & Palmer, 1975; Davidson *et al.*, 1976). The activity in these fibres is characterised by its excitatory input from arterial chemo-receptors and baroreceptors, and a marked expiratory related firing pattern, the fibres being silenced during inspiration. Indeed, these excitatory inputs are only seen when the fibres are active, i.e. during expiration; stimulation of the arterial baroreceptors during inspiration being ineffective (Davidson *et al.*, 1976) (Fig. 17.1). Koepchen *et al.* (1961a, b) proposed three possible mechanisms by which such modulation of the baroreceptor–cardiac reflex might occur. First, respiratory activity could modulate the baroreceptor afferent input on its path to the cardiomotor neurones. Secondly, the respiratory effect could act on the cardiomotor neurones themselves. The third possibility was a combination of the first two. In a series of investigations in our, and other, laboratories over the last ten years, evidence has been accumulating in favour of the last of these hypotheses.

One series of experiments tested the possibility that respiratory drive could block the baroreceptor input at its first synapse, by a presynaptic action. This was considered as a possibility since baroreceptor afferents are known to terminate within the nucleus of the tractus solitarius (NTS) (Spyer, 1981; Jordan & Spyer, 1986, for review) and this nucleus also contains a group of respiratory neurones (von Baumgarten & Kanzow, 1958). The occurrence of such synaptic modification as a result of presynaptic actions on a variety of afferent terminals within the NTS has been reviewed recently (Jordan & Spyer, 1986). In summary, measurements of terminal excitability have indicated that certain vagal afferents which travel in the superior laryngeal nerve (SLN) are presynaptically influenced by other vagal afferents, the slowly adapting lung stretch afferents (SARs) and aortic baroreceptor afferents (Rudomin, 1967; Barillot, 1970). Also SARs are themselves affected by conditioning stimuli applied to the SLN (Barillot, 1970). This has been

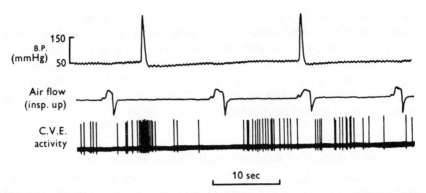

Fig. 17.1.   Dog. Records of carotid sinus blood pressure, respiratory airflow and the activity of a single cardiac vagal efferent nerve fibre (CVE). A burst of firing in the fibre was evoked by a baroreceptor stimulus timed to occur in the expiratory pause. No firing was evoked when a similar stimulus was given during inspiration (amplitude of the recorded action potentials in the range 100–300 µV). (Reproduced with permission from Davidson *et al.*, 1976).

confirmed by direct measurement of the membrane potential of SAR fibres close to their point of termination in the NTS (Richter *et al.*, 1986). However, in addition to the small waves of the membrane depolarisation in phase with lung inflation, these intracellular recordings revealed a wave of depolarisation in phase with central inspiratory activity, confirming the respiratory modulation of SARs previously inferred from excitability studies (Jordan *et al.*, 1981).

Whereas there is clear evidence that afferents from the lungs and airways are amenable to presynaptic influences, no such evidence is available for afferents in the CSN or aortic depressor nerve (ADN). Neither changes in terminal excitability (Rudomin, 1967, 1968; Barillot, 1970; Jordan & Spyer, 1979) nor membrane potential (Richter *et al.*, 1986) could be detected in such afferents, which include the arterial baroreceptors and chemoreceptors. Clearly then, respiratory modulation of these reflexes must occur later in the reflex pathway, and a postsynaptic site within the NTS is one possibility. In this nucleus some neurones show both a cardiac and respiratory rhythm (Stroh-Werz *et al.*, 1977) but in both extracellular (Lipski, *et al.*, 1975) and intracellular (Donoghue *et al.*, 1985, Mifflin *et al.*, 1986) studies the majority of cells receiving a baroreceptor input showed no evidence of receiving a major respiratory input. This absence of such convergence of baroreceptor and respiratory activity makes the NTS an unlikely site for a major 'gating' of the baroreceptor reflex.

It has been argued that the anterior depressor area of the hypothalamus forms a suprabulbar arm of the baroreceptor reflex since neurones here receive a baroreceptor input (Spyer, 1972) and stimulation initiates cardiovascular responses qualitatively identical to the baroreceptor reflex (Hilton &

Spyer, 1971). Since the latency of the baroreceptor input to this region is longer than that to the NTS, it is argued that neurones in this region receive a synaptic input from the NTS (Spyer, 1981). However, Lopes & Palmer (1978) have shown that the cardiac component of the response to anterior hypothalamic stimulation is modified by respiration in the same manner as a baroreceptor stimulus, so that it appears only during expiration. This again would argue for a site of respiratory modulation acting late in the reflex pathway.

A series of experiments carried out in our laboratory have led to the conclusion that the generation of sinus arrhythmia, and the respiratory 'gating' of the baroreceptor–cardiac reflex, can be accounted for by a direct inhibitory action of respiratory inputs on to the vagal preganglionic cardiomotor neurones (CVMs) themselves. We were led to this conclusion by a variety of different pieces of evidence from different experiments, but all involved recording from the cell bodies of those CVMs.

The location of the vagal motoneurones innervating the heart has been a matter of controversy over many years. Anatomical studies have shown such motoneurones in the dorsal vagal motor nucleus (DVN), the nucleus ambiguus (nA) and the region of the reticular formation lying between these. However, the relative importance of these nuclei varies between species (see Withington-Wray *et al.*, Chapter 16 of this volume, for review). Electrophysiological studies have shown that those vagal motoneurones with a cardioinhibitory function are located exclusively in the DVN in the pigeon (Schwaber & Cohen, 1978a, b), in the nA of the cat (McAllen & Spyer, 1976, 1978a) and in both these nuclei in the rabbit (Schwaber & Schneiderman, 1975; Jordan *et al.*, 1982).

CVMs were identified as described previously (McAllen & Spyer, 1976, 1978a, b). Briefly, this was by their antidromic response to electrical stimulation of the cardiac branches of the vagus in the chest of cats. In the anaesthetised cat these neurones have little, if any, spontaneous discharge, and hence recordings from CVM axons in this species are rare and difficult to study (Calaresu & Pearce, 1965; Kunze, 1972). The use of multi-barrelled micropipettes in some of our recordings allowed drugs to be applied to the immediate vicinity of the cell bodies. Application of small amounts of an excitant amino acid DL-homocysteic acid (DLH) depolarises the cell membrane, inducing the neurones to fire, discharge occurring predominantly in expiration. Spontaneous, and DLH-evoked, discharge can be augmented by CSN stimulation and shows a pulse modulation originating from both carotid sinus and aortic arch baroreceptors (McAllen & Spyer, 1978b). This artificial method of increasing vagal tone, if large enough, can induce the neurones to fire even during the period of inspiration, when they are normally silent. In this situation, both the CSN excitatory input and the pulse modulation of the discharge are present not only during expiration (Fig. 17.2B), as described previously, but also during inspiration

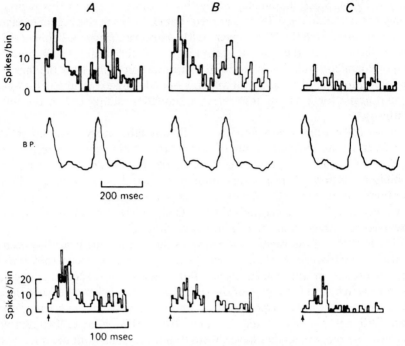

Fig. 17.2.   Cat. Cardiac rhythm of a CVM and its response to electrical stimulation of the CSN. Traces from above: pulse-triggered histograms of CVM activity (120 cycles, 10 ms bins), femoral pulse wave on same time scale, post-stimulus time histograms of the response to CSN stimulation (0.1 ms pulse at 2V; 5 ms bins, 128 cycles). A: Analysed throughout respiratory cycle; B: only in expiration; C: only in inspiration. Unit firing in response to 60 nA DLH. (Reproduced with permission from McAllen & Spyer, 1978b.)

(Fig. 17.2C), when normally it would have evoked no change in CVM activity and no change in heart rate. Clearly, then, if any respiratory 'gate' is acting early in the baroreceptor reflex pathway, it cannot be of major importance since the baroreceptor input reaches the CVM throughout the respiratory cycle but it is usually subliminal during inspiration due to processes acting at the level of the preganglionic neurone. We have recently provided further direct evidence for this suggestion.

First, we have identified acetylcholine as a putative inhibitory neurotransmitter in the nA since its iontophoretic application reduces the discharge of CVMs through a muscarinic receptor, atropine sulphate, simultaneously applied, blocking the action of acetylcholine (Garcia *et al.*, 1978; Gilbey *et al.*, 1984) (Fig. 17.3). This proposed cholinergic input appears to act both tonically and phasically since atropine applied alone enhanced neuronal discharge, particularly during inspiration when the cell is normally silent. The effect of this atropine application was a reduction, or complete

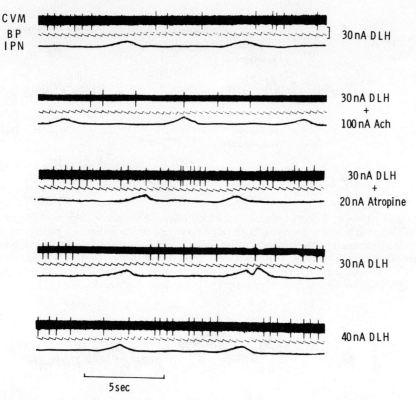

Fig. 17.3.   Cat. Effect of *DL*-homocysteic acid (DLH), acetylcholine (Ach) and atropine on the discharge of a CVM. In each panel traces from above: CVM activity, arterial blood pressure and integrated phrenic nerve activity (IPN). (Reproduced with permission from Gilbey *et al.*, 1984.)

suppression, of the respiratory modulation of CVM discharge (Fig. 17.4a). This is quite unlike the general excitant action of DLH, which has a greater effect on the discharge in expiration, maintaining the cells' repiratory modulation (Fig. 17.3). These data confirm earlier suggestions of a central action of atropine, at doses lower than those that produce peripheral blocking actions (McGuigan, 1921; Heinekamp, 1922; Morton & Thomas, 1958; Averill & Lamb, 1959). Indeed, more recently, Katona *et al.* (1977) showed in dogs that such minute doses of atropine given i.v. resulted in an augmentation of CVE fibre discharge, but only when the animals had spontaneous respiratory discharge, and experiments in man have demonstrated an augmentation of vagal outflow and baroreflex–cardiac slowing after intravenous infusions of atropine (Raczkowska *et al.*, 1983).

   The diffusion of drugs during iontophoretic application in the above experiments does not allow us to distinguish between a direct inhibitory effect of acetylcholine on CVMs and a cholinergic inhibition of a local excitatory

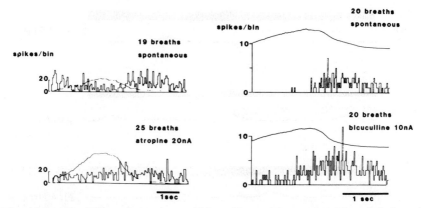

Fig. 17.4.   Cat. Effect of atropine and bicuculline on the respiratory modulation of CVMs. Each of the four panels shows an average of the integrated phrenic nerve discharge superimposed upon a histogram of CVM discharge triggered from the rise in phrenic nerve activity. The two panels on the left show the respiratory modulation of CVM discharge prior to, and during, application of atropine sulphate; those on the right prior to, and during, application of bicuculline methiodide.

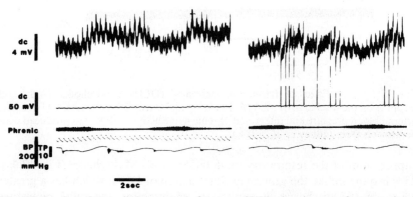

Fig. 17.5.   Cat. Intracellular record from a CVM showing respiratory-related changes in membrane potential. Five minutes after penetration the cell stopped firing action potentials (1st panel) but could be made to fire by injecting low depolarising currents (2nd panel). In each panel traces from above: high and low gain records of membrane potential, phrenic nerve activity, arterial blood pressure and tracheal pressure. (Reproduced with permission from Jordan *et al.*, 1985.)

interneurone. Any proposed interneurone, however, would have to show an inspiratory-related discharge to be effective, and in a parallel study we were unable to find a significant population of inspiratory neurones in this region which were affected by acetylcholine (Jordan & Spyer, 1981). On the balance of the available evidence, and the fact that CVMs are located in a region containing the ventral group of inspiratory neurones, we considered it most

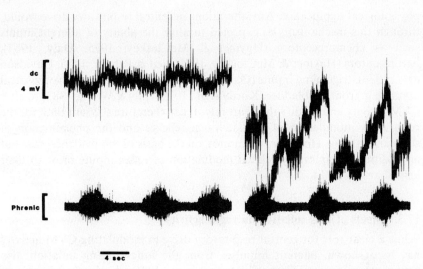

Fig. 17.6. Cat. Intracellular record from a CVM showing respiratory-related changes in membrane potential (1st panel). After passage of negative hyperpolarising current (1 nA for 3 min) hyperpolarising waves reversed (2nd panel). In each panel traces from above: high gain d.c. recording of membrane potential and phrenic nerve activity. (Reproduced with permission from Jordan *et al.*, 1985.)

likely that the major effect of central respiratory drive on cardiac activity is mediated by a cholinergic inhibitory input to CVMs which is active during inspiration. This has been confirmed in our intracellular recordings of the membrane potential of CVMs (Gilbey *et al.*, 1984). The neurones received depolarising potentials 110–120 ms after the onset of each femoral pressure wave, which is consistent with the latency of the baroreceptor input to CVMs (McAllen & Spyer, 1978b). These depolarisations were superimposed upon slower fluctuations of membrane potential occurring in phase with the central respiratory cycle, the membrane of CVMs being relatively hyper-polarised during inspiration when the phrenic nerve was active (Fig. 17.5). Measurements of membrane input resistance and the reversal of the hyperpolarisations to waves of depolarisation during inspiration by Cl⁻ injection (Fig. 17.6) confirmed our hypothesis that these cells were receiving i.p.s.p.s at a time when phrenic nerve activity was greatest. During this period membrane resistance is lowered and shunts any excitatory input reaching the neurone, including pulse-rhythmical e.p.s.p.s. The cells were at their most excitable immediately after the end of inspiration (phase I expiration or post-inspiration, Richter & Ballantyne, 1983) and relatively less excitable during phase II expiration when they appeared to receive a variable but less effective period of inhibitory input from an, as yet, unidentified source.

The mechanism described is clearly one that can contribute significantly to the excitability of CVMs, and so would be expected to have considerable physiological significance. Any alterations in central respiratory drive would, through this mechanism, be expected to alter the ability of afferent inputs such as chemoreceptors (Haymet & McCloskey, 1975; Daly, 1983), baroreceptors (Haymet & McCloskey, 1975; Neil & Palmer, 1975; Davidson *et al.*, 1976), trigeminal inputs (Gandevia *et al.*, 1978b; Daly, 1984) or visceral inputs, e.g. from the bladder (Kordy *et al.*, 1975; Daly & Wood, 1982) to alter CVM activity and modify the heart rate. It can therefore account both for the respiratory modulation of cardiac vagal reflexes and the phenomenon of sinus arrhythmia. However, we cannot, on the basis of this evidence, rule out an additional respiratory-related modulation of reflex inputs prior to their arrival at the CVM.

## 17.3. Effects of lung inflation on vagal activity

While a clear role for central respiratory drive in modulating CVM activity has been shown, afferent impulses from the lungs during inflation also contribute to sinus arrhythmia (Anrep *et al.*, 1936a, b). In the absence of respiratory-centre activity sinus arrhythmia is abolished by denervation of the lungs (Angell-James & Daly, 1978). Inflation of the lungs has also been shown to inhibit CVE fibre activity in dogs (Jewett, 1964; Iriuchijima, 1972) and to produce tachycardia (Daly & Scott, 1958; Hainsworth, 1974; Gandevia *et al.*, 1978a; Angell-James *et al.*, 1981; Daly *et al.*, 1983) but only when vagal tone was high (Jewett, 1964; Iriuchijima, 1972; Potter, 1981; Daly *et al.*, 1983). Indeed, the effects of lung inflation can be so powerful that they can reverse the bradycardia evoked by chemoreceptor stimulation to a tachycardia (Daly & Scott, 1958). A recent study (Gandevia *et al.*, 1978a) has shown that lung inflation itself can inhibit the cardiac effects of brief chemoreceptor or baroreceptor stimuli and that this is more powerful during rapid inflations than during slow ramp inflations. During maintained inflations, however, the blockade of these reflex responses soon accommodates, though the Hering–Breuer apnoea is maintained. Deflation had no effect on the reflex responses. The receptors responsible for these responses are unknown, but it has been suggested that SARs could mediate the effects (Angell-James *et al.*, 1981). These afferents certainly respond to inflation, but not to deflation, and show a sensitivity to the rate of inflation (Knowlton & Larrabee, 1946). However, their afferent response adapts only slowly, as was seen for the Hering–Breuer apnoea, whereas the suppression of the cardiac reflexes was transient. Other pulmonary afferents — the 'irritant receptors' — may also be considered. They too respond to lung inflation in a roughly rate-sensitive manner and they adapt rapidly to maintained inflation. However, these receptors also fire in response to lung deflation (Widdicombe, 1954). Thus, it appears more likely that SARs are indeed responsible for this response, but it must be postulated that their activity is modified by some central mechanism such that there is adaptation of a maintained afferent input. Recently, an elegant study by Potter (1981) has shown that whereas CVE activity was totally abolished when the phrenic nerve was active, moderate lung inflations had relatively little effect on CVE discharge until vagal tone was raised by increasing arterial blood pressure. Even with this increased background tone the effect of lung inflation was not large, though similar lung inflations were most effective in blocking baroreceptor-evoked increases in CVE activity. This dissociation of effect on background as opposed to reflexly evoked discharge has led to the suggestion that whilst central respiratory drive acts primarily at the level of the CVM, to decrease its excitability and therefore reduce background tone, the major effect of lung inflation is to suppress reflex inputs before they arrive at the CVM.

The site of such actions of lung inflation remains to be resolved. Lopes & Palmer (1976) suggested that the Rβ neurones of the dorsal medulla, which fire in response to lung inflation as well as central respiratory drive (von Baumgarten & Kanzow, 1958), may act as one site of the respiratory gate. This was based on the assumption that lung inflation effects and central respiratory drive acted through the same mechanism. These neurones may well be the integrating site of the lung stretch input since the response of these neurones is known to adapt to maintained lung inflation (Berger, 1977; Lipski *et al.*, 1977b). This could then account for the transient suppressive effect of maintained lung inflation on reflex bradycardia. However, since lung inflation and central respiratory drive can act independently (Potter, 1981), a role for Rβ neurones as a convergent site is not necessary to explain the observed results. Recent studies in fact would argue against such a role. The majority of Rβ neurones are now thought to have axons projecting to the contralateral spinal cord (Berger, 1977; Lipski *et al.*, 1979, 1983) and lung stretch afferents terminate in other regions of the NTS as well (Donoghue *et al.*, 1982) where they excite many non-respiratory neurones (Donoghue *et al.*, 1985) some of which also show cardiovascular rhythms (Stroh-Werz *et al.*, 1977).

## 17.4. The origin of vagal 'tone'

At this point it may well be worth considering the origin of background 'tone' in CVMs. It is clear that anaesthesia tends to cause a rise in heart rate due to removal of vagal tone, and indeed Inoue & Arndt (1982) have shown in cats a clear depression of the activity of CVE fibres by a variety of anaesthetics. Indeed, in the anaesthetised cat vagal tone is notoriously low (Katona *et al.*, 1970; Kunze, 1972; McAllen & Spyer, 1976, 1978a, b) and may well explain the inability to find cardioinhibitory fibres in the cervical vagus (Calaresu & Pearce, 1965). Vagal tone in anaesthetised dogs, however, is said to be higher than in cats (Jewett, 1964; Katona *et al.*, 1970; Iriuchijima, 1972; Davidson *et al.*, 1976), and this is probably true. However, it must be kept in mind that in the majority of experiments on dogs the animals were pretreated with morphine. Microinjections of enkephalins and opiate agonists into the nA cause profound bradycardia (Laubie *et al.*, 1979), and intravenous or intracerebroventricular injections of these drugs excite cardioinhibitory fibres (Inoue *et al.*, 1980, 1985).

Clearly, an important tonically active excitatory drive to CVMs arises from the arterial baroreceptors, the level of vagal discharge being related to the prevailing level of arterial blood pressure. However, impulses from baroreceptors are not the sole source of vagal tone since removal of both sets of baroreceptor nerves does not remove ongoing discharge in all CVE fibres (Iriuchijima, 1972).

Ongoing discharges in peripheral arterial chemoreceptors would also be expected to produce a level of excitatory drive to CVMs. Indeed artificial ventilation producing hypocapnia causes tachycardia and a fall in CVE fibre activity (Daly & Hazzledine, 1963; Haymet & McCloskey, 1975; Sutton, 1981). However, whether this is due to an effect on peripheral or central chemoreceptors or is independent of these remains to be determined. Interestingly, during similar levels of hyperventilation the cardiac effects of chemoreceptor stimulation were blocked if the animal was hypocapnic, but only attenuated if isocapnia was maintained (Daly & Hazzledine, 1963). Similarly, Haymet & McCloskey (1975) were unable to produce baroreceptor or chemoreceptor cardiac reflexes early in a period of hyperventilatory apnoea, though the reflexes gradually reappeared as the apnoea progressed, these effects being independent of the degree of lung inflation. This would indicate that a certain level of activity in the chemorespiratory system is required to produce a level of tone for the reflexes to exert themselves.

In experimental studies a common method for inducing extra vagal tone is stimulation of the SLN. This induces apnoea by inhibiting both inspiratory activity and the consequent lung inflation, these factors then acting together to raise CVE activity (Kordy, *et al.*, 1975). Indeed the effect of SLN stimulation is so powerful that any other reflex input concomitantly producing bradycardia would be markedly facilitated, even to the level of cardiac arrest (see Daly *et al.*, 1979; Daly, 1983, 1984). This apnoeic disinhibition of CVE activity would only be effective if a certain level of tone was already present in the fibres. Indeed, in cats, which have a low level of vagal tone, Lopes & Palmer (1976) claimed that SLN stimulation only induced bradycardia if both CSN and ADN were intact. However, in dogs, Iriuchijima & Kumada (1968) argue against disinhibition of the CSN input being the major effect of SLN stimulation since not only could CVE fibres be activated by SLN stimulation at a shorter latency than by CSN stimulation but also SLN stimulation could still induce bradycardia, though of smaller magnitude, during a hyperventilatory apnoea. On the basis of this, it is postulated that SLN may directly excite CVMs (see Fig. 17.8). Also, it is known that laryngeal stimulation is a powerful excitant of postinspiratory neurones (Remmers *et al.*, 1985), and the firing pattern of CVMs resembles that of postinspiratory neurones (Gilbey *et al.*, 1984). Hence SLN and other synaptic inputs may also excite CVMs via a subpopulation of the post-inspiratory group of neurones.

Although these brainstem afferent systems clearly contribute to the ongoing level of vagal discharge, the fact that anaesthetics alter such tone may indicate that suprabulbar areas are also involved. Indeed, decerebration produces a fall in heart rate by increasing vagal tone (Glaser, 1962; Barman & Gebber, 1979).

Stimulation in the perifornical area of the cat elicits a pattern of response known as the hypothalamic defence response (Abrahams *et al.*, 1960) which includes tachycardia, increased inspiratory drive, and blockade of the baroreceptor reflex (Coote *et al.*, 1979). Such a suppression of the baroreceptor-induced bradycardia could be explained by an overriding inhibition of vagal activity evoked by the increased respiratory drive. Indeed, concomitant stimulation of the SLN, which abolishes any effect of in-spiratory changes, removes in part the hypothalamic inhibition of CSN-induced bradycardia (Lopes & Palmer, 1978). However, stimulation of this same hypothalamic area has been shown to have an inhibitory action on CVMs independent of respiration (Jordan *et al.*, 1980; Spyer, 1984) for up to 200 ms following a single shock to the hypothalamus. The simultaneous application of atropine in these experiments blocked any simultaneous inhibitory effect of increased inspiratory drive.

Descending inputs from this region appear to tonically inhibit vagal outflow since small knife cuts which disconnect this region from the brainstem immediately produce a fall in heart rate (Lopes & Palmer, 1978). The neurotransmitter used by this pathway in the brainstem appears to be the inhibitory amino acid GABA. Barman & Gebber (1979) demonstrated that the tachycardia produced by hypothalamic stimulation was attenuated by drugs which had GABA-antagonist actions (picrotoxin and bicuculline) but not by other stimulants (strychnine and pentylentetrazol). Indeed, the GABA antagonists produced a fall in basal heart rate only in intact animals, not in decerebrate preparations. This work also suggested that the GABA inhibition was acting close to the vagal outflow since other inputs from the inferior olive and peripheral nerves, which also block reflex vagal brady-cardia, were also blocked by picrotoxin. Microinjections of the GABA antagonist bicuculline into the region of the nA, the site of CVMs, evokes a dose-related bradycardia (DiMicco *et al.*, 1979) whereas injections of the GABA agonist muscimol inhibit baroreceptor-induced bradycardia (Wil-liford *et al.*, 1980). Most recently, iontophoretic application has shown that GABA inhibits CVM activity in cats, an effect blocked by bicuculline which, when applied alone, induced CVM discharge (Fig. 17.7) (Gilbey *et al.*, 1985b; Jordan *et al.*, 1985). Interestingly, the excitatory effect of the antagonist bicuculline had no effect on the respiratory discharge of the cell, in contrast to the effect of the cholinergic antagonist atropine sulphate (Fig. 17.4).

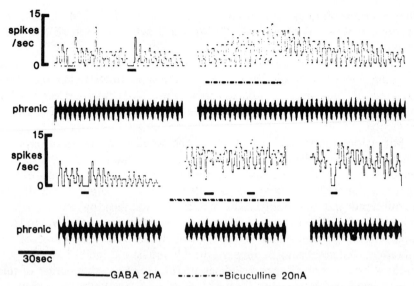

Fig. 17.7. Cat. Effect of iontophoretic application of GABA (2 nA) and bicuculline (20 nA) on the discharge rate of a CVM. Each panel shows a ratemeter record of CVM activity and, below, phrenic nerve activity. (Reproduced with permission from Jordan *et al.*, 1985.)

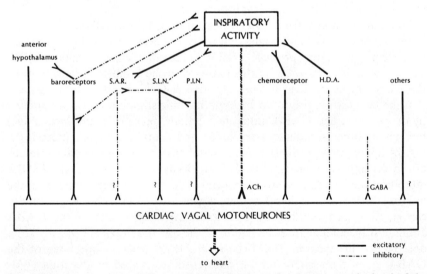

Fig. 17.8. A summary of the possible mechanisms that interact at the level of the CVM based on the foregoing discussion. Excitatory mechanisms are shown as solid lines, inhibitory mechanisms as dotted lines. The lines indicate pathways, not individual neurones, and say nothing of the number of synapses involved. Abbreviations: ACh, acetylcholine; GABA, gamma-aminobutyric acid; H.D.A., hypothalamic defence area; P.I.N., subpopulation of postinspiratory neurones; S.A.R., slow-adapting lung stretch receptors; S.L.N., superior laryngeal nerve afferents; ?, postulated pathways.

A summary of the synaptic processes determining cardiac vagal activity which have been discussed are shown in Fig. 17.8. This should be read as a whole, such that the simultaneous activation of more than one system will interact with the other systems. It should be noted that pathways, not individual neurones, are depicted, and postulated pathways are marked with a '?'.

## 17.5. Respiratory modulation of sympathetic nerve activity

Although sinus arrhythmia and control of the heart is primarily via the vagus nerves, a degree of sinus arrhythmia still appears in dogs after vagotomy (Davis *et al.*, 1977), and in these same animals there is still a respiratory-related modulation of the baroreceptor and chemoreceptor cardiac reflexes. Indeed, a respiratory-related component has been identified in many sympathetic nerves since the original studies in 1932 of Adrian, Bronk & Phillips, maximal sympathetic discharge occurring during the period of phrenic activity, with a minimum in early expiration (Seller & Richter, 1971; Gootman & Cohen, 1980). The mechanisms producing such variations in sympathetic discharge are sufficient to modulate the duration of baroreceptor-induced sympatho-inhibition which is maximal during early expiration and minimal during inspiration (Seller & Richter, 1971).

The synaptic processes underlying such respiratory modulation of sympathetic discharge are more a matter of debate. Barman & Gebber (1976) argue that the respiratory rhythm in the phrenic and sympathetic nerves is generated by two independent oscillators which are normally coupled to one another since changes in respiratory rate were able to alter the phase relations between phrenic and sympathetic nerve activity.

Other recordings by Polosa and his colleagues on single preganglionic fibres in the cervical sympathetic nerve of cats have produced a different conclusion. Such fibres showed three types of firing pattern: inspiratory peak (with or without a superimposed tonic drive), expiratory peak, or no respiratory rhythm (Preiss *et al.*, 1975). Any procedure which decreased central respiratory drive such as hypocapnia (Preiss & Polosa, 1977), lung inflation (Gerber & Polosa, 1978) or SLN stimulation (Gerber & Polosa, 1979) simultaneously reduced the inspiratory-related component of sympathetic discharge, whilst hyperventilation produced tonic firing in expiratory-related fibres (Preiss *et al.*, 1975). These results would suggest that sympathetic preganglionic neurones receive an input which is a direct copy of the central respiratory drive potentials delivered to respiratory motoneurones. A similar conclusion was reached in a recent study involving the recording of the respiratory modulation of cervical sympathetic preganglionic neurones in rats (Gilbey *et al.*, 1985a).

The end organ responses of those fibres recorded in the previous studies are unknown. However, similar inspiratory-related discharge has been identified in sudomotor neurones and in vasoconstrictor neurones supplying skeletal muscle and skin in both cats and humans (Jänig *et al.*, 1980, 1983). However, although part of the modulation could be accounted for by respiratory drive potentials, another component appeared to be due to baroreceptor unloading during respiratory-related blood-pressure waves. This may simply reflect the varying degree of baroreceptor control of the various sympathetic outflows.

Whilst changes in central respiratory drive can explain much of the respiratory modulation of sympathetic discharge, it is clear that lung inflation can have an action independent of central respiratory changes. Lipski *et al.* (1977a) noted subliminal changes in the excitability of silent sympathetic preganglionic neurones during lung inflation in the absence of phrenic nerve discharges. In the majority of cases these indicated an inhibitory input. Cohen *et al.* (1980) showed a similar inhibitory effect of lung expansion on cervical sympathetic and greater splanchnic nerves during the phase of phrenic silence. Similarly, SLN stimulation in addition to inhibiting inspiratory-related sympathetic discharge can also excite any tonic background discharge in these neurones (Gerber & Polosa, 1979).

Clearly, the synaptic mechanisms underlying respiratory modulation of the sympathetic outflow are not as clearly defined as those for vagal motoneurones, though with similar techniques it should be possible to provide a clearer picture.

### Acknowledgements

The original studies described here were supported by grants from the Medical Research Council and the British Heart Foundation. Thanks are due to Dr M. P. Gilbey and Dr L. M. Wood for their constructive discussions and criticisms during the writing of the manuscript, and to Marion Roper and Virginia Scott for their skilful typing and patience.

### References

Abrahams, V. C., Hilton, S. M. & Zbrożyna, A. (1960). Active muscle vasodilatation produced by stimulation of the brain stem: its significance in the defence reaction. *J. Physiol.* **154**, 491–513.

Adrian, E. D., Bronk, D. W. & Phillips, G. (1932). Discharges in mammalian sympathetic nerves. *J. Physiol.* **74**, 115–33.

Angell-James, J. E. & Daly, M. de B. (1978). The effects of artificial lung inflation on reflexly induced bradycardia associated with apnoea in the dog. *J. Physiol.* **274**, 349–66.

Angell-James, J. E., Elsner, R. & Daly, M. de B. (1981). Lung inflation: effects on heart rate, respiration and vagal afferent activity in seals. *Am. J. Physiol.* **240**, H190–8.

Anrep, G. V., Pascual, W. & Rössler, R. (1936a). Respiratory variations of the heart rate. I. The reflex mechanism of the respiratory arrhythmia. *Proc. R. Soc. Lond. (Biol.)* **119**, 191–217.

Anrep, G. V., Pascual, W. & Rössler, R. (1936b). Respiratory variations of the heart rate. II. The central mechanism of respiratory arrhythmia and the inter-relationships between central and reflex mechanisms. *Proc. R. Soc. Lond. (Biol.)* **119**, 218–30.

Averill, K. H. & Lamb, L. E. (1959). Less commonly recognised actions of atropine on cardiac rhythm. *Am. J. Med. Sci.* **237**, 304–18.

Barillot, J.-C. (1970). Dépolarisation présynaptique des fibres sensitives vagales et laryngées. *J. Physiol. (Paris)* **62**, 273–94.

Barman, S. M. & Gebber, G. L. (1976). Basis for synchronization of sympathetic and phrenic nerve discharges. *Am. J. Physiol.* **231**, 1601–7.

Barman, S. M. & Gebber, G. L. (1979). Picrotoxin- and bicuculline-sensitive inhibition of cardiac vagal reflexes. *J. Pharmacol. Exp. Ther.* **209**, 67–72.

Berger, A. J. (1977). Dorsal respiratory group neurones in the medulla of cat: spinal projections, responses to lung inflation and superior laryngeal nerve stimulation. *Brain Res.* **135**, 231–54.

Butler, P. J. & Jones, D. R. (1982). The comparative physiology of diving in vertebrates. *Adv. Comp. Physiol. Biochem.* **8**, 179–364.

Calaresu, F. R. & Pearce, J. W. (1965). Electrical activity of efferent vagal fibres and dorsal nucleus of the vagus during reflex bradycardia in the cat. *J. Physiol.* **176**, 228–39.

Cohen, M. I., Gootman, P. M. & Feldman, J. L. (1980). Inhibition of sympathetic discharge by lung inflation. In *Arterial Baroreceptors and Hypertension*, pp. 161–7 (ed. P. Sleight). Oxford: Oxford Medical Publications.

Coote, J. H., Hilton, S. M. & Perez-Gonzalez, J. F. (1979). Inhibition of the baroreceptor reflex on stimulation in the brainstem defence centre. *J. Physiol.* **288**, 549–60.

Daly, M. de B. (1983). Peripheral arterial chemoreceptors and the cardiovascular system. In *Physiology of the Peripheral Arterial Chemoreceptors*, pp. 325–93 (eds H. Acker & R. G. O'Regan). Amsterdam: Elsevier/North Holland Biomedical Press BV.

Daly, M. de B. (1984). Breath-hold diving: mechanisms of cardiovascular adjust-ments in the mammal. In *Recent Advances in Physiology*, *10* pp. 201–45 (ed. P. F. Baker). Edinburgh: Churchill Livingstone.

Daly, M. de B., Angell-James, J. E. & Elsner, R. (1979). Role of carotid body chemoreceptors and their reflex interactions in bradycardia and cardiac arrest. *Lancet* **i**, 764–7.

Daly, M. de B. & Hazzledine, J. L. (1963). The effects of artificially induced hyperventilation on the primary cardiac reflex response to stimulation of the carotid bodies in the dog. *J. Physiol.* **168**, 872–89.

Daly, M. de B., Litherland, A. S. & Wood, L. M. (1983). The reflex effects of inflation of the lungs on heart rate and hind limb vascular resistance in the cat. *I.R.C.S. Med. Sci.* **11**, 859–60.

Daly, M. de B. & Scott, M. J. (1958). The effects of stimulation of the carotid body chemoreceptors on heart rate in the dog. *J. Physiol.* **144**, 148–66.

Daly, M. de B. & Wood, L. M. (1982). Effects of distension of the urinary bladder on the carotid sinus baroreceptor reflex in the dog. *J. Physiol.* **325**, 16P.

Davidson, N. S., Goldner, S. & McCloskey, D. I. (1976). Respiratory modulation of baroreceptor and chemoreceptor reflexes affecting heart-rate and cardiac vagal efferent nerve activity. *J. Physiol.* **259**, 523–30.

Davis, A. L., McCloskey, D. I. & Potter, E. K. (1977). Respiratory modulation of baroreceptor and chemoreceptor reflexes affecting heart rate through the sym-pathetic nervous system. *J. Physiol.* **272**, 691–703.

DiMicco, J. A., Gale, K., Hamilton, B. L. & Gillis, R. A. (1979) GABA receptor control of parasympathetic outflow to heart: characterization and brainstem location. *Science* **204**, 1106–9.

Donoghue, S., Felder, R. B., Gilbey, M. P., Jordan, D. & Spyer, K. M. (1985). Postsynaptic activity evoked in the nucleus tractus solitarius by carotid sinus and aortic nerve afferents in the cat. *J. Physiol.* **360**, 261–73.

Donoghue, S., Garcia, M., Jordan, D. & Spyer, K. M. (1982). The brain-stem projections of pulmonary stretch afferent neurones in cats and rabbits. *J. Physiol.* **322**, 353–63.

Eckberg, D. L. & Orshan, C. R. (1980). Central respiratory–baroreceptor reflex interaction in man. In *Central Interaction between Respiratory and Cardiovascular Control Systems*, pp. 206–15 (eds H. P. Koepchen, S. M. Hilton & A. Trzebski). Berlin: Springer-Verlag.

Gandevia, S. C., McCloskey, D. I. & Potter, E. K. (1978a). Inhibition of baroreceptor and chemoreceptor reflexes on heart rate by afferents from the lungs. *J. Physiol.* **276**, 369–81.

Gandevia, S. C., McCloskey, D. I. & Potter, E. K. (1978b). Reflex bradycardia occurring in response to diving, nasopharyngeal stimulation and ocular pressure, and its modification by respiraction and swallowing. *J. Physiol.* **276**, 383–94.

Garcia, M., Jordan, D. & Spyer, K. M. (1978). Studies on the properties of cardiac vagal neurones. *Neurosci. Lett.* Suppl. 1, S16.

Gerber, U. & Polosa, C. (1978). Effects of pulmonary stretch receptor afferent stimulation on sympathetic preganglionic neuron firing. *Can. J. Physiol. Pharmacol.* **56**, 191–8.

Gerber, U. & Polosa, C. (1979). Some effects of superior laryngeal nerve stimulation on sympathetic preganglionic neuron firing. *Can. J. Physiol. Pharmacol.* **57**, 1073–81.

Gilbey, M. P., Jordan, D., Numao, Y., Spyer, K. M. & Wood, L. M. (1985a). Respiratory modulation of cervical sympathetic preganglionic neurones in the anaesthetised rat. *J. Physiol.* **369**, 145P.

Gilbey, M. P., Jordan, D., Richter, D. W. & Spyer, K. M. (1984). Synaptic mechanisms involved in the inspiratory modulation of vagal cardio-inhibitory neurones in the cat. *J. Physiol.* **356**, 65–78.

Gilbey, M. P., Jordan, D., Spyer, K. M. & Wood, L. M. (1985b). The inhibitory actions of GABA on cardiac vagal motoneurones in the cat. *J. Physiol.* **361**, 49P.

Glaser, R. L. (1962). Vagal inhibition of cardiovascular activity in the decerebrate cat. *Am. J. Physiol.* **203**, 449–52.

Gootman, P. M. & Cohen, M. I. (1980). Origin of rhythms common to sympathetic outflows at different spinal levels. In *Arterial Baroreceptors and Hypertension*, pp. 154–60 (ed. P. Sleight). Oxford: Oxford Medical Publications.

Hainsworth, R. (1974). Circulatory responses from lung inflation in anesthetized dogs. *Am. J. Physiol.* **226**, 247–55.

Haymet, B. T. & McCloskey, D. I. (1975). Baroreceptor and chemoreceptor infuences on heart-rate during the respiratory cycle in the dog. *J. Physiol.* **245**, 699–712.

Heinekamp, W. J. R. (1922). The central influence of atropine and lyoscine on the heart rate. *J. Lab. Clin. Med.* **8**, 104–11.

Hilton, S. M. & Spyer, K. M. (1971). Participation of the anterior hypothalamus in the baroreceptor reflex. *J. Physiol.* **218**, 271–93.

Inoue, K. & Arndt, J. O. (1982). Efferent vagal discharge and heart rate in response to methohexitone, althesin, ketamine and etomidate in cats. *Br. J. Anaesth.* **54**, 1105–16.

Inoue, K., Nashan, B. & Arndt, J. O. (1985). [D-met$^2$, pro$^5$] enkephalinamide activates cardioinhibitory efferents in anaesthetized dogs. *Eur. J. Pharmacol.* **110**, 233-9.

Inoue, K., Samodelov, L. F. & Arndt, J. O. (1980). Fentanyl activates a particular population of vagal efferents which are cardioinhibitory. *Naunyn-Schmiedebergs's Arch. Pharmacol.* **312**, 57-61.

Iriuchijima, J. (1972). Cardiac vagal efferent discharge. In *Cardiovascular Physiology*, pp. 1-25 (ed. J. Iriuchijima). Tokyo: Igaku Shoin.

Iriuchijima, J. & Kumada, M. (1963). Efferent cardiac vagal discharge of the dog in response to electrical stimulation of sensory nerves. *Jpn. J. Physiol.* **13**, 599-605.

Iriuchijima, J. & Kumada, M. (1965). Activity in single vagal efferent fibres to the heart. *Jpn. J. Physiol.* **14**, 479-87.

Iriuchijima, J. & Kumada, M. (1968). On the cardioinhibitory reflex originating from the superior laryngeal nerve. *Jpn. J. Physiol.* **18**, 453-61.

Jänig, W., Kummel, H. & Wiprich, L. (1980). Respiratory rhythmicities in vaso-constrictor and sudomotor neurones supplying the cat's hindlimb. In *Central Interaction between Respiratory and Cardiovascular Control Systems*, pp. 128-36 (eds H. P. Koepchen, S. M. Hilton & A. Trzebski). Berlin: Springer-Verlag.

Jänig, W., Sundlöf, G. & Wallin, B. G. (1983). Discharge patterns of sympathetic neurones supplying skeletal muscle and skin in man and cat. *J. Auton. Nerv. Syst.* **7**, 239-56.

Jewett, D. L. (1964). Activity of single efferent fibres in the cervical vagus nerve of the dog with special reference to possible cardioinhibitory fibres. *J. Physiol.* **175**, 321-57.

Jordan, D., Donoghue, S. & Spyer, K. M. (1981). Respiratory modulation of afferent terminal excitability in the nucleus tractus solitarius. *J. Auton. Nerv. Syst.* **3**, 291-7.

Jordan, D., Gilbey, M. P., Richter, D. W., Spyer, K. M. & Wood, L. M. (1985). Respiratory-vagal interactions in the nucleus ambiguus of the cat. In *Neurogenesis of Central Respiratory Rhythm*, pp. 370-8 (eds A. L. Bianchi & M. Denavit-Saubié). Lancaster: MTP Press.

Jordan, D., Khalid, M. E. M., Schneiderman, N. & Spyer, K. M. (1980). The inhibitory control of vagal cardiomotor neurones. *J. Physiol.* **301**, 54-5P.

Jordan, D., Khalid, M. E. M., Schniederman, N. & Spyer, K. M. (1982). The location and properties of preganglionic vagal cardiomotor neurones in the rabbit. *Pflügers Archiv.* **395**, 244-50.

Jordan, D. & Spyer, K. M. (1979). Studies on the excitability of sinus nerve afferent terminals. *J. Physiol.* **297**, 123-34.

Jordan, D. & Spyer, K. M. (1981). Effects of acetylcholine on respiratory neurones in the nucleus ambiguus-retroambigualis complex of the cat. *J. Physiol.* **320**, 103-11.

Jordan, D. & Spyer, K. M. (1986). Brainstem integration of cardiovascular and pulmonary afferent activity. *Prog. Brain Res.* **67**, 295-314.

Katona, P. G., Lipson, D. & Dauchot, P. J. (1977). Opposing central and peripheral effects of atropine on parasympathetic cardiac control. *Am. J. Physiol.* **232**, H146-51.

Katona, P. G., Poitras, J. W., Barnett, G. O. & Terry, B. S. (1970). Cardiac vagal efferent activity and heart period in the carotid sinus reflex. *Am. J. Physiol.* **218**, 1030-7.

Knowlton, G. C. & Larrabee, M. F. (1946). A unitary analysis of pulmonary volume receptors. *Am. J. Physiol.* **147**, 100-14.

Koepchen, H. P., Lux, H. D. & Wagner, P. H. (1961a). Untersuchungen über Zeitbedarf und zentrale Verarbeitung des Pressoreceptischen Herz-reflexes. *Pflügers Arch.* **273**, 413-30.

Koepchen, H. P., Wagner, P. H. & Lux, H. D. (1961b). Uber die Zusammenhange zwischen zentraler Erregbarkeit reflektorischen Atemrhythmus bei der nervosen Steuerung der Herzfrequenz. *Pflügers Arch.* **273**, 443–65.

Kordy, M. T., Neil, E. & Palmer, J. F. (1975). The influence of laryngeal afferent stimulation on cardiac vagal responses to carotid chemoreceptor excitation. *J. Physiol.* **247**, 24–5P.

Kunze, D. L. (1972). Reflex discharge patterns of cardiac vagal efferent fibres. *J. Physiol.* **222**, 1–15.

Laubie, M., Schmitt, H. & Vincent, M. (1979). Vagal bradycardia produced by microinjections of morphine-like drugs into the nucleus ambiguus in anaesthetized dogs. *Eur. J. Pharmacol.* **59**, 287–91.

Lipski, J., Coote, J. H. & Trzebski, A. (1977a). Temporal patterns of antidromic invasion latencies of sympathetic preganglionic neurons related to central inspiratory activity and pulmonary stretch receptor reflex. *Brain Res.* **135**, 162–6.

Lipski, J., Kubin, L. & Jodkowski, J. (1983). Synaptic action of Rβ neurones on phrenic motoneurones studied with spike-triggered averaging. *Brain Res.* **288**, 105–18.

Lipski, J., McAllen, R. M. & Spyer, K. M. (1975). The sinus nerve and baroreceptor input to the medulla of the cat. *J. Physiol.* **251**, 61–78.

Lipski, J., McAllen, R. M. & Spyer, K. M. (1977b). The carotid chemoreceptor input to the respiratory neurones of the nucleus of tractus solitarius. *J. Physiol.* **269**, 797–810.

Lipski, J., Trzebski, A. & Kubin, L. (1979). Excitability changes of dorsal inspiratory neurones during lung inflations as studied by measurement of antidromic invasion latencies. *Brain Res.* **161**, 25–38.

Lopes, O. U. & Palmer, J. F. (1976). Proposed respiratory 'gating' mechanism for cardiac slowing. *Nature* **264**, 454–6.

Lopes, O. U. & Palmer, J. F. (1978). Mechanism of hypothalamic control of cardiac component of sinus nerve reflex. *Quart. J. Exp. Physiol.* **63**, 231–54.

McAllen, R. M. & Spyer, K. M. (1976). The location of cardiac vagal preganglionic motoneurones in the medulla of the cat. *J. Physiol.* **258**, 187–204.

McAllen, R. M. & Spyer, K. M. (1978a). Two types of vagal preganglionic motoneurones projecting to the heart and lungs. *J. Physiol.* **282**, 353–64.

McAllen, R. M. & Spyer, K. M. (1978b). The baroreceptor input to cardiac vagal motoneurones. *J. Physiol.* **282**, 365–74.

McGuigan, H. (1921). The effect of small doses of atropine on the heart rate. *J.A.M.A.* **76**, 1338–40.

Mifflin, S. W., Spyer, K. M. & Withington-Wray, D. J. (1986). Lack of respiratory modulation of baroreceptor inputs in the nucleus of the tractus solitarius of the cat. *J. Physiol.* **376**, 33P.

Morton, H. J. V. & Thomas, E. T. (1958). Effect of atropine on the heart rate. *Lancet* **ii**, 1313–15.

Neil, E. & Palmer, J. F. (1975). Effects of spontaneous respiration on the latency of reflex cardiac chronotropic responses to baroreceptor stimulation. *J. Physiol.* **247**, 16P.

Potter, E. K. (1981). Inspiratory inhibition of vagal responses to baroreceptor and chemoreceptor stimuli in the dog. *J. Physiol.* **316**, 177–90.

Preiss, G., Kirchner, F. & Polosa, C. (1975). Patterning of sympathetic preganglionic neuron firing by the central respiratory drive. *Brain Res.* **87**, 363–74.

Preiss, G. & Polosa, C. (1977). The relation between end-tidal $CO_2$ and discharge patterns of sympathetic preganglionic neurones. *Brain Res.* **122**, 255–67.

Raczkowska, M., Eckberg, D. L. & Ebert, T. J. (1983). Muscarinic cholinergic receptors modulate vagal cardiac responses in man. *J. Auton. Nerv. Syst.* **7**, 271–8.

Remmers, J. E., Richter, D. W., Ballantyne, D., Bainton, C. R. & Klein, J. P. (1985). Activation of bulbar post-inspiratory neurones by upper airway stimulation. In *Neurogenesis of Central Respiratory Rhythm*, pp. 290–1 (eds A. L. Bianchi & M. Denavit-Saubié). Lancaster: MTP Press.

Richter, D. W. & Ballantyne, D. (1983). A three phase theory about the basic respiratory pattern generator. In *Central Neurone Environment*, pp. 164–74 (eds M. E. Schläfke, H. P. Koepchen & W. R. See). Berlin, Heidelberg: Springer-Verlag.

Richter, D. W., Jordan, D., Ballantyne, D., Meesmann, M. & Spyer, K. M. (1986). Presynaptic depolarization in myelinated vagal afferent fibres terminating in the nucleus of the tractus solitarius in the cat. *Pflügers Arch.* **406**, 12–19.

Rudomin, P. (1967). Presynaptic inhibition induced by vagal afferent volleys. *J. Neurophysiol.* **30**, 964–81.

Rudomin, P. (1968). Excitability changes of superior laryngeal, vagal and depressor afferent terminals produced by stimulation of the solitary tract nucleus. *Exptl. Brain Res.* **6**, 156–70.

Schwaber, J. S. & Cohen, D. H. (1978a). Field potential and single unit analyses of the avian dorsal motor nucleus of the vagus and criteria for identifying vagal cardiac cells of origin. *Brain Res.* **147**, 79–90.

Schwaber, J. S. & Cohen, D. H. (1978b). Electrophysiological and electron microscopic analysis of the vagus nerve of the pigeon, with particular reference to the cardiac innervation. *Brain Res.* **147**, 65–78.

Schwaber, J. S. & Schneiderman, N. (1975). Aortic nerve-activated cardioinhibitory neurons and interneurones. *Am. J. Physiol.* **229**, 783–9.

Seller, H. & Richter, D. W. (1971). Some quantitative aspects of the central transmission of the baroreceptor activity. In *Research in Physiology*, pp. 541–9 (eds F. F. Kao, K. Koizumi & M. Vassalle). Bologna: Auto Craggi.

Spyer, K. M. (1972). Baroreceptor sensitive neurones in the anterior hypothalamus of the cat. *J. Physiol.* **224**, 245–57.

Spyer, K. M. (1981). Neural organisation and control of the baroreceptor reflex. *Rev. Physiol. Biochem. Pharmacol.* **88**, 23–124.

Spyer, K. M. (1984). Central control of the cardiovascular system. In *Recent Advances in Physiology*, 10, pp. 163–200 (ed. P. F. Baker). Edinburgh: Churchill Livingstone.

Stroh-Werz, M., Langhorst, P. & Camerer, H. (1977). Neuronal activity with cardiac rhythm in the nucleus of the solitary tract in cats and dogs. II. Activity modulation in relationship to the respiratory cycle. *Brain Res.* **133**, 81–93.

Sutton, P. M. I. (1981). The effect of hypocapnia and hyperventilation on reflex cardiac vagal efferent activity in dogs. *J. Physiol.* **315**, 35P.

Trzebski, A., Raczkowska, M. & Kubin, L. (1980). Influence of respiratory activity and hypocapnia on the carotid baroreceptor reflex in man. In *Arterial Baroreceptors and Hypertension*, pp. 282–90 (ed. P. Sleight). Oxford: Oxford Medical Publications.

von Baumgarten, R. & Kanzow, E. (1958). The interaction of two types of inspiratory neurones in the region of the tractus solitarius of the cat. *Arch. ital Biol.* **96**, 361–73.

Whipp, B. J. & Ward, S. A. (1982). Cardiopulmonary coupling during exercise. *J. Exp. Biol.* **100**, 175–93.

Widdicombe, J. E. (1954). Receptors in the trachea and bronchi of the cat. *J. Physiol.* **123**, 71–104.

Williford, D. J., Hamilton, B. L. & Gillis, R. A. (1980). Evidence that a GABAergic mechanism at nucleus ambiguus influences reflex-induced vagal activity. *Brain Res.* **193**, 584–8.

# 18

# The peripheral chemoreceptors and cardiovascular–respiratory integration

M. de Burgh Daly,[1] J. Ward[2] and L. M. Wood[3]

*Departments of Physiology of [1] Royal Free Hospital School of Medicine, Rowland Hill Street, London NW3 2PF, UK, [2] the United Medical and Dental Schools of Guy's and St Thomas's Hospitals, St Thomas's Street, London SE1 9RT, UK, and [3] Department of Pharmacology, Smith Kline and French Research Ltd, The Frythe, Welwyn, Herts AL6 9AR, UK*

## 18.1. Introduction

### 18.1.1. *Morphology*

The peripheral arterial chemoreceptors are situated in two main areas: the carotid bodies located in the carotid bifurcation regions and the thoracic chemoreceptors, commonly referred to as the aortic bodies, which are widely distributed in the subclavian and aortic arch regions. Their morphology is complex, the functional unit consisting of clusters of cells comprising glomus or type I cells which make extensive synaptic contact with sensory axons, surrounded by sustentacular or type II cells, and a dense capillary network (see Verna, 1979). In the carotid bifurcation region the type I and II cells are largely distributed in a division of connective tissue with definable but irregular borders, comprising the principal mass of the carotid body. They also exist in many animal species as small isolated groups of cells in the connective tissue and have been termed *corpuscles aberrants* or 'Periadventitial cells' (de Castro, 1962; Clarke & Daly, 1982, 1983; Clarke *et al.*, 1986). Similar islets of tissue occur along the length of the common carotid artery in the cat ('mini-glomera'; Matsuura, 1973). The distribution of the aortic bodies in the cat and dog has been classified by Howe (1956) (see also Coleridge *et al.* (1979)). However, the rabbit, rat and mouse have no functional aortic bodies.

Chemoreceptors are highly vascular structures and their arterial blood supply and venous drainage have been described in detail for the cartoid (Chungcharoen *et al.*, 1952) and aortic bodies (Howe, 1956; Coleridge *et al.*, 1970). The specific blood flow for the carotid body in the cat is in excess of 2000 ml min$^{-1}$ 100 g$^{-1}$ tissue (Daly *et al.*, 1954; Clarke *et al.*, 1986), the highest figure for any organ in the body, and comparable values have been obtained in other species (see Clarke *et al.*, 1986).

### 18.1.2. *Nature of stimulus*

The carotid and aortic bodies are stimulated by a reduction in arterial $PO_2$, and by an increase in arterial $PCO_2$ and hydrogen ion concentration. The activity of the chemoreceptors, as indicated by the discharge frequency in single or multifibre strands of chemoreceptor afferents in the carotid sinus nerve, increases as the arterial $PO_2$ falls, the relationship being nearly hyperbolic. The responses of the aortic bodies are in general smaller than those of the carotid bodies to all three stimuli. There is a continuous interaction between hypoxia and hypercapnia, one stimulus augmenting the response of the other. For further details of the stimulus–response curves and the respiratory-linked variations that occur in chemoreceptor discharge, the reader should consult the review by Lahiri *et al.* (1983).

The carotid and aortic bodies are also stimulated by local stagnant hypoxia. This can occur through a reduction in blood flow resulting from arterial hypotension and/or local vasoconstriction of sympathetic origin. The responses of the aortic bodies are greater than those from the carotid bodies at any given level of blood pressure, and in the case of both groups of chemoreceptors, the responses are larger in the presence of arterial hypoxaemia (Lahiri *et al.*, 1980).

A wide variety of exogenous chemical agents are capable of stimulating the carotid and aortic bodies. It is important, however, when using such stimuli to elicit reflex responses, to select one which, in the doses used, does not have any effect on other types of receptor to which the agent has access, because many chemical agents are not specific to the chemoreceptors. Cyanide, physiological saline solution saturated with $CO_2$ and phosphate, injected into a common carotid artery, are probably the best solutions to use.

### 18.1.3. *Functions*

The role of the carotid and aortic chemoreceptors in the reflex regulation of respiration has been reviewed by Heymans *et al.* (1933) and Heymans & Neil (1958). In this respect the carotid bodies are the more important group of receptors (Comroe & Mortimer, 1964; Daly & Ungar, 1966), while in those species which have no aortic bodies they are entirely responsible for this peripheral chemoreceptor function (Neil *et al.*, 1949; Chalmers *et al.*, 1967; Sapru & Krieger, 1977).

There is now clear evidence that the carotid and aortic chemoreceptors are also important in the control of the cardiovascular system. Thus in such conditions as sleep, haemorrhagic hypotension, systemic (arterial) hypoxia, asphyxia and breath-hold diving, they play a role in the control of heart rate and peripheral vascular resistance (see Daly, 1983, 1984). The mechanisms by which they achieve this control are, however, complex, and it is the purpose of this chapter to review briefly the integrative nature of the chemoreceptor control of the cardiovascular system with particular reference to the role of the concomitant changes in pulmonary ventilation.

In any disturbance of the circulation in which the peripheral chemoreceptors are involved it is inevitable that several receptor groups with different reflex functions, such as arterial baroreceptors in the carotid sinuses and aortic arch, are affected simultaneously so that the sum total of all information reaching the central nervous system evokes a pattern of autonomic effector activity. In addition the effectiveness of incoming chemoreceptor impulses to the nervous system can be influenced by activity of the hypothalamic defence area (see Marshall, 1986; and also Chapter 12). Furthermore, if there are accompanying changes in respiration, then the observed response pattern will be determined by mechanisms arising from the direction and magnitude of the change in pulmonary ventilation. These respiratory mechanisms include alterations in central respiratory neuronal activity, pulmonary receptor activity and the level of arterial $PCO_2$. They can modify the autonomic outflow directly and by modifying centrally the effectiveness of the reflex responses engendered by excitation of specific groups of receptors, including the peripheral chemoreceptors.

## 18.2. Cardiovascular responses

### 18.2.1. *Carotid bodies*
In spontaneously breathing animals anaesthetised with chloralose, urethane or a barbiturate, sustained stimulations of the carotid bodies by hypoxic blood or brief stimulations by chemical agents injected into a common carotid artery invariably cause an increase in pulmonary ventilation. The changes in heart rate, cardiac output and peripheral vascular resistance are, however, difficult to predict. This can be illustrated by responses observed in the dog and monkey. The effects of sustained stimulations are: predominantly tachycardia, and occasionally no change in heart rate or bradycardia, accompanied by no change in mean arterial blood pressure or hypotension, an increase in cardiac output, and transient increases followed by reductions in total peripheral and hindlimb vascular resistances. Brief stimulations with cyanide cause, initially, bradycardia followed by tachycardia, a reduction in cardiac output and an increase in hindlimb vascular resistance (Bernthal *et al.*, 1951; Daly & Scott, 1958, 1962, 1963; Daly *et al.*, 1978a). In the cat, on the other hand, sustained stimulations have different effects: bradycardia, hypertension, little or no change in cardiac output and an increase in total

peripheral vascular resistance and hindlimb vascular resistance (Macleod & Scott, 1964; Carmody & Scott, 1974; Daly *et al.*, 1983b).

Although it is possible that these variable responses represent a true species difference, this explanation seems unlikely because the variations occurred in the same species and even at different times in the experiment in the same animal. It is more probable that the observed responses were in some instances complicated by other reflex or humoral effects secondary to the stimulation of the carotid bodies. However, on examination it was found that the variable cardiac and vascular responses could not be attributed solely to the concomitant change in arterial blood pressure resulting in activation of an arterial baroreceptor reflex. The evidence reviewed below from different types of experiment indicated that the increase in pulmonary ventilation played an important role in determining the final response.

### 18.2.2. *Role of changes in pulmonary ventilation*

When the carotid bodies were stimulated in the spontaneously breathing dog there was a close correlation between the size of the increase in pulmonary ventilation and the direction of the change in heart rate, tachycardia being associated with the larger increases in ventilation, bradycardia with the small increases (Daly & Scott, 1958). These results were consistent with the finding that when ventilation was held constant by a mechanical respirator, stimulation of the carotid chemoreceptors invariably caused bradycardia (Bernthal *et al.*, 1951; Daly & Scott, 1958, 1962, 1963; Angell-James & Daly, 1969a). Likewise peripheral vasoconstriction was the only response seen during carotid body stimulation when respiration was controlled, and vasodilation only occurred when respiration was allowed to increase spontaneously (Bernthal, 1938; Daly & Scott, 1962, 1963; Daly & Ungar, 1966; Angell-James & Daly, 1969a; Hainsworth *et al.*, 1983). In some species, the heart slows when the carotid bodies are stimulated, independently of the size of the ventilatory response, e.g. in the cat (Macleod & Scott, 1964; Daly *et al.*, 1983b) and seal (Elsner *et al.*, 1977), whereas in the monkey the predominant response of tachycardia in the spontaneously breathing animal is converted to bradycardia when pulmonary ventilation is held constant (Daly *et al.*, 1978b).

Using another experimental approach the contribution of the carotid bodies to the cardiac response to systemic hypoxia was studied. Ventilation with an inspired gas mixture of low oxygen content usually causes tachycardia. If the carotid body 'drive' was withdrawn by perfusion of the chemoreceptors with oxygenated blood, no change in heart rate or a further acceleration of the heart occurred independently of the change in breathing (Neil, 1956; Daly & Scott, 1959, 1964). This means that the tachycardia of systemic hypoxia could not have been the direct effect of carotid chemoreceptor stimulation.

Consistent with these observations are those of Rutherford & Vatner (1978) who showed in the conscious dog that the immediate bradycardia and peripheral vasoconstrictor responses to brief stimulations of the carotid bodies were potentiated when pulmonary ventilation was maintained constant; the later cardioaccelerator and vasodilator effects were abolished. The interpretation is that these latter responses were the result of the accompanying hyperventilation in the spontaneously breathing animal.

### 18.2.3. *Aortic bodies*

The control of the circulation by the aortic bodies has received less attention, probably because of their relative inaccessibility for carrying out controlled experiments. A method for vascular isolation of the aortic bodies for selective stimulation with hypoxic blood was first devised by Daly *et al.* (1965). Histological examination of the perfused area revealed perfused aortic bodies along the caudal border of the aortic arch corresponding to group 3 of Howe's (1956) classification. In dogs with controlled pulmonary ventilation, stimulation of the aortic bodies caused variable effects on heart rate but consistent peripheral vasoconstrictor responses (Daly *et al.*, 1965; Daly & Ungar, 1966; Karim *et al.*, 1980). Quantitatively the primary vascular responses elicited by the aortic and carotid bodies were similar (Daly & Ungar, 1966). Stimulation of the aortic bodies also causes vasoconstriction in the sheep fetus and newborn lamb (Dawes *et al.*, 1968).

In the spontaneously breathing adult dog, stimulation of the aortic bodies invariably caused vasoconstriction at a time when the same hypoxic blood stimulus to the carotid bodies may have either no effect or cause vasodilatation (Daly & Ungar, 1966). This difference is probably related to the contrasting responses of respiration to stimulation of the two groups of chemoreceptors in that a hypoxic blood stimulus to the carotid bodies produces an increase in respiratory minute volume which in the dog at least is, on average, seven times greater than that elicited by the same stimulus to the aortic bodies. Thus the secondary respiratory effects counteracting the primary vascular responses from the aortic bodies would be expected to be considerably less.

### 18.3. **The effects of respiration on the cardiovascular system**

The several ways in which the cyclic changes in breathing can affect the cardiovascular system have been debated for over a century (see Daly, 1986). It is now evident that at least two mechanisms are responsible for the respiratory-related changes in heart rate (respiratory sinus arrhythmia; acceleration of the heart accompanying the phase of inspiration): a centrally generated respiratory drive affecting the activity of the medullary cardiac vagal motoneurones, and a sensory input from the lungs related to stretch and rate of change of stretch of the lungs. Central inspiratory neuronal activity and the pulmonary input can also affect systemic vascular resistance. The evidence for these mechanisms will now be discussed, together with the possibility that they play a role in determining the cardiovascular responses to stimulation of the carotid and aortic bodies.

### 18.3.1. *Inspiratory neuronal activity*

Traube (1865) showed that respiratory sinus arrhythmia persisted after curarisation of the animal and so was due to a central effect. This finding has been confirmed by numerous workers and is due largely to changes in cardiac vagus nerve activity (see Spyer, 1981; Daly, 1983, 1986).

### 18.3.2. *Pulmonary reflex*

When the lungs are inflated, an increase in heart rate occurs which is reflex in origin. It is due largely to a reduction in activity in cardiac fibres in the vagus nerves and is abolished by selective denervation of the lungs (Hering, 1871; Anrep *et al.*, 1936; Daly & Scott, 1958; Angell-James & Daly, 1969a, 1978; Hainsworth, 1974; Daly *et al.*, 1983a). When the arterial baroreceptor input is controlled, lung inflation also causes reflex vasodilatation (Salisbury *et al.*, 1959; Daly *et al.*, 1967, 1983a, 1986; Daly & Robinson, 1968; Angell-James & Daly, 1969a) due to a reduction in activity in sympathetic α-adrenergic fibres (Adrian *et al.*, 1932; Bronk *et al.*, 1936; Polosa *et al.*, 1980; see also Daly, 1986). These responses are produced by a single inflation of the lungs and also by increasing the tidal volume of lungs rhythmically ventilated at a constant frequency. There is a direct relationship between the increase in lung volume and size of the vasodilator responses (Daly *et al.*, 1967, 1986).

There have been reports by Hainsworth and his colleagues (Hainsworth, 1974; Wood *et al.*, 1985) that tachycardia in response to lung inflation is usually accompanied by vasoconstriction, and bradycardia by vasodilatation, although the reason for this discrepancy between these results and those described above is not at present clear.

In experiments carried out to test the effects of a reduction in lung volume, cardiovascular responses opposite to those elicited by lung inflation were observed, namely, bradycardia and vasoconstriction. It was concluded therefore that, by inference, the lungs at their normal functional residual capacity are a source of afferent impulses inhibiting the sympathetic vasoconstrictor outflow (Daly *et al.*, 1967, 1986) and the cardiac vagal motoneurones (Anrep *et al.*, 1936; Daly & Scott, 1958).

The cardioaccelerator and vasodilator responses to lung inflation were abolished by selective surgical denervation of the lungs by a method which did not affect the functional integrity of cardiac efferent fibres (Daly & Scott, 1958; Daly *et al.*, 1983a, 1986). This means that these responses must be elicited by intrapulmonary receptors (Anrep *et al.*, 1936; Daly & Scott, 1958; Daly *et al.*, 1967; Daly & Robinson, 1968; Angell-James & Daly, 1969a; Daly *et al.*, 1983a, 1986). The site of the receptors responsible for the variable cardiac chronotropic and vascular responses observed by others was not determined (Greenwood *et al.*, 1980; Wood *et al.*, 1985), although, in the preparations used, secondary reflex effects of lung inflation from arterial baroreceptors and chemoreceptors were minimised.

The histological and physiological properties of the three groups of receptor found in the lungs have been reviewed elsewhere (Widdicombe, 1982). Those responsible for the cardiovascular effects of inflation and deflation of the lungs, at least in the dog, were probably the pulmonary stretch receptors. This conclusion is based on the properties of the reflex responses they evoke. The receptors are low threshold in that the responses can be produced by changes in volume well within the eupnoeic tidal volume; they are rate sensitive; they are slowly adapting in that the responses to sustained increases in lung volume are well maintained, provided the input from the arterial baroreceptors and the arterial blood gases are held constant; and thermal studies on the afferent fibres in the cervical vagus are consistent with myelinated fibres being involved (Daly & Scott, 1958; Anrep *et al.*, 1936; Davis *et al.*, 1956; Daly *et al.*, 1967; Daly & Robinson, 1968; Angell-James & Daly, 1969a; Hainsworth, 1974; Gandevia *et al.*, 1978). This conclusion is consistent with the findings relating to the properties of pulmonary stretch receptors based on electroneurographic studies of their afferent innervation (Adrian, 1933; Davis *et al.*, 1956). The possibility that rapidly adapting pulmonary irritant receptors are involved, as in the muscle vasodilatation occurring in the rat during periodic gasps or 'augmented breaths' (Marshall & Metcalfe, 1986), cannot be excluded. Biologically active substances, such as histamine and prostaglandins, released from the lungs by their inflation and acting on pulmonary afferent nerves may also be involved (Wood *et al.*, 1985).

### 18.3.3. *Changes in $P_aCO_2$*

The effects of changes in $P_aCO_2$ on heart rate and peripheral vascular resistance by an action on the brain and spinal cord have been reviewed elsewhere (Daly, 1986). Hypocapnia causes tachycardia and vasodilatation (see also Ford *et al.*, 1985).

### 18.4. **Respiratory modulation of reflex responses**

### 18.4.1. *Respiration*

The effects of brief selective stimulations of the carotid bodies are dependent on the phase of the respiratory cycle at which such stimuli are applied. Those timed to reach the carotid bodies during the inspiratory phase of the cycle increase the size of the ongoing inspiratory activity; those delivered during the expiratory phase either have no effect, prolong the expiratory pause or sometimes evoke an active expiratory effort (Black & Torrance, 1971; Eldridge, 1972; Haymet & McCloskey, 1975).

### 18.4.2. *Heart rate*

The important role played by a pulmonary reflex in the integration of cardiac reflexes elicited by stimulation of the carotid chemoreceptors has been stressed previously. In the artificially ventilated animal, sustained chemoreceptor stimulation caused bradycardia. When the test was repeated during mechanical hyperventilation, which itself resulted in tachycardia, the cardio-inhibitory response was either reduced in size or abolished (Daly & Hazzledine, 1963) (Figs 18.1 and 18.2). This suppression of the chemoreceptor bradycardia by hyperventilation is partly or wholly abolished by denervation of the lungs (Daly & Scott, 1958; Daly & Hazzledine, 1963).

A representative result is shown in Fig. 18.1. The carotid bodies were stimulated by hypoxic blood during normal artificial ventilation and during artificial hyperventilation. Artificial hyperventilation itself resulted in tachycardia and suppressed the bradycardia of carotid-body stimulation. Both these effects of artificial hyperventilation were abolished by denervation of the lungs. This interaction between the inputs from the carotid bodies and receptors in the lungs goes some way to explaining how it is that in the spontaneously breathing dog, with a control value of heart rate during eupnoeic breathing corresponding to point $X$, acceleration of the heart during stimulation of the carotid bodies occurs when accompanied by hyperventilation $(Y)$; this response is converted to bradycardia after denervation of the lungs $(X'-Y')$.

Brief chemoreceptor stimuli slow the heart, but only when they are applied during the expiratory phase of the respiratory cycle. When delivered during the inspiratory phase, they have little or no effect (Haymet & McCloskey, 1975; Davidson *et al.*, 1976; Davis *et al.*, 1977), or cause tachycardia due to an overriding effect of the secondary respiratory mechanisms (M. de B. Daly, unpublished observations). This suppression of the chemoreceptor reflex bradycardia during the inspiratory phase of the respiratory cycle was interpreted as being due to a combination of the central inspiratory neuronal drive and a pulmonary vagal reflex on to cardiac vagal motoneurones (Davidson *et al.*, 1976; Gandevia *et al.*, 1978; Potter, 1981).

### 18.4.3. *Central mechanisms*

The central mechanisms involved in the integration of respiratory–vagal effects have been reviewed by Spyer (1981, 1982). Briefly, primary afferent

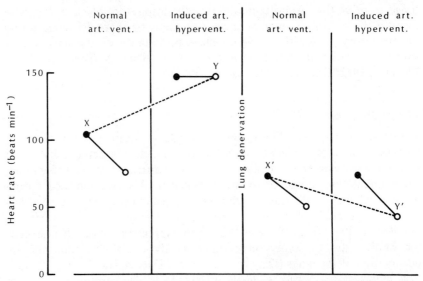

Fig. 18.1. The effects of stimulation of the carotid bodies by hypoxic blood on the heart rate during normal artificial ventilation (*art. vent.*) and during an induced artificial hyperventilation (*art. hypervent.*), the $P_aCO_2$ being maintained constant, before and after denervation of the lungs by the method of Daly & Scott (1958). Dog anaesthetised with a mixture of chloralose and urethane. Filled circles (●), control values; open circules (○), values during stimulation of the carotid bodies. Note: (1) Before lung denervation the primary reflex bradycardia elicited by chemoreceptor stimulation is abolished during artificial hyperventilation, and that hyperventilation *per se* caused acceleration of the heart; and (2) after denervation of the lungs the primary cardiac response to stimulation of the carotid bodies is relatively unaffected by artificial hyperventilation, and the hyperventilation *per se* has no effect on heart rate. These data can be used to mimic events occurring on stimulation of the carotid bodies in the spontaneously breathing dog: the control value of heart rate during eupnoeic breathing, the carotid bodies being perfused with oxygenated blood, corresponds to point X; point Y represents the value during chemoreceptor stimulation associated with spontaneous hyperventilation. The interrupted line X–Y indicates that carotid body stimulation causes acceleration of the heart. This response in converted to bradycardia after denervation of the lungs (X'–Y'). (From Daly & Hazzledine, 1963.)

neurones from chemoreceptors, baroreceptors and pulmonary stretch receptors terminate in the nucleus of the tractus solitarius (NTS) (see also Donoghue *et al.*, 1982, 1984). The cardiac vagal motoneurones (CVMs) are situated in the nucleus ambiguus (NA) in the cat and also in the dorsal vagal motor nucleus in the rabbit and dog, and send small myelinated and unmyelinated axons to innervate the heart.

Ventral and ventrolateral to the tractus solitarius is one of the major groups of brainstem respiratory neurones (Richter, 1982), which have been differentiated into two types, α and β, on the basis of their response to stimulation of pulmonary stretch receptors during lung inflation. Whereas both types of neurone are excited by central inspiratory activity and discharge with phrenic nerve activity, only the β neurones are excited by lung inflation (Baumgarten & Kanzow, 1958; Backman *et al.*, 1985). A second major group of brainstem respiratory neurones lie in the region of the NA. The normal respiratory rhythm is assumed to arise from synaptic interactions within the network of respiratory neurones (see Richter, 1982).

Cardiac vagal efferent fibres have been shown to discharge primarily during expiration and have a conspicuous respiratory-related rhythm (see Spyer, 1981). Recordings from CVMs have a very similar pattern of discharge provided there is a reasonable degree of cardiac 'vagal tone', which is dependent largely on the input from arterial baroreceptors, and this proviso applies as well to the cardiac vagal efferent discharge. The site of interaction of respiration and cardiac vagal control is largely on the CVMs rather than earlier in the reflex pathway, since the afferent terminals in the NTS are unaffected presynaptically by central respiratory activity (Mifflin *et al.*, 1986). The excitability of the CVMs determines whether or not they respond to a baroreceptor or chemoreceptor input, and this excitability is reduced during inspiration by brainstem inspiratory neurones through a cholinergic mechanism (Spyer, 1982; Gilbey *et al.*, 1984). The involvement of central *expiratory* neurones is unlikely because the recruiting pattern of their discharge does not resemble the pattern of firing of CVMs (Spyer, 1981). Thus the efficacy of baroreceptor and chemoreceptor reflexes on to the CVMs is maximal during expiration which is at the height of excitability of the CVMs; during inspiration the CVMs are partially or totally refractory to excitatory inputs.

Another inspiratory-related mechanism affecting the CVMs results from excitation of pulmonary stretch receptors. Lopes & Palmer (1976) postulated that the inhibitory effect of lung inflation was due to excitation of the Rβ group of inspiratory neurones which are also excited by the central inspiratory drive (Baumgarten & Kanzow, 1958). These neurones are located in the NTS and project to the NA (Merrill, 1975). When comparing the inhibitory effects of lung inflation and of central inspiratory activity, Potter (1981) found that whereas both tonic and reflexly evoked cardiac vagal activity were inhibited during central inspiratory activity, lung inflation was more effective in inhibiting the reflexly evoked vagal discharge than the tonic vagal discharge. She suggested that lung inflation had its main actions on phasic inputs, leaving responses to sustained inputs relatively unaffected. Different central synaptic pathways may be involved. The powerful inspiratory-related inhibition of the CVMs, both centrally and reflexly engendered, is clearly an important mechanism determining the cardiac responses to stimulation of the chemoreceptors, as reviewed here.

18.4.4. *Vascular resistance*

Angell-James & Daly (1969a) showed that the increase in vascular resistance elicited by asphyxia in the absence of movements of the lungs was due to stimulation of the carotid and aortic bodies. When, however, spontaneous breathing was allowed to increase commensurate with a degree of hypoxia and hypercapnia, asphyxia then had no effect on vascular resistance. This suppression of the vasoconstrictor response to asphyxia was dependent on the innervation to the lungs, and this result suggested that because the vascular response was mediated through the arterial chemoreceptors, there was an interaction between the inputs from the chemoreceptors and pulmonary receptors.

This has now been examined in detail in experiments in which the effects were studied of step increases in pulmonary ventilation on the responses of hindlimb and systemic vascular resistances to stimulation of the carotid body chemoreceptors (Daly *et al.*, 1986). In an investigation of this sort it was necessary to control certain physiological variables which might otherwise complicate the interpretation of the results. A preparation in the dog was therefore used which incorporated:

(1) cardiopulmonary bypass, with oxygenation of the systemic venous blood by extracorporeal isolated perfused donor lungs;
(2) separate pulsatile perfusion of the vascularly isolated carotid bifurcation regions, provision being made for maintaining constant the systolic, diastolic and mean pressures, and for temporarily perfusing the carotid bodies with hypoxic hypercapnic blood; and
(3) separate perfusions of the arch of the aorta and cerebral circulation, the abdominal circulation and right hindlimb, and the left hindlimb.

The abdominal circulation and right hindlimb ('systemic circulation') and the left hindlimb were each perfused at constant blood flow so that changes in perfusion pressures indicated similar directional changes in systemic and hindlimb vascular resistances respectively. Thus during stimulation of the carotid bodies by hypoxic hypercapnic blood, or during mechanical alternations of pulmonary ventilation by varying the tidal volume at constant frequency, or during a combination of the two inputs, the following variables were held constant: the arterial $PO_2$, $PCO_2$ and pH, the inputs from the carotid sinus and aortic arch baroreceptors by maintaining the phasic and mean pressures unchanged, and the cerebral perfusion pressure.

When pulmonary ventilation was increased in steps, chosen at random, from 0·095 to 0·665 litre $min^{-1}$ $kg^{-1}$ body weight, a significant progressive reduction in hindlimb and systemic vascular resistances occurred. The typical responses are shown in Fig. 18.2, and the results occurring in the hindlimb are summarised in Figure 18.3. These were similar to those seen in the systemic vascular resistance. All the vascular responses to increasing ventilation were abolished by surgical denervation of the lungs by the method of

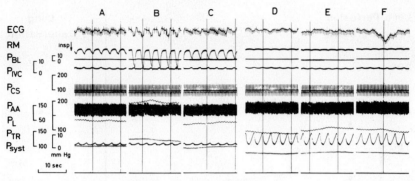

Fig. 18.2. The effects of stimulation of the carotid body chemoreceptors at two levels of pulmonary ventilation. Dog on cardiopulmonary bypass. Artifical respiration, frequency 19 cycles min$^{-1}$. The following variables were held constant: arterial blood gases, urinary bladder pressure, carotid sinus perfusion pressure, aortic arch and cerebral perfusion pressures, and inferior vena caval pressure. Systemic circulation and left hind limb each perfused at constant blood flow. A–C, Pulmonary ventilation of test lung 0·095 litre min$^{-1}$ kg$^{-1}$. D–F, pulmonary ventilation 0·665 litre min$^{-1}$ kg$^{-1}$. In B and E, stimulation of carotid bodies by substituting mixed venous blood for arterial blood perfusion of the vascularly isolated carotid bifurcation regions. Arterial blood/mixed venous blood composition: $PO_2$ 107·8 ± 21·7/41·3 ± 0·2 mmHg; $PCO_2$ 37·9 ± 3·7/45·9 ± 0·7 mmHg; pH 7·419 ± 0·036/7·372 ± 0·004). Note the smaller rises in systemic and hindlimb perfusion pressures in response to carotid body stimulation in D–F compared with A–C. Records from above downwards: ECG, electrocardiogram; RM, rib measurements (inspiration downwards); $P_{BL}$, urinary bladder pressure; $P_{IVC}$, inferior vena caval pressure; $P_{CS}$, phasic and mean carotid sinus pressures; $P_{AA}$, phasic pressure in aortic arch and cerebral circulation; $P_L$, hindlimb mean perfusion pressure; $P_{TR}$, tracheal pressure; $P_{syst}$, systemic mean perfusion pressure. Time marker and calibration, 10 s. (From Daly *et al.*, 1986.)

Daly & Scott (1958). Similar results were observed on single inflations of the lungs and therefore confirm previous observations (Daly *et al.*, 1967, 1983a; Daly & Robinson, 1968; Angell-James & Daly, 1969a).

Stimulation of the carotid bodies by changing the composition of the blood perfusing the carotid bifurcation regions from arterial blood to hypoxic hypercapnic (venous) blood invariably caused an increase in hindlimb and systemic perfusion pressures, indicating vasoconstriction, at all four levels of pulmonary ventilation (Figs 18.2 and 18.3). The size of the vascular responses were, however, not the same at all levels of ventilation. The response at the lowest level of ventilation of 0·095 litre min$^{-1}$ kg$^{-1}$ was greater than the responses at all other levels of ventilation. After denervation of the lungs these differences disappeared and the vasoconstrictor response occurring on stimulation of the carotid bodies became the same at all levels of pulmonary ventilation, the size of the response being approximately equal to that occurring at the lowest level of ventilation with the pulmonary nerves intact (Fig. 18.3).

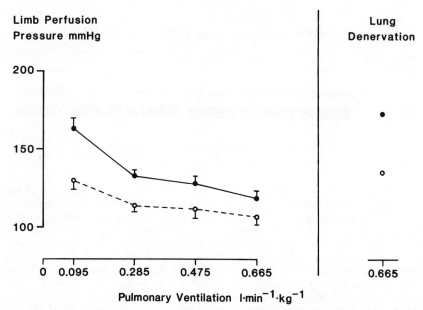

Fig. 18.3. The effects of stimulation of the carotid bodies on hindlimb perfusion pressure (constant blood flow) at four levels of pulmonary ventilation, 0·095, 0·285, 0·475 and 0·665 litre $min^{-1}$ $kg^{-1}$, respiratory frequency 19 cycles $min^{-1}$. Dogs on total cardiopulmonary bypass. Arterial blood $PO_2$, $PCO_2$ and pH, and the carotid sinus, aortic arch and cerebral perfusion pressures held constant. Left-hand panel: lower curve shows the effects of increasing pulmonary ventilation *per se* with arterial blood perfusion of the carotid bodies; upper curve: stimulation of the carotid bodies at different levels of pulmonary ventilation. Mean values ± SEM; 21 tests in 9 dogs. Right-hand panel: effects after surgical denervation of the lungs (method of Daly & Scott, 1958); mean values for 3 tests in 3 dogs. (From Daly *et al.*, 1986.)

This interaction between the inputs from the carotid bodies and receptors in the lungs goes some way to explaining how it is that in the spontaneously breathing dog selective stimulation of the carotid bodies may cause reflex vasodilatation (Daly & Scott, 1962, 1963; Daly & Ungar, 1966). With reference to Fig. 18.4, which is a diagrammatic representation of the results contained in Fig. 18.3, the lower curve indicates the vascular response to increasing respiratory minute volume *per se*, and the upper curve the effects of stimulating the carotid bodies, e.g. at an eupnoeic level of ventilation (a) and at an increased level (b). The respective sizes of the primary vasoconstrictor responses to chemoreceptor excitation are shown by the vertical interrupted lines. Considering now the respiratory and vascular responses occurring in the *spontaneously breathing* animal: the point corresponding to the eupnoeic level of pulmonary ventilation and vascular resistance without chemoreceptor stimulation will lie on the lower curve at point X. During stimulation of the chemoreceptors in which there is a potential reflex

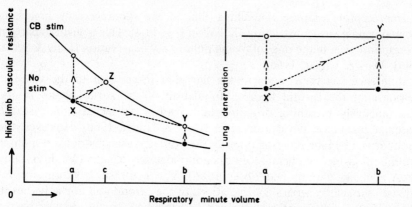

Fig. 18.4. Diagrammatic representation of the effects of stimulation of the carotid bodies on hindlimb vascular resistance at constant artificial ventilation and during spontaneous hyperventilation with the $P_aCO_2$ held constant. Before lung denervation the lower curve shows the effects of increasing pulmonary ventilation *per se* causing reflex vasodilation; the upper curve during chemoreceptor stimulation. Stimulation of the carotid bodies at a constant level of ventilation (a) causes hindlimb vasoconstriction (left vertical interrupted line), and a smaller response at increased level of ventilation (b) (right vertical interrupted line). In the events mimicking those occurring in the spontaneously breathing animal, the eupnoeic level of ventilation and vascular resistance is represented by point X on lower curve. During stimulation of the carotid bodies, ventilation increases to (b) and the corresponding level of vascular resistance is point Y on the upper curve. Thus carotid body stimulation associated with a spontaneous increase in pulmonary ventilation causes vasodilatation (interrupted X–Y). After lung denervation, the vasodilator response to an increase in pulmonary ventilation *per se* is abolished (lower curve), and the carotid body vasoconstrictor responses are all the same size as that occurring at the lowest level of pulmonary ventilation, 0·095 litre min⁻¹ kg⁻¹. The response to chemoreceptor stimulation occurring in the spontaneously breathing animal is now vasoconstriction (X′–Y′). The *upper curve* also represents the relationship between hindlimb vascular resistance and pulmonary ventilation during stimulation of the aortic bodies; the primary vascular responses are quantitatively the same as those elicited by stimulation of the carotid bodies (Daly & Ungar, 1966). The ventilatory response to stimulation of the aortic bodies in the dog (c) is only one-seventh that of stimulation of the carotid bodies (b). The response of the aortic bodies mimicking that in the spontaneously breathing dog is therefore represented by X–Z. For further details see text.

vasoconstrictor response associated with an increase in respiratory minute volume, the corresponding levels of ventilation and vascular resistance will now lie on the upper curve at point Y. Thus, under these conditions, stimulation of the carotid bodies results in hyperventilation and vasodilatation (X–Y).

After lung denervation which abolishes the vasodilator response to an increase in pulmonary ventilation, the vasoconstrictor response to carotid body stimulation becomes the same at all levels of ventilation. The chemoreceptor response mimicking that in the spontaneously breathing animal is now vasoconstriction (X′–Y′ in Fig. 18.4). This is just the pattern of response seen in the dog following pulmonary denervation (Daly & Scott, 1963; Daly & Ungar, 1966).

Reference has been made to the fact that in contrast to the vascular response of the carotid bodies, stimulation of the aortic bodies in the spontaneously breathing dog invariably causes an increase in systemic vascular resistance, never a decrease (Daly & Ungar, 1966). However, the input driven by lung inflation opposes the primary vasoconstrictor responses from both groups of chemoreceptors approximately equally (M. de B. Daly & A. Ungar, unpublished observation). The contrasting vasomotor responses evoked by separate stimulations of the carotid and aortic bodies in the spontaneously breathing dog can be explained, partly at least, by the differing respiratory responses, the increase in respiratory minute volume resulting from excitation of the aortic bodies being on average only one-seventh that from the carotid bodies (Comroe & Mortimer, 1964; Daly & Ungar, 1966). With reference to Fig. 18.4, point X represents the control level of hindlimb vascular resistance during eupnoeic respiration (a). Assuming, on the evidence cited above, that the upper curve, representing the hindlimb resistance–pulmonary ventilation relationship, is the same for the aortic bodies as for the carotid bodies in response to the same stimulus, then point Z on the upper curve corresponds to the hindlimb vascular resistance during aortic body excitation in the spontaneously breathing dog at a correspondingly smaller increase in pulmonary ventilation (c) than that evoked by stimulation of the carotid bodies (b). Thus excitation of the aortic bodies in the spontaneously breathing animal causes hyperventilation and vasoconstriction (X–Z).

By contrast with the spontaneously breathing dog, carotid body stimulation in the spontaneously breathing cat invariably causes an increase in systemic vascular resistance and in hindlimb vascular resistance (Carmody & Scott, 1974; Daly *et al.*, 1983b). As in the dog, the input resulting from lung inflation causes reflex vasodilatation and opposes the vasoconstrictor response evoked by stimulation of the carotid bodies (Daly *et al.*, 1983a). Since the respiratory responses are smaller in the cat than in the dog at comparable levels of $P_aO_2$ and $P_aCO_2$ (see Fig. 2 in Daly, 1983), the explanation for the predominance of vasoconstrictor responses from the carotid bodies might be considered similar to that for the aortic bodies in the dog (Fig. 18.4). However, the exact relationship between respiration and vascular resistance during carotid body stimulation in the cat is at present unknown. An alternative explanation is that, compared with the dog, the vascular resistance response during carotid body stimulation is greater at any given value of respiratory minute volume.

### 18.4.5. *Central mechanisms*

The central mechanisms by which the sympathetic nervous system is involved in the interaction between the inputs from the carotid bodies and pulmonary receptors driven by lung inflation are still poorly understood. However, the pathways involved must be different to those involved in the vascular responses evoked by inputs from the carotid sinus baroreceptors and urinary bladder receptors on the one hand, and on the other from pulmonary receptors, because the combination of these inputs causes responses that are purely additive (Daly *et al.*, 1986).

The traditional concept that the tonic discharge in preganglionic sympathetic neurones is dependent on the activity of a 'vasomotor centre' in the medulla is no longer tenable in the light of evidence that has accumulated over the last decade (Hilton, 1975; Spyer, 1982). Even so, a fairly discrete region on the ventral surface of the medulla, the 'glycine-sensitive area', has been described by Guertzenstein & Silver (1974), which contributes significantly to 'background' vascular tone, besides mediating excitatory drives from the hypothalamus and midbrain and from the input from arterial baroreceptors to sympathetic preganglionic neurones (Loewy *et al.*, 1981; Spyer, 1982; Yamada *et al.*, 1984; McAllen, 1985). However, when stimulation of the carotid bodies causes vasoconstriction, this response is at least partly mediated via pathways which do not synapse in the glycine-sensitive area (Marshall, 1986).

There is abundant evidence that the discharge in sympathetic pre- and postganglionic nerves is modulated by respiration in laboratory animals (Adrian *et al.*, 1932; Tang *et al.*, 1957; Polosa *et al.*, 1980) and man (Eckberg *et al.*, 1985). The respiratory modulation of the firing rate is also synchronous with oscillations in hindlimb blood flow (Koepchen *et al.*, 1968). The pattern of firing is thought to be due to an excitatory synaptic input from brainstem inspiratory neurones (Preiss *et al.*, 1975; Gerber & Polosa, 1978) that can be suppressed by activation of pulmonary stretch receptors which inhibit inspiratory neurones (Gerber & Polosa, 1978; Gootman *et al.*, 1980; Polosa *et al.*, 1980). The reflex vasodilatation resulting from lung inflation reported here and elsewhere (Daly & Robinson, 1968; Daly *et al.*, 1983a, 1986) could be due to a decrease of sympathetic preganglionic activity through selective suppression of the inspiratory synchronous component. This cannot be the whole explanation, however, because when the inspiratory synchronous activity in sympathetic nerves is suppressed by lowering the arterial $PCO_2$, which also abolishes spontaneous respiratory movements, lung inflation still causes reflex vasodilatation (Daly *et al.*, 1967), indicating that there is another synaptic pathway mediating the reduction of sympathetic activity. Although the arterial baroreceptor reflex can be evoked whether or not inspiratory synchronicity of the sympathetic discharge is present (Gerber & Polosa, 1978), there is no comparable information about carotid chemoreceptor reflexes and still less about the exact sites of integration of sympathetic effects between inputs from chemoreceptors and pulmonary receptors driven by lung inflation. These sites may occur not only in the brainstem but also at the level of the spinal cord. Several excitatory and inhibitory pathways are known to converge on to the sympathetic preganglionic neurones in the spinal cord (Coote, 1980).

The fact that the vasoconstrictor response occurring on carotid chemoreceptor stimulation was partly suppressed by lung inflation, whereas that elicited by inputs from carotid baroreceptors and urinary bladder receptors was not (Daly *et al.*, 1986), lends further support to the concept that the sympathetic nervous system is organised in a way which allows selective control of the postganglionic innervation.

### 18.4.6. *Changes in $P_aCO_2$*

When the $P_aCO_2$ is lowered, such as during the hypeventilatory response to chemoreceptor stimulation, hypocapnia *per se* is a mechanism whereby the primary cardiac and vascular responses resulting from stimulation of the carotid and aortic bodies are partly suppressed (Daly & Hazzledine, 1963; Daly & Scott, 1963; Daly & Ungar, 1966). Furthermore the cardiac negative inotropic response (left ventricular d$P$/d$t$ max) to stimulation of the carotid bodies was reduced by decreasing the cephalic $PCO_2$ from 56 to 34 mmHg (Hainsworth *et al.*, 1985).

### 18.4.7. *Role of mechanisms secondary to hyperventilation in acute hypoxia*

Further evidence for the participation of these secondary respiratory mechanisms has been obtained in studies of acute hypoxia. The tachycardia and peripheral vasodilatation occurring under these conditions are to a large extent secondary to overriding respiratory mechanisms because they are reversed by maintaining pulmonary ventilation constant (Kontos *et al.*, 1965) and attenuated or reversed by denervation of the lungs (Kontos, 1967).

In man, withdrawal of a carotid body drive by breathing oxygen from a steady state of normocapnic hypoxia caused a transient tachycardia after a latency approximately the same as the average lung–ear circulation time (Drysdale & Petersen, 1977). Thus the primary cardiac effect of stimulation of the carotid bodies is the same in man as in laboratory animals.

### 18.5. **Role of brainstem defence areas**

This aspect of cardiovascular control by the carotid bodies is fully described in Chapter 12 by Janice M. Marshall. Briefly, anaesthetics such as chloralose, urethane and barbiturates undoubtedly have some depressant action on synaptic transmission in parts of the central nervous system such as the hypothalamus and midbrain. Transmission through the defence areas is less distorted in high decerebrate cats and cats under Althesin (Glaxo) anaesthesia. Under these conditions the effects of brief stimulations of the carotid bodies resemble those of the autonomic components of the alerting stage of the defence reaction evoked by excitation of the hypothalamic and brainstem defence areas (Abrahams *et al.*, 1960, 1964; Marshall, 1981; Hilton & Marshall, 1982). These include hyperventilation, usually tachycardia, vasoconstriction in the renal and mesenteric circulations and in the skin of the paw, and vasodilatation in skeletal muscle. The vasodilatation in skeletal muscle is due to activation of sympathetic cholinergic fibres and to inhibition of sympathetic noradrenergic tone. The cardiac and vascular responses are not secondary to the hyperventilation.

These experiments demonstrate that the hypothalamic and brainstem defence areas are important sites in the integration of the cardiovascular responses evoked by stimulation of the carotid bodies. There is still too little information on the pattern of responses produced by stimulation of the chemoreceptors in the conscious animal. In this connection Rutherford & Vatner (1978) showed in the conscious dog that brief stimulations of the carotid bodies evoked an immediate bradycardia and vasoconstriction in the mesenteric and iliac vascular beds followed about 12s later by tachycardia and vasodilatation. These latter responses did not occur when the accompanying hyperventilation was prevented by maintaining respiration constant by means of a mechanical respirator. From this it was concluded that they were secondary to the increase in respiration.

The prominence of the cardio-inhibitory and vasoconstrictor responses to excitation of the carotid bodies in the conscious animal compared with those elicited in high decerebrate cats without anaesthesia and in cats under Althesin anaesthesia is difficult to explain at present. It is possible that the bulbopontine respiratory and cardiovascular motoneurones have a lower threshold to carotid chemoreceptor afferent impulses than the diencephalic mechanisms for rage (Bizzi *et al.*, 1961). An alternative explanation is that in the cats under Althesin anaesthesia and in high decerebrate preparations without anaesthesia, synaptic transmission in descending inhibitory inputs is impaired or removed, thereby enabling full expression of the responses of defence areas to take place.

### 18.6. Modulation of chemoreceptor responses by apnoea

The foregoing evidence indicates that the primary cardiac and vascular responses from the carotid bodies are diminished, abolished or even reversed by the accompanying mechanisms arising from the concomitant increase in pulmonary ventilation. It would be expected therefore that they would be prepotent under conditions in which the secondary respiratory mechanisms evoked by hyperventilation were suppressed, and the following experiments showed this to be the case.

The bradycardia and increase in peripheral vascular resistance occurring in response to asphyxia during apnoea are due entirely to excitation of the carotid and aortic bodies (Angell-James & Daly, 1969a). The effectiveness of these chemoreceptor responses is contingent upon there being a reduction in the input from pulmonary receptors associated with apnoea. In the absence of alterations of the arterial blood gases or of the input from the arterial baroreceptors, restoration of spontaneous lung movements corresponding to a respiratory minute volume commensurate with the degree of arterial hypoxaemia and hypercapnia abolished the chemo receptor bradycardia and vasoconstriction by initiating a pulmonary reflex (Angell-James & Daly, 1969a).

Reflex apnoea can be produced by excitation of receptors in the skin of the face, in the nasal mucosa and larynx, and by electrical stimulation of the central cut end of a superior laryngeal nerve (see Angell-James & Daly, 1969b, 1972; Daly, 1986). Respiration is inhibited in the end-expiratory position so that there is cessation of the inspiratory neuronal activity and a diminution in activity of pulmonary stretch receptors.

The effects of stimulation of the carotid bodies during a reflexly induced apnoea are quite different from those elicited during normal breathing.

(1) The normal carotid body respiratory excitatory response is wholly or partly suppressed (Angell-James & Daly, 1973, 1978; Elsner *et al.*, 1977; Daly *et al.*, 1978b, 1983b). This is consistent with the finding that brief stimulation of the carotid bodies during the normal expiratory phase of the respiratory cycle does not cause inspiration but may prolong expiration (Black & Torrance, 1971; Eldridge, 1972).

(2) The primary cardiac response to stimulation of the carotid bodies is revealed, so that the control cardio-accelerator response during spontaneous ventilation is converted to bradycardia during an induced apnoea, or a bradycardia during spontaneous ventilation is potentiated (Angell-James & Daly, 1973; Elsner *et al.*, 1977; Daly *et al.*, 1978b, 1983b; Daly & Taton, 1979a, b). The explanation for these responses is that during a reflexly induced apnoea the cardiac vagal motoneurones become less refractory to incoming excitatory stimuli through a combination of a reduction in central inspiratory neuronal drive and a reduction in activity of pulmonary stretch receptors (see Spyer, 1981, 1982).

(3) The primary vasoconstrictor response to carotid body stimulation becomes more evident in that a vasodilatation occurring during normal breathing is reversed to vasoconstriction during an induced apnoea, while vasoconstrictor responses are potentiated (Daly *et al.*, 1978b, 1983b).

The important role of a pulmonary reflex in these integrative mechanisms is also demonstrated by artificially inflating the lungs during the period of apnoea; tachycardia and vasodilatation then result, responses which are dependent on the innervation to the lungs (Angell-James & Daly, 1978; Daly *et al.*, 1983a).

The integration of these cardiovascular responses to carotid body stimulation with changes in respiration, and in particular during reflexly induced periods of apnoea, have important implications with regard to the mechanisms underlying the responses in breath-hold diving. The literature has been fully reviewed elsewhere (Angell-James & Daly, 1972; Elsner & Gooden, 1983; Daly, 1984, 1986). In breath-hold diving, apnoea occurs, usually in the end-expiratory position, accompanied by bradycardia and selective vasoconstriction. The cardiovascular responses are due, at least in part, to excitation of the carotid body chemoreceptors and the concomitant cessation of respiration. The apnoea is maintained since the excitatory input from the chemoreceptors to the inspiratory neurones is suppressed by the inhibitory input from the trigeminal receptors stimulated by water (see Daly, 1984).

## 18.7. Conclusions

The cardiovascular responses to stimulation of the peripheral arterial chemoreceptors are dependent on the direction and size of the concomitant respiratory effect mediated through changes in the central inspiratory drive and in the input from pulmonary vagal receptors on to cardiac vagal motoneurones and sympathetic motoneurones, and on the changes in $P_aCO_2$. Under steady-state conditions the overal response will depend on a number of factors:

(1) the magnitude of the inputs from the carotid and aortic bodies and pulmonary receptors, the latter being determined by the hyperventilatory response;
(2) the activity of the central inspiratory neurones which, together with the input from pulmonary receptors driven by lung inflation, determines the effectiveness of the excitatory input from chemoreceptors on to cardiac vagal motoneurones and central sympathetic neurones; and
(3) the prevailing level of $P_aCO_2$ which again determines the effectiveness of excitatory inputs to the nervous system.

These are in addition to other mechanisms, e.g. changes in the input from arterial baroreceptors, which might influence the final observed response (see Daly, 1983). The reflex cardiac and vascular responses to chemoreceptor stimulation at any moment will depend on a balance of all these various mechanisms.

The cardiovascular responses to systemic hypoxia are known to vary with increasing levels of hypoxia. The explanation probably lies in the fact that the balance of the various factors listed above are not the same at all levels of $P_aO_2$. From the evidence available the gain of the primary cardiac and vascular reflex responses from the chemoreceptors varies with the $P_aCO_2$, the gain increasing the lower the $P_aCO_2$. The hyperventilation, on the other hand, also increases as the $P_aO_2$ falls, but less in some species than in others. Under these conditions, at the lower levels of $P_aO_2$ the balance of the various factors involved would be expected to shift towards those promoting bradycardia and vasoconstriction, as in the rabbit (Korner, 1965).

## Acknowledgements

Financial support from the British Heart Foundation and Medical Research Council is gratefully acknowledged. We wish to thank Mr D. R. Bacon for expert technical assistance.

## References

Abrahams, V. C., Hilton, S. M. & Zbrożyna, A. (1960). Active muscle vasodilatation produced by stimulation of the brain stem: its significance in the defence reaction. *J. Physiol.* **154**, 491–513.

Abrahams, V. C., Hilton, S. M. & Zbrożyna, A. W. (1964). The role of active muscle vasodilatation in the alerting stage of the defence reaction. *J. Physiol.* **171**, 189–202.

Adrian, E. D. (1933). Afferent impulses in the vagus and their effect on respiration. *J. Physiol.* **79**, 332–58.

Adrian, E. D., Bronk, D. W. & Phillips, G. (1932). Discharges in mammalian sympathetic nerves. *J. Physiol.* **74**, 115–33.

Angell-James, J. E. & Daly, M. de B. (1969a). Cardiovascular responses in apnoeic asphyxia: role of arterial chemoreceptors and the modification of their effects by a pulmonary vagal inflation reflex. *J. Physiol.* **201**, 87–104.

Angell-James, J. E. & Daly, M. de B. (1969b). Nasal reflexes. *Proc. Roy. Soc. Med.* **62**, 1287–93.

Angell-James, J. E. & Daly, M. de B. (1972). Some mechamisms involved in the cardiovascular adaptations to diving. In *The Effects of Pressure on Organisms* (eds M. A. Sleigh & A. G. MacDonald). *Symp. Soc. Exp. Biol.* **26**, 313–41. Cambridge: Cambridge University Press.

Angell-James, J. E. & Daly, M. de B. (1973). The interaction of reflexes elicited by stimulation of carotid body chemoreceptors and receptors in the nasal mucosa affecting respiration and pulse interval in the dog. *J. Physiol.* **229**, 133–49.

Angell-James, J. E. & Daly, M. de B. (1978). The effects of artificial lung inflation on reflexly induced bradycardia associated with apnoea in the dog. *J. Physiol.* **274**, 349–66.

Anrep, G. V., Pascual, W. & Rössler, R. (1936). Respiratory variations of the heart rate. I. The reflex mechanism of the respiratory arrhythmia. *Proc. R. Soc. Lond. (Biol.)* **119**, 191–217.

Backman, S. B., Ballantyne, D., Mifflin, S., Anders, K., Jordan, D., Spyer, K. M. & Richter, D. W. (1985). Analysis of the connection between slowly adapting pulmonary stretch receptor afferents and inspiratory neurones within the tractus solitarius region in cats. In *Neurogenesis of Central Respiratory Rhythm*, (pp. 258–61 eds A. L. Bianchi & M. Denavit-Saubié). Lancaster: MTP Press.

Baumgarten, R. von & Kanzow, E. (1958). The interaction of two types of inspiratory neurones in the region of the tractus solitarius of the cat. *Arch. Ital. Biol.* **96**, 361–73.

Bernthal, T. (1938). Chemo-reflex control of vascular reactions through the carotid body. *Am. J. Physiol.* **121**, 1–20.

Bernthal, T., Greene, W., Jr & Revzin, A. M. (1951). Role of carotid chemoreceptors in hypoxic cardiac acceleration. *Proc. Soc. Exp. Biol. N.Y.* **76**, 121–4.

Bizzi, E., Libretti, A., Malliani, A. & Zanchetti, A. (1961). Reflex chemoceptive excitation of diencephalic sham rage behavior. *Am. J. Physiol.* **200**, 923–6.

Black, A. M. S. & Torrance, R. W. (1971). Respiratory oscillations in chemoreceptor discharge in the control of breathing. *Resp. Physiol.* **13**, 221–37.

Bronk, D. W., Ferguson, L. K., Margaria, R. & Solandt, D. Y. (1936). The activity of the cardiac sympathetic centers. *Am. J. Physiol.* **117**, 237–49.

Carmody, J. J. & Scott, M. J. (1974). Respiratory and cardiovascular responses to prolonged stimulation of the carotid body chemoreceptors in the cat. *Aust. J. Exp. Biol. Med. Sci.* **52**, 271–83.

Chalmers, J. P., Korner, P. I. & White, S. W. (1967). The relative roles of the aortic and carotid sinus nerves in the rabbit in the control of respiration and circulation during arterial hypoxia and hypercapnia. *J. Physiol.* **188**, 435–50.

Chungcharoen, D., Daly, M. de B. & Schweitzer, A. (1952). The blood supply of the carotid body in cats, dogs and rabbits. *J. Physiol.* **117**, 347–58.

Clarke, J. A. & Daly, M. de B. (1982). The distribution of carotid body type-I cells and periadventitial type-I cells in the carotid bifurcation regions of the dog. *Acta Anat.* **113**, 352–70.

Clarke, J. A. & Daly, M. de B. (1983). Distribution of carotid body type-I cells and other periadventitial type-I cells in the carotid bifurcation regions of the cat. *Anat. Embryol.* **166**, 169–89.

Clarke, J. A., Daly, M. de B. & Ead, H. W. (1986). Dimensions and volume of the carotid body in the adult cat, and their relation to the organ's specific blood flow. *Acta Anat.* **126**, 84–6.

Coleridge, H. M., Coleridge, J. C. G. & Howe, A. (1970). Thoracic chemoreceptors in the dog. A histological and electrophysiological study of the location, innervation and blood supply of the aortic bodies. *Circ. Res.* **26**, 235–47.

Comroe, J. H., Jr & Mortimer, L. (1964). The respiratory and cardiovascular responses of temporally separated aortic and carotid bodies to cyanide, nicotine, phenyldiguanide and serotonin. *J. Pharmacol.* **146**, 33–41.

Coote, J. H. (1980). The integrative role of the sympathetic neurone. In *Central Interaction between Respiratory and Cardiovascular Control Systems*, pp. 15–20 (eds H. P. Koepchen, S. M. Hilton & A. Trzebski). Berlin, Heidelberg, New York: Springer-Verlag.

Daly, M. de B. (1983). Peripheral arterial chemoreceptors and the cardiovascular system. In *Physiology of the Peripheral Arterial Chemoreceptors*, pp. 325–93. (Eds H. Acker & R. G. O'Regan). Amsterdam: Elsevier/Holland Biomedical Press BV.

Daly, M. de B. (1984). Breath-hold diving: mechanisms of cardiovascular adjustments in the mammal. In *Recent Advances in Physiology*, *10*, pp. 201–45 (ed. P. F. Baker). Edinburgh: Churchill Livingstone.

Daly, M. de B. (1986). Interactions between respiration and circulation. In *Handbook of Physiology, Section 3, The Respiratory System, vol. 2, Control of Breathing, Part II*, pp. 529–94. Bethesda, MD: American Physiological Society.

Daly, M. de B. & Hazzledine, J. L. (1963). The effects of artificially induced hyperventilation on the primary cardiac reflex response to stimulation of the carotid bodies in the dog. *J. Physiol.* **168**, 872–89.

Daly, M. de B., Hazzledine, J. L. & Howe, A. (1965). Reflex respiratory and peripheral vascular responses to stimulation of the isolated perfused aortic arch chemoreceptors of the dog. *J. Physiol.* **177**, 300–22.

Daly, M. de B., Hazzledine, J. L. & Ungar, A. (1967). The reflex effects of alterations in lung volume on systemic vascular resistance in the dog. *J. Physiol.* **188**, 331–51.

Daly, M. de B., Korner, P. I., Angell-James, J. E. & Oliver, J. A. (1978a). Cardiovascular and respiratory effects of carotid body stimulation in the monkey. *Clin. Exp. Pharmacol. Physiol.* **5**, 511–24.

Daly, M. de B., Korner, P. I., Angell-James, J. E. & Oliver, J. A. (1978b). Cardiovascular–respiratory reflex interactions between the carotid bodies and upper airways receptors in the monkey. *Am. J. Physiol.* **234**, H293–9.

Daly, M. de B., Lambertsen, C. J. & Schweitzer, A. (1954). Observations on the volume of blood flow and oxygen utilization of the carotid body in the cat. *J. Physiol.* **125**, 67–89.

Daly, M. de B., Litherland, A. S. & Wood, L. M. (1983a). The reflex effects of inflation of the lungs on heart rate and hind limb vascular resistance in the cat. *IRCS Med. Sci.* **11**, 859–60.

Daly, M. de B., Litherland, A. S. & Wood, L. M. (1983b). The modification of the respiratory, cardiac and vascular responses to stimulation of the carotid body chemoreceptors by a laryngeal input in the cat. *IRCS Med. Sci.* **11**, 861–2.

Daly, M. de B. & Robinson, B. H. (1968). An analysis of the reflex systemic vasodilator response elicited by lung inflation in the dog. *J. Physiol.* **195**, 387–406.

Daly, M. de B. & Scott, M. J. (1958). The effects of stimulation of the carotid body chemoreceptors on heart rate in the dog. *J. Physiol.* **144**, 148–66.

Daly, M. de B. & Scott, M. J. (1959). The effect of hypoxia on the heart rate of the dog with special reference to the contribution of the carotid body chemoreceptors. *J. Physiol.* **145**, 440–6.

Daly, M. de B. & Scott, M. J. (1962). An analysis of the primary cardiovascular reflex effects of stimulation of the carotid body chemoreceptors in the dog. *J. Physiol.* **162**, 555–73.

Daly, M. de B. & Scott, M. J. (1963). The cardiovascular responses to stimulation of the carotid body chemoreceptors in the dog. *J. Physiol.* **165**, 179–97.

Daly, M. de B. & Scott, M. J. (1964). The cardiovascular effects of hypoxia in the dog with special reference to the contribution of the carotid body chemoreceptors. *J. Physiol.* **173**, 210–14.

Daly, M. de B. & Taton, A. (1979a). Interactions of cardiorespiratory reflexes elicited from the carotid bodies and upper airways receptors in the conscious rabbit. *J. Physiol.* **291**, 34P.

Daly, M. de B. & Taton, A. (1979b). Upper airways reflexes evoked by broncho-dilator drugs administered in pressurized aerosol form in the conscious rabbit. *IRCS Med. Sci.* **7**, 255.

Daly, M. de B. & Ungar, A. (1966). Comparison of the reflex responses elicited by stimulation of the separately perfused carotid and aortic body chemoreceptors in the dog. *J. Physiol.* **182**, 379–403.

Daly, M. de B., Ward, J. & Wood, L. M. (1986). Modification by lung inflation of the vascular responses from the carotid body chemoreceptors and other receptors in dogs. *J. Physiol.* **375**, 13–20.

Davidson, N. S., Goldner, S. & McCloskey, D. I. (1976). Respiratory modulation of baroreceptor and chemoreceptor reflexes affecting heart rate and cardiac vagal efferent nerve activity. *J. Physiol.* **259**, 523–30.

Davis, A. L., McCloskey, D. I. & Potter, E. K. (1977). Respiratory modulation of baroreceptor and chemoreceptor reflexes affecting heart rate through the sympathetic nervous system. *J. Physiol.* **272**, 691–703.

Davis, H. L., Fowler, W. S. & Lambert, E. H. (1956). Effect of volume and rate of inflation and deflation on transpulmonary pressure and response of pulmonary stretch receptors. *Am. J. Physiol.* **187**, 558–66.

Dawes, G. S., Lewis, B. V., Milligan, J. E., Roach, M. R. & Talner, N. S. (1968). Vasomotor responses in the hind limbs of foetal and new-born lambs to asphyxia and aortic chemoreceptor stimulation. *J. Physiol.* **195**, 55–81.

de Castro, F. (1962). Sur la vascularisation et l'innervation des corpuscles carotidiens aberrants. *Arch. int. Pharmacodyn. Thèr.* **89**, 212–24.

Donoghue, S., Felder, R. B., Jordan, D. & Spyer, K. M. (1984). The central projections of carotid baroreceptors and chemoreceptors in the cat: a neuro-physiological study. *J. Physiol.* **347**, 397–409.

Donoghue, S., Garcia, M., Jordan, D. & Spyer, K. M. (1982). The brain-stem projections of pulmonary stretch afferent neurones in cats and rabbits. *J. Physiol.* **322**, 353–63.

Drysdale, D. B. & Petersen, E. S. (1977). Arterial chemoreceptors, ventilation and heart rate in man. *J. Physiol.* **273**, 109–20.

Eckberg, D. L., Nerhed, C. & Wallin, B. G. (1985). Respiratory modulation of muscle sympathetic and vagal outflow in man. *J. Physiol.* **365**, 181–96.

Eldridge, F. L. (1972). The importance of timing on the respiratory effects of intermittent carotid body chemoreceptor stimulation. *J. Physiol.* **222**, 319–33.

Elsner, R., Angell-James, J. E. & Daly, M. de B. (1977). Carotid body chemoreceptor reflexes and their interactions in the seal. *Am. J. Physiol.* **232**, H517–25.

Elsner, R. & Gooden, B. A. (1983). *Diving and Asphyxia.* Cambridge: Cambridge University Press.

Ford, R., Hainsworth, R., Rankin, A. J. & Soladoye, A. D. (1985). Abdominal vascular responses to changes in carbon dioxide tension in the cephalic circulation of anaesthetized dogs. *J. Physiol.* **358**, 417–31.

Gandevia, S. C., McCloskey, D. I. & Potter, E. K. (1978). Inhibition of baroreceptor and chemoreceptor reflexes on heart rate by afferents from the lungs. *J. Physiol.* **276**, 369–82.

Greenwood, P. V., Hainsworth, R., Karim, F., Morrison, G. W. & Sofola, O. A. (1980). Reflex inotropic responses of the heart from lung inflation in anaesthetized dogs. *Pflügers Arch.* **386**, 199–205.

Gerber, U. & Polosa, C. (1978). Effects of pulmonary stretch receptor afferent stimulation on sympathetic preganglionic neuron firing. *Can. J. Physiol. Pharmacol.* **56**, 191–8.

Gilbey, M. P., Jordan, D., Richter, D. W. & Spyer, K. M. (1984). Synaptic mechanisms involved in the inspiratory modulation of vagal cardio-inhibitory neurones in the cat. *J. Physiol.* **356**, 65–78.

Gootman, P. M., Feldman, J. L. & Cohen, M. I. (1980). Pulmonary afferent influences on respiratory modulation of sympathetic discharge. In *Central Interaction between Respiratory and Cardiovascular Control Systems*, pp. 172–78 (eds H. P. Koepchen, S. M. Hilton & A. Trzebski). Berlin: Springer-Verlag.

Guertzenstein, P. G. & Silver, A. (1974). Fall in blood pressure produced from discrete regions of the ventral surface of the medulla by glycine and lesions. *J. Physiol.* **242**, 489–503.

Hainsworth, R. (1974). Circulatory responses from lung inflation in anesthetized dogs. *Am. J. Physiol.* **226**, 247–55.

Hainsworth, R., Karim, F., McGregor, K. H. & Wood, L. M. (1983). Responses of abdominal vascular resistance and capacitance to stimulation of carotid chemoreceptors in anaesthetized dogs. *J. Physiol.* **334**, 409–19.

Hainsworth, R., Rankin, A. J. & Soladoye, A. O. (1985). Effect of cephalic carbon dioxide tension on the cardiac inotropic response to carotid chemoreceptor stimulation in dogs. *J. Physiol.* **358**, 405–16.

Haymet, B. T. & McCloskey, D. I. (1975). Baroreceptor and chemoreceptor influences on heart rate during the respiratory cycle in the dog. *J. Physiol.* **245**, 699–712.

Hering, E. (1871). Uber den Einfluss der Athmung auf den Kreislauf. Zweite Mittheilung. Uber die reflectorische Beziehung zwischen Lunge und Herz. *S. B. Akad. Wiss. Wein* **64**, 333–53.

Heymans, C., Bouckaert, J. J. & Regniers, P. (1933). *Le Sinus Carotidien et la Zone Homologue Cardio-aortique.* Paris, Doin.

Heymans, C. & Neil, E. (1958). *Reflexogenic Areas of the Cardiovascular System.* London: Churchill.

Hilton, S. M. (1975). Ways of viewing the central nervous control of the circulation — old and new. *Brain Res.* **87**, 213–19.

Hilton, S. M. & Marshall, J. M. (1982). The pattern of cardiovascular response to carotid chemoreceptor stimulation in the cat. *J. Physiol.* **326**, 495–513.

Howe, A. (1956). The vasculature of the aortic bodies in the cat. *J. Physiol.* **134**, 311–18.

Karim, F., Hainsworth, R., Sofola, O. A. & Wood, L. M. (1980). Responses of the heart to stimulation of the aortic body chemoreceptors in dogs. *Circ. Res.* **46**, 77–83.

Koepchen, H. P., Seller, H., Polster, J. & Langhorst, P. (1968). Uber die Fein-Vasomotorik der Muskelstrohmbahn und ihre Beziehung zur Ateminnervation. *Pflügers Archiv,* **302**, 285–99.

Kontos, H. A., Goldin, D., Richardson, D. W. & Patterson, J. L., Jr (1967). Contribution of pulmonary vagal reflexes to circulatory response to hypoxia. *Am. J. Physiol.* **212**, 1441–6.

Kontos, H. A., Mauck, H. P., Jr, Richardson, D. W. & Patterson, J. L., Jr (1965). Mechanism of circulatory responses to systemic hypoxia in the anesthetized dog. *Am. J. Physiol.* **209**, 397–403.

Korner, P. I. (1965). The role of the arterial chemoreceptors and baroreceptors in the circulatory response to hypoxia of the rabbit. *J. Physiol.* **180**, 279–303.

Lahiri, S., Nishino, T., Mokashi, A. & Mulligan, E. (1980). Relative responses of aortic and carotid body chemoreceptors to hypotension. *J. Appl. Physiol.* **48**, 781–8.

Lahiri, S., Smatresk, N. J. & Mulligan, E. (1983). Responses of peripheral chemoreceptors to natural stimuli. In *Physiology of the Peripheral Arterial Chemoreceptors*, pp. 221–56 (eds H. Acker & R. G. O'Regan). Amsterdam: Elsevier Science Publishers BV.

Loewy, A. D., Wallach, J. H. & McKellar, S. (1981). Efferent connections of the ventral medulla oblongata in the rat. *Brain Res. (Reviews)* **3**, 63–80.

Lopes, O. U. & Palmer, J. F. (1976). Proposed respiratory 'gating' mechanism for cardiac slowing. *Nature* **264**, 454–6.

Macleod, R. D. M. & Scott, M. J. (1964). The heart rate responses to carotid body chemoreceptor stimulation in the cat. *J. Physiol.* **175**, 193–202.

Marshall, J. M. (1981). Interaction between the responses to stimulation of peripheral chemoreceptors and baroreceptors: The importance of chemoreceptor activation of the defence areas. *J. Auton. Nerv. Syst.* **3**, 389–400.

Marshall, J. M. (1986). The role of the glycine sensitive area of the ventral medulla in cardiovascular responses to carotid chemoreceptor and peripheral nerve stimulation. *Pflügers Arch.* **406**, 225–31.

Marshall, J. & Metcalfe, J. D. (1986). Cardiovascular changes associated with augmented breaths during normoxia and hypoxia in the rat. *J. Physiol.* **373**, 77P.

Matsuura, S. (1973). Chemoreceptor properties of glomus tissue found in the carotid region of the cat. *J. Physiol.* **235**, 57–73.

McAllen, R. M. (1985). Mediation of the fastigial pressor response and a somato-sympathetic reflex by ventral medullary neurones in the cat. *J. Physiol.* **368**, 423–33.

Merrill, E. G. (1975). Preliminary studies on nucleus retroambigualis — nucleus of the solitary tract interactions in cats. *J. Physiol.* **244**, 54–5P.

Mifflin, S. W., Spyer, K. M. & Withington-Wray, D. J. (1986). Lack of respiratory modulation of baroreceptor inputs in the nucleus of the tractus solitarius. *J. Physiol.* **373**, 58P.

Neil, E. (1956). Influence of the carotid chemoreceptor reflexes on the heart rate in systemic anoxia. *Arch. Int. Pharmacodyn. Thèr.*, **105**, 477–88.

Neil, E., Redwood, C. R. M. & Schweitzer, A. (1949). Effects of electrical stimulation of the aortic nerve on blood pressure and respiration in cats and rabbits under chloralose and nembutal anaesthesia. *J. Physiol.* **109**, 392–401.

Polosa, C., Gerber, U. & Schondorf, R. (1980). Central mechanisms of interaction between sympathetic preganglionic neurones and the respiratory oscillator. In *Central Interaction between Respiratory and Cardiovascular Control Systems*, pp. 137–42 (eds H. P. Koepchen, S. M. Hilton & A. Trzebski). Berlin: Springer-Verlag.

Potter, E. K. (1981). Inspiratory inhibition of vagal responses to baroreceptor and chemoreceptor stimuli in the dog. *J. Physiol.* **316**, 177–90.

Preiss, G., Kirchner, F. & Polosa, C. (1975). Patterning of sympathetic preganglionic neuron firing by the central respiratory drive. *Brain Res.* **87**, 363–74.

Richter, D. (1982). Generation and maintenance of the respiratory rhythm. In *Control and Co-ordination of Respiration and Circulation* (ed P. J. Butler). *J. Exp. Biol.* **100**, 93–107. Cambridge: Cambridge University Press.

Rutherford, J. D. & Vatner, S. F. (1978). Integrated carotid chemoreceptor and pulmonary inflation reflex control of peripheral vasoactivity in conscious dogs. *Circ. Res.* **43**, 200–8.

Salisbury, P. F., Galletti, P.-M., Lewin, R. J. & Rieben, P. A. (1959). Stretch reflexes from the dog's lungs to the systemic circulation. *Circ. Res.* **7**, 62–7.

Sapru, H. N. & Krieger, A. J. (1977). Carotid and aortic chemoreceptor function in the rat. *J. Appl. Physiol.* **42**, 344–8.

Spyer, K. M. (1981). Neural organisation and control of the baroreceptor reflex. *Rev. Physiol. Biochem. Pharmacol.* **88**, 24–124.

Spyer, K. M. (1982). Central nervous integration of cardiovascular control. In *Control and Co-ordination of Respiration and Circulation* (ed. P. J. Butler). *J. Exp. Biol.* **100**, 109–28. Cambridge: Cambridge University Press.

Tang, P. C., Maire, F. W. & Amassian, V. E. (1957). Respiratory influence on the vasomotor center. *Am. J. Physiol.* **191**, 218–24.

Traube, L. (1865). Ueber periodische Thatigkeits-Aeusserungen des vasomotorischen und Hemmungs-Nervencentrums. *Zentbl. med. Wiss.* **56**, 881–5.

Verna, A. (1979). Ultrastructure of the carotid body in mammals. *Int. Rev. Cytol.* **60**, 271–330.

Widdicombe, J. G. (1982). Pulmonary and respiratory tract receptors. In *Control and Co-ordination of Respiration and Circulation* (ed. P. J. Butler). *J. Exp. Biol.* **100**, 41–57. Cambridge: Cambridge University Press.

Wood, L. M., Hainsworth, R. & McGregor, K. H. (1985). Effects of lung inflation on abdominal vascular resistance in anaesthetized dogs. *Quart. J. Exp. Physiol.* **70**, 575–84.

Yamada, K. A., McAllen, R. M. & Loewy, A. D. (1984). GABA antagonists applied to the ventral surface of the medulla oblongata block the baroreceptor reflex. *Brain Res.* **297**, 175–80.

# 19

# Nervous control of the diving response in birds and mammals

**R. Stephenson**[†] **and P. J. Butler**

*Department of Zoology and Comparative Physiology, University of Birmingham, Birmingham B15 2TT, UK*

## 19.1. Introduction

When fully submerged in water, air-breathing homeotherms must rely upon oxygen stored within the body to support all aerobic processes and tolerate or reduce any deleterious effects of end-products of metabolism until the resumption of lung ventilation (Hochachka & Somero, 1984). The logical solution to the problem of survival for prolonged periods of submersion, first suggested by Irving (1934, 1939), is to reduce overall metabolic rate and in particular to reduce the level of aerobic metabolism or, in other words, to invoke an oxygen-conserving response. Such a response occurs during involuntary submersions (e.g. Scholander, 1940; Andersen, 1959; Pickwell, 1968). Naturally diving animals, however, are usually physically active, and the exercising muscles therefore elevate overall metabolic rate, increasing the demand for oxygen. Thus, an actively diving animal faces a metabolic dilemma: the need to use oxygen as slowly as possible in order to extend the period of submersion and at the same time to increase aerobic metabolism to do work. In unrestrained, naturally behaving aquatic animals the problem is solved by behavioural control of lung ventilation, and through anatomical and biochemical adaptations that enhance oxygen storage capacity and thereby increase the efficacy of cardiovascular adjustments which in turn are designed to optimise oxygen utilisation by balancing the opposing requirements of submersion and exercise.

A comprehensive comparative review of responses to voluntary and involuntary submersion in all classes of aquatic air-breathing vertebrates is given by Butler & Jones (1982). Physiological adjustments in response to submersion of non-aquatic mammals, including humans, are reviewed by Lin (1982), and are qualitatively similar to those in natural divers. The emphasis here is on the variability of cardiorespiratory responses under

[†]*Present address:* Department of Zoology, University of British Columbia, BC, Canada V6T 2A9.

different experimental conditions, and an attempt is made to explain this variability in terms of possible neural mechanisms.

The controlled submersion of restrained animals is usually the only practical way to investigate the neural control of the cardiorespiratory system during submersion, and consequently relatively little neurophysiological information is available from freely diving animals. For this reason there follows a very brief description of neural control of the cardiorespiratory system during involuntary submersion, and this is followed by a discussion of the possible role of suprabulbar and peripheral nervous influences in unrestrained diving animals, and, in particular, of the roles of the defence-arousal system and exercise. Much of the information which is used to support or refute hypotheses is derived from experiments that were not designed specifically to investigate the responses to submersion and often involved the use of anaesthetised, non-aquatic animals. Obviously, extrapolation from one experimental situation and from one species of animal to another must be done with caution.

## 19.2. Involuntary submersion

The cardiorespiratory response to involuntary submersion basically consists of apnoea accompanied by bradycardia, reduced cardiac output and increased total peripheral resistance with maintained arterial blood pressure. Perfusion of the skeletal musculature and viscera is markedly reduced, whereas blood supply to the CNS, eyes, heart and adrenal glands is maintained (see, for example, Jones *et al.*, 1979; Blix *et al.*, 1983).

### 19.2.1. *Reflex apnoea*

Immediately upon head immersion, receptors in the exposed skin of the face and in the nasal mucosa (innervated by branches of the trigeminal (V) nerves) and in the upper respiratory tract (innervated by branches of the glossopharyngeal (IX) and vagus (X) nerves) are stimulated by water and evoke a reflex apnoea. These facial and nasopharyngeal receptors have been reported to be sensitive to thermal, mechanical and chemical stimuli in ducks (Gregory, 1973; Bamford & Jones, 1974).

Apnoea, which is usually (though not always) in the expiratory position, is maintained, despite increasing excitatory inputs, until head emersion. The nasopharyngeal and facial receptors in ducks are slowly adapting (Bamford & Jones, 1974), and work on cats has shown that stimulation of the central and peripheral chemoreceptors during expiration enhances expiratory duration and effort (e.g. Black & Torrance, 1971; Marek *et al.*, 1985). Since stimulation of nasophrayngeal and facial receptors causes apnoea in the expiratory position in most diving animals, this effect of chemoreceptor activation during apnoeic asphyxia could contribute to maintenance of apnoea. A further mechanism which may contribute to maintenance of submersion apnoea is a suppression of activity in central respiratory neurones (CRN) by increased $P_aCO_2$ in the absence of pulmonary afferent feedback, which has been demonstrated in cats (Cohen, 1964) and ducks though not in chickens (Jones & Bamford, 1976). Furthermore, most experiments involving involuntary submersion use fully conscious animals and it is likely that cortical influences exert an inhibitory effect on respiration under these circumstances (Bamford & Jones, 1974; Florin-Christensen *et al.*, 1986). Certainly, motivation is an important factor determining breaking-point during voluntary breath-hold in humans (Lin, 1982).

### 19.2.2. *Redistribution of blood flow*

As well as apnoea, involuntary submersion also evokes the 'classical' oxygen-conserving cardiovascular response (Fig. 19.1). Upon immersion there is a reflex redistribution of blood away from the hypoxia-tolerant tissues and into the capacitance vessels in ducks and seals (e.g. Jones *et al.*, 1979; Zapol *et al.*, 1979; Blix *et al.*, 1983). Absolute blood flow to the inactive skeletal muscles, lungs, liver, spleen, pancreas, kidney and intestines is significantly reduced, in some cases to very low levels, whereas blood flow to the brain, eyes and adrenal glands is maintained close to or increased above pre-submersion values.

Coronary blood flow is reduced in the harbour seal, *Phoca vitulina*, in proportion to the decrease in myocardial work (Kjekshus *et al.*, 1982). This reduction occurs, probably as a result of increased sympathetic vasomotor activity, despite the fall in $P_aO_2$ and increase in diastolic period, which would tend to increases flow in a non-diving situation (Klocke & Ellis, 1980). Coronary blood flow does not change during submersion in domestic ducks (*Anas platyrhynchos*), however, despite a marked reduction in cardiac work (Jones *et al.*, 1979).

Cerebral blood flow (CBF) is maintained at, or increased above, pre-immersion levels in spotted and grey seals, *Phoca vitulina largha* and *Halichoerus grypus*, and in the domestic duck (Jones *et al.*, 1979; Blix *et al.*, 1983). CBF is initially relatively low, probably as a result of the weak action of sympathetic cerebral vasoconstrictor fibres, but increases gradually as the 'dive' progresses. In ducks this is the result of the local vasodilator action of decreased $P_aO_2$ and increased $P_aCO_2$ whose effects are additive (Grubb *et al.*, 1977, 1978). Cerebral vasodilatation may involve a reflex from the arterial chemoreceptors (Ponte & Purves, 1974; Neubauer *et al.*, 1978) though this is not effected by cranial parasympathetic nerves in rabbits (Scremin *et al.*, 1983).

The venous oxygen stores in domestic ducks are mobilised by venoconstriction (Djojosugito *et al.*, 1969; Langille, 1983). The diluting effect of the deoxygenated blood from the brain is reduced in the harp seal, *Pagophilus groenlandicus*, by the cessation of blood flow in the cervical vertebral venous

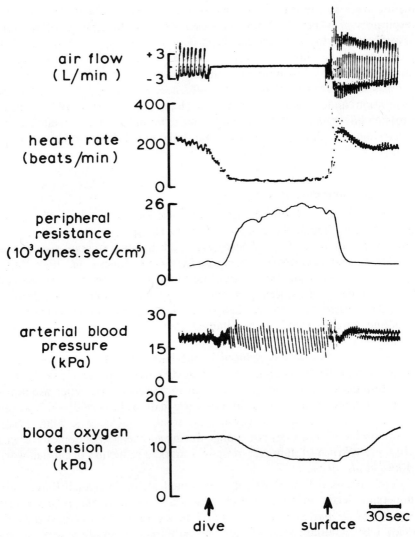

air flow
(L/min)
+3
-3

heart rate
(beats/min)
400
200
0

peripheral
resistance
(10³dynes.sec/cm⁵)
26
0

arterial blood
pressure
(kPa)
30
15
0

blood oxygen
tension
(kPa)
20
10
0

dive          surface      30sec

Fig. 19.1. Cardiovascular responses to involuntary submergence of the head of a domestic duck (*Anas platyrhynchos*). 'Peripheral resistance' refers to the resistance to blood flow through the sciatic vascular bed of one leg. (From Butler & Jones, 1982.)

system with a consequent reduction in blood flow in the anterior vena cava — the blood being returned to the main venous system (posterior vena cava) as far from the heart as possible via the extradural intervertebral veins (Ronald *et al.*, 1977).

These widespread vascular adjustments are effected by the sympathetic nervous system and blood-borne catecholamines. Innervation of large arteries in ducks is much denser than the corresponding arteries in non-divers (turkeys and cats, Folkow *et al.*, 1966; Gooden, 1980), and duck arteries are also more sensitive to plasma noradrenaline than those of the chicken (Gooden 1980; Wilson & West, 1986). These nervous and endocrine vasoconstrictor influences must overrule metabolic vasodilatation during involuntary submersion, and the increased constriction of large vessels in divers is probably important in this respect since they are situated away from the perfused tissue and therefore will not be affected by metabolites. Plasma concentrations of adrenaline and noradrenaline are considerably elevated during involuntary submersion (Hudson & Jones, 1982; Hance *et al.*, 1982), though they can only act on those vessels where blood flow remains great enough to allow their delivery.

Sympathetic efferent activity (to the external carotid, renal and splanchnic blood vessels) can be generated in spinalised cats in the intermediolateral cell column (IML) of the spinal cord from which the preganglionic fibres arise (Ardell *et al.*, 1982). However, under normal circumstances, this tonic outflow probably originates in the medulla and hypothalamus (Gebber & Barman, 1981; Barman & Gebber, 1982, 1983). The intrinsic sympathetic rhythm is modulated by inputs from higher levels of the CNS and various peripheral afferent inputs (see Jordan & Spyer, 1987), all of which are important during submersion.

### 19.2.3. Cardiac output

In concert with the increased in peripheral resistance is a reduction in cardiac output which is proportional to the fall in heart rate. There is very little change in stroke volume, despite cardiac distension resulting from increased pre-load, as a result of the powerful negatively inotropic influence of vagal input (e.g. Jones & Holeton, 1972; Blix *et al.*, 1983). Cardiac output is almost exclusively under parasympathetic (vagal) control during involuntary submersion as demonstrated by nerve section, cold blockade, and atropinisation (e.g. Butler & Jones, 1968, 1981). A reduction in sympathetic tone may (Folkow *et al.*, 1967) or may not (Butler & Jones, 1971) be involved. The cardiac vagal preganglionic fibres originate mainly in the nucleus ambiguus (NA) and also in the dorsal motor nucleus (DMN) of the vagus in the medulla of birds and mammals (Cabot & Cohen, 1980; Ellenberger *et al.*, 1983). Mean arterial blood pressure is maintained during involuntary submersion as a direct result of the opposing effects of bradycardia and vasoconstriction.

### 19.2.4. Sensory afferent inputs

Several groups of sensory receptors are actively involved in cardiovascular control during involuntary submersion, the most important of which are the facial and nasopharyngeal receptors, arterial and central chemoreceptors (particularly the carotid body chemoreceptors), and arterial and cardiac baroreceptors. Though a large amount of relevant data have been obtained from open-loop experiments, it has become clear over recent years that when these reflexes are activated simultaneously, as they are during submersion, they interact with each other as well as being profoundly affected by changes in respiration (mammalian cardiovascular and respiratory reflex interactions are reviewed by Abboud & Thames, 1983, and Daly, 1986).

### 19.2.4.1. *Respiratory–cardiovascular interaction*

As mentioned earlier, reflex apnoea is the first event that occurs upon head immersion, and the cardiovascular system is affected by changes in respiration in two ways: by reflexes initiated in the lungs, and by changes in CRN activity (see Daly, 1986; Jordan & Spyer, 1987). There are at least three groups of receptors in the mammalian lung which may play a role in circulatory control. One of these is the slowly adapting stretch receptors (SARs) which are innervated by myelinated vagal A fibres, are stimulated by low levels of lung inflation, and are believed to mediate reflex tachycardia and vasodilatation (see Daly, 1986). The tachycardia is caused by withdrawal of vagal efferent activity and occurs independently of any central inspiratory activity. The vasodilatation is caused by reduction of sympathetic vasomotor tone and is not uniform between vascular beds. In the relatively inexpansible avian lung the functionally equivalent receptors are sensitive to $P_aCO_2$: they are inhibited by a build-up of $CO_2$ in the lung air (Fedde *et al.*, 1974a, b). Thus, the activity of these intrapulmonary chemoreceptors (IPCs), like that of the SARs of the mammalian lung, is reduced during expiration. A single lung influation/deflation cycle with air during head immersion evokes an immediate reflex tachycardia in intact ducks but not in pulmonary denervated ducks nor when 10% $CO_2$ is added to the inflating gas in intact animals (Fig. 19.2). Cardiovascular effects of CRN activity are inferred from observations of cardiac sinus arrhythmia in pulmonary denervated animals, and studies in which reflex effects of other afferent inputs (such as those from arterial chemoreceptors) continue to be dependent upon the phase of respiration when lung reflexes are abolished or artificially controlled. Briefly, the cardiac vagal preganglionic neurones are fully accessible to afferent input only during expiration, whereas during the inspiratory phase they are refractory to afferent inputs. Sympathetic preganglionic efferent nerve activity also usually exhibits respiratory-related rhythmicity, though the situation is less clear, with some fibres showing inspiratory peak and others expiratory peak activities. The central nervous mechanisms are discussed by Jordan & Spyer (1987).

Apnoea itself is therefore essential for the full development of the cardiovascular responses to involuntary submersion. The pulmonary SAR

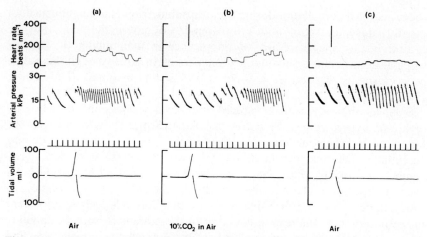

Fig. 19.2. Effects of a single inflation/deflation of the respiratory system with air, or 10% $CO_2$ in air, on heart rate and arterial blood pressure of intact (a, b) or pulmonary denervated (c) mallard ducks (*Anas platyrhynchos*) 30–40 s after submersion of the head in water (head still submerged). Inflation volume was similar to that of the first inspiratory effort upon surfacing from 60 s of head submersion. Vertical line above each heart-rate trace indicates beginning of inflation. Inflation upwards on trace. Time marker, 1 s. (a, b) 1·05 kg, (c) 0·9 kg. (From Butler & Taylor, 1983.)

(or IPC) and CRN effects on the circulation make it difficult to determine whether stimulation of nasopharyngeal and facial receptors has a direct effect on the cardiovascular system as opposed to a secondary effect via apnoea. The evidence available suggests that there is a direct effect, though the magnitude appears to be species-specific. The potency of the direct cardiovascular response (bradycardia and vasoconstriction in most vascular beds) is markedly diminished by artificial lung inflation and spontaneous inspiration (through a tracheal cannula), and bradycardia develops relatively slowly in animals which submerge on inspiration (Gandevia *et al.*, 1978; Butler & Taylor, 1983).

### 19.2.4.2. *Chemoreceptor input*

In normally ventilating birds and mammals, stimulation of the carotid body chemoreceptors results in hyperventilation and tachycardia (or sometimes mild bradycardia), and reduced total peripheral vascular resistance. It was found, however, that these cardiovascular responses are effects of reflexes secondary to the hyperventilation (Daly, 1983) and possibly also a result of activation of the defence-arousal system (Marshall, 1987). When ventilation is prevented from increasing, the primary cardiovascular effects of carotid body chemoreceptor stimulation — bradycardia and peripheral vasoconstriction — are unmasked. Thus, the primary effect of carotid body chemoreceptor stimulation during apnoeic submersion is to augment both vagal (parasympathetic) and sympathetic vasomotor outputs, and the carotid bodies are, therefore, of importance in maintaining the cardio-vascular adjustments to involuntary submersion in birds (though this varies between species, e.g. Butler & Woakes, 1982a) and mammals (Daly *et al.*, 1977; Jones *et al.*, 1982a; Fig. 19.3).

Submersion bradycardia is reduced or delayed in ducks and seals by pre-breathing hyperoxic gas, by perfusion of the carotid sinus with hyperoxic blood or by chemodenervation. Conversely, pre-breathing hypoxic gas accentuates the bradycardia in the following submersion in ducks (e.g. Jones *et al.*, 1982b; Mangalam & Jones, 1984). The effect of carotid body chemoreceptor stimulation increases during the period of submersion as asphyxia develops, and these receptors are therefore relatively unimportant in the initiation of the response, except in those animals, such as dabbling ducks, in which the nasophrayngeal reflexes are relatively ineffective and which therefore exhibit a slowly developing cardiovascular response (Daly *et al.*, 1977; Jones *et al.*, 1982a).

### 19.2.4.3. *Baroreceptor input*

Open-loop experiments have led to conflicting conclusions regarding the role of the arterial baroreceptors during involuntary submersion (Jones, 1973; Jones *et al.*, 1983). It now appears that the baroreceptors, although active, do not directly effect either the bradycardia or the peripheral vasoconstriction. Bradycardia will occur in the absence of peripheral vasoconstriction (result-ing in a decrease in blood pressure: Kobinger & Oda, 1969; Butler & Jones, 1971) and vasoconstriction will occur in the absence of bradycardia (result-ing in increased blood pressure: Murdaugh *et al.*, 1968; Butler & Jones, 1971; Blix *et al.*, 1974). In the harbour seal, *Phoca vitulina*, the contribution of the baroreceptors to the 'diving' responses is by way of a shift in the set-point towards bradycardia and vasoconstriction together with an increase in the gain of the reflex; for a given change in arteral blood pressure, there is a greater change in heart rate (Angell-James *et al.*, 1978). Thus, baroreceptors continue to buffer changes in blood pressure during submersion, but around new set-points for heart rate and vasoconstriction. These changes in baroreceptor activity are probably due to central facilitation brought about by apnoea and by interactions of the baroreceptor input with inputs from chemoreceptors and from nasopharyngeal and facial receptors (Angell-James & Daly, 1969; Wennergren *et al.*, 1976) though a proportion of the alteration between mean arterial pressure and heart rate is probably independent of baroreceptors (Jones *et al.*, 1983).

In addition to the arterial baroreceptors, avian and mammalian hearts contain receptors sensitive to stretch and contraction of the myocardium (see Bishop *et al.*, 1983). These receptors, innervated by unmyelinated vagal

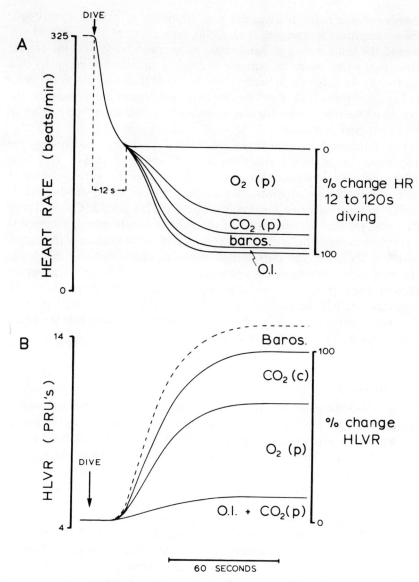

Fig. 19.3. The estimated contribution of central (c) and peripheral (p) chemoreceptors, baroreceptors ('baros') and other unidentified inputs (O.I.) to the bradycardia
and increased hindlimb vascular resistance (HLVR) in domestic ducks during the
period from 12 to 120 s of involuntary head submersion. (From Jones *et al.*, 1982a.)

C-fibres, evoke reflex bradycardia and inhibition of cardiac sympathetic chemoreceptors (Wennergren *et al.*, 1976). As mentioned, the increased pre-load to the heart during an involuntary submersion tends to cause cardiac distension, which would be expected to activate these cardiac receptors thus reinforcing the submersion bradycardia. Evidence both for (Blix *et al.*, 1976) and against (Jones *et al.*, 1980) the role of these receptors in the control of the oxygen-conserving cardiovascular response to involuntary submersion in ducks has been presented.

The functional neuroanatomy of central pathways controlling the mammalian circulation is described by Calaresu *et al.* (1984). Very little information is available concerning central neural cardiorespiratory control mechanisms in birds, though they appear to be fundamentally similar to mammals (see Jones & Johansen, 1972; Cabot & Cohen, 1980). Basically, the central integration of the afferent inputs during submersion takes place in the medulla. Particularly important is the nucleus of the tractus solitarius (NTS) in the dorsomedial medulla, which contains the dorsal group of inspiratory neurones and which is the site of the first synapse for afferent fibres from the peripheral receptors described above. The NTS projects to the NA and the DMN as well as to the IML (Sawchenko, 1983). It does not function simply as a relay nucleus though its precise role in sensory afferent integration is not clear at present.

### 19.3. Recovery

On emersion, all animals hyperventilate, and the duration and intensity of this appears to depend upon the duration of the preceding period of submersion (Kooyman *et al.*, 1971; Bamford & Jones, 1976a; Lillo & Jones, 1982). The first breath following involuntary submersion initiates the cardiovascular recovery process, which is essentially a reversal of the submersion events, i.e. tachycardia and peripheral vasodilatation.

The rapid onset of the cardiorespiratory recovery process is dependent upon the integrity of the pulmonary afferent nerves in the mallard duck, the responses being markedly reduced in pulmonary denervated animals (Fig. 19.4). When breathing recommences it is augmented in the early stages of recovery by stimulation of the central and peripheral chemoreceptors (Lillo & Jones, 1982; Milsom *et al.*, 1983). Hyperpnoea persists, however, after blood gas partial pressures have returned to normal, both in intact ducks and in those whose carotid bodies have been denervated (Butler & Jones, 1971; Lillo & Jones, 1982). The duration of post-dive hyperpnoea in ducks is dependent upon the changes in blood gases (particularly oxygen) that occur during the 'dive' rather than during recovery, and it appears that hypoxia has its effect via receptors other than the carotid body chemoreceptors (Milsom *et al.*, 1983). Persistence of hyperpnoea could be due to the activation of the

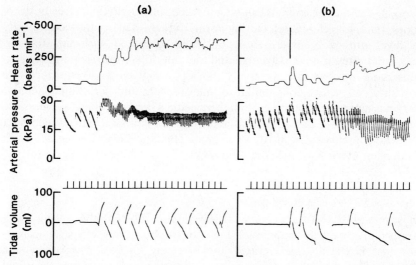

Fig. 19.4. Heart rate, arterial blood pressure and ventilation in intact (a) and pulmonary denervated (b) mallard ducks (*Anas platyrhynchos*) upon surfacing after 60 s of head submersion. Vertical line above each heart rate trace indicates beginning of first inspiration. Inspiration, upwards on trace. Time marker, 1 s. (a) 0·77 kg, (b) 0·7 kg. (From Butler & Taylor, 1983.)

defence-arousal system, though this remains untested at present. The chemoreceptor involvement in the cardiovascular adjustments upon recovery also appears to be minimal since surfacing into nitrogen does not affect the immediate tachycardia in birds (Bamford & Jones, 1976a) and artificially maintaining chemoreceptor stimulation has little or no effect on recovery tachycardia in the seal (Daly *et al.*, 1977).

Upon surfacing, the ventilation volume in ducks in no greater than that caused by a level of hypercapnic hypoxia that is similar to that at the time of surfacing, yet heart rate is much higher (Butler & Taylor, 1973). Butler & Jones (1982) have suggested that the IPCs are sensitised during the apnoeic period of submersion since there is an increased pulmonary afferent discharge during the first inflations terminating apnoea, even if ventilation rate and volume are maintained at pre-apnoeic levels (Bamford & Jones, 1976b).

## 19.4. Voluntary submersion

Recent studies on unrestrained diving animals have demonstrated that rather than the cardiovascular and metabolic responses to submersion being the predictable results of an orchestrated series of stereotyped reflexes, they seem to be extremely variable.

The amphibians, reptiles, and several fully aquatic birds and mammals respire intermittently at rest — lung ventilation is punctuated by apnoeic periods — and these animals exhibit a marked sinus arrhythmia (see Butler & Jones, 1982, for references). During normal aquatic activity the vast majority of dives are of relatively short duration compared with the animals' maximum breath-hold capacity, and do not, therefore, require oxygen-conserving mechanisms. In many cases, during short dives, heart rate remains at a level which is similar to that observed during resting apnoea. It has been suggested that rather than there being a bradycardia on submersion, the low heart rate during normal aerobic dives is instead interrupted by a 'breathing tachycardia' in these animals (Belkin, 1964; Lin *et al.*, 1972; Kooyman, 1985; Kanwisher & Gabrielsen, 1986; Gallivan *et al.*, 1986).

### 19.4.1. *Exercise and diving*

In semi-aquatic birds, where work levels rise substantially during unre-strained diving due to the animals' high positive buoyancy, oxygen consump-tion and heart rate are elevated above resting levels during submersion (Woakes & Butler, 1983). A similar cardiac response also occurs in the initial stages of submerged swimming with breath-hold in humans (Butler & Woakes, 1987). This observation has led to the suggestion that in these cases the metabolic and cardiovascular adjustments to diving are a balance between those of exercise (increased cardiac output and redistribution of blood flow in favour of the exercising muscles) and those of the 'classical' response to involuntary submersion, with the bias towards the exercise response (Butler, 1982).

Two neural mechanisms have been proposed to mediate the hyperpnoea and cardiovascular changes during exercise in normally ventilating mammals (see Mitchell & Schmidt, 1983, for a review). The first is a feedback mechanism involving the stimulation of fine afferent nerves in the working muscles and moving joints, and the second is a feedforward mechanism which involves a 'central command' issued by suprapontine brain structures which drive both the locomotion and the cardiorespiratory adjustments in parallel.

The fine diameter Gp III (myelinated) and Gp IV (unmyelinated) afferent fibres, which constitute by far the larger proportion of total afferent fibres from skeletal muscle, are stimulated by muscle contraction (McCloskey & Mitchell, 1972). Some units appear to be primarily mechanoreceptors (Kniffki *et al.*, 1981) while others are apparently chemoreceptors, being sensitive to substances, such as lactate, bradykinin and potassium ions, produced by the active muscle tissue (Thimm *et al.*, 1984; Rybicki *et al.*, 1985; Stebbins & Longhurst, 1985). The exact pattern of cardiovascular responses to evoked muscular activity is dependent upon the mode of contraction, the level of tension developed and the muscle mass involved (e.g. Iwamoto & Botterman, 1985; Lewis *et al.*, 1985). Isometric contraction (tetanus) induced by stimulation of the appropriate ventral roots, rhythmic contractions evoked by intermittent tetanic stimulation, and actual static and dynamic exercise all result in reflex tachycardia, increased myocardial contractility and hypertension, a response which is potentiated by restricting blood supply to the muscle during contractions (Coote *et al.*, 1971; McCloskey & Mitchell, 1972).

Several studies in humans and laboratory mammals have provided supporting data for the concept of a 'central command' component of cardiovascular control during exercise (e.g. Goodwin *et al.*, 1972; Eldridge *et al.*, 1985). Central command appears to be independent of cortical input since it may be evoked by electrical stimulation of the subthalamic or mesencephalic locomotory areas in the cat (Eldridge *et al.*, 1985).

It has been suggested that the central mechanism represents the primary drive for both locomotion and the cardiorespiratory adjustments during exercise whereas the feedback mechanism provides a fine modulation (Eldridge *et al.*, 1985). The somatic reflex may be responsible for the entrainment of cardiorespiratory parameters with limb motion during exercise (Eldridge *et al.*, 1985). In this connection, leg-beat frequency in freely diving tufted ducks, *Aythya fuligula*, is entrained to heart rate in a 1:1 ratio (Butler & Woakes, 1982b), and it would be interesting to know the role, if any, that the muscle afferent fibres play in this phenomenon.

### 19.4.2. *The defence reaction and diving*

A suggested explanation for the differences in the responses to involuntary and voluntary submersion is that the 'classical diving response' is a fear-induced artefact of the experimental conditions (Kanwisher *et al.*, 1981; Smith & Tobey, 1983; Kanwisher & Gabrielsen, 1986). It has been claimed that a proportion of the response to involuntary submersion is the result of an orienting response (a response to a novel experience, see Sokolov, 1963), or a passive defence reaction (see Blix, 1986; Kanwisher & Gabrielsen, 1986). However, arguments for and against this suggestion — hypothesis (a) — are inconclusive, being based mainly on indirect and circumstantial evidence. It has also been suggested — hypothesis (b) — that the oxygen-conserving response is the basic reflex response to submersion, independent of the defence-arousal system, and is suppressed (possibly by habituation or conditioning) during unrestrained voluntary diving behaviour.

In favour of hypothesis (a) is the observation that in restrained animals pain, abrupt noise or threatening gestures can elicit a typical bradycardia without submersion (Scholander, 1940; Irving *et al.*, 1942; Elsner *et al.*, 1966), while a bradycardia also occurs in response to threatening gestures or flashing lights in unrestrained diving penguins and manatees (Butler & Woakes, 1984; Gallivan *et al.*, 1986). Also, a very similar series of cardiovascular adjustments occurs in those amphibians, reptiles, birds and mammals which have been observed to adopt a strategy of 'freezing' or 'playing dead' in response to a threatening stimulus (see Gabrielsen & Smith, 1985 for references). This response is characterised by physical immobility, and reductions in heart rate, minute ventilation, core body temperature, and rate of oxygen consumption (Smith et al., 1981). It is possible that the cardiovascular and metabolic adjustments occur secondarily to the respiratory depression.

Feigl & Folkow (1963) and Folkow & Rubinstein (1965) described an area in the mesencephalon and ventral hypothalamus ('area A') of the domestic duck which, when stimulated, causes apnoea in the expiratory position, bradycardia, general vasoconstriction, and hypertension (i.e. a response closely resembling that to involuntary submersion). It is noteworthy that the given coordinates of the areas of the brain of the domestic duck, Anas boscas, stimulated by Feigl & Folkow (1963) and Folkow & Rubinstein (1965; Fig. 19.5) do not correspond to the coordinates of the respective brain areas given in the stereotactic atlas of the mallard, A. platyrhynchos (Zweers, 1971). The discrepancy may result from differences in the orientation of the head, since Zweers (1971) used a stereotaxic apparatus which was specially designed for Anatidae (ducks), whereas Feigl & Folkow (1963) and Folkow & Rubinstein (1965) used a modified cat stereotaxic instrument. Using the nucleus rotundus as a reference point, it is estimated that, according to the brainstem orientation used by Zweers (1971), 'area B' described by Folkow & Rubinstein (1965) lies approximately 4–6 mm rostral to the zero point in the sagittal plane. Insufficient data are provided to estimate usefully the positions of 'areas A' (Feigel & Folkow, 1963; Folkow & Rubinstein, 1965) or 'areas B' (Feigl & Folkow, 1963). It is important that the exact location and functional significance of these areas of the brainstem is re-evaluated experimentally.

Electrical stimulation of part of the periventricular area of the anterior hypothalamus in the northern elephant seal, Mirounga angustirostris, also evokes cardiovascular responses which mimic those to involuntary submersion (Van Citters et al., 1965). Furthermore, in chronically implanted conscious ducks, stimulation of 'area A' potentiates the cardiorespiratory responses to immersion and also causes phyiscal immobility ('huddling up') both in and out of water. These observations suggest that 'area A' may be responsible for the onset of the passive defence reaction. It was found that in anaesthetised ducks the reflexogenic effects of apnoea and asphyxia as well as stimulation of 'area A' are necessary for maximum development of the response to immerse. Electrical stimulation of an area in the diencephalon ('area B'; Feigl & Folkow, 1963) evokes a cardiovascular response which is reminiscent of a conventional 'flight' reaction, i.e. tachycardia, peripheral vasoconstriction, hypertension and a cholinergically mediated skeletal muscle vasodilatation. Stimulation of another 'area B' described by Folkow & Rubinstein (1965) in the thalamus, ventromedial to the nucleus rotundus, elicits typical feeding behaviour in chronically implanted ducks (dabbling on

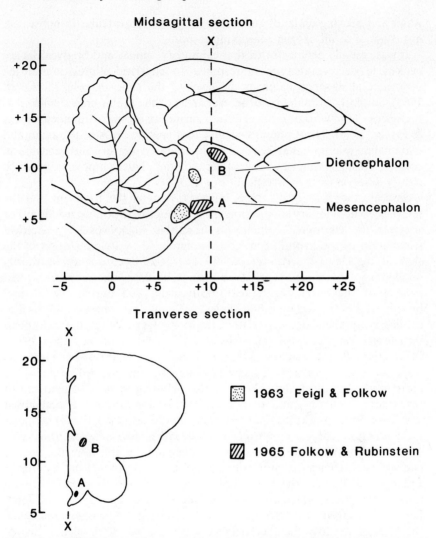

Fig. 19.5. Midsagittal and transverse sections of the brain of the domestic duck (*Anas boscas*) illustrating the positions of the mesencephalic/hypothalamic 'areas A' and diencephalic 'areas B' which, when electrically stimulated, elicited cardiorespiratory and behavioural responses very similar to those during a passive defence reaction, involuntary head immersion and unrestrained feeding behaviour. The coordinates are those of the original authors but do not correspond to those of Zweers (1971) — see text for details. (Modified from Feigl & Folkow, 1963, and Folkow & Rubinstein, 1965).

water and pecking on land) and, interestingly, cardiovascular responses are not those of a full oxygen-conserving response.

It was recently demonstrated that expiratory apnoea and bradycardia are evoked in decerebrate rats in response to electrical stimulation of the ventrolateral mesencephalon at the level of the superior colliculi (Coles, 1986). Similarly, stimulation of several areas of the rabbit brainstem evokes respiratory (and cardiovascular) effects, including expiratory apnoea (Evans & Pepler, 1974). These findings suggest that specific areas of the avian and mammalian midbrain may be involved in cardiorespiratory and behavioural control, during diving as well as other activities. This is a possibility which clearly deserves further investigation.

Several other lines of evidence, however, counter the argument that the response to involuntary submersion is a type of passive defence reaction. For example, the 'emotional' response in the rabbit, when evoked by electrical stimulation of the hypothalamus, is accompanied by vasodilatation in the skeletal muscles (Azevedo *et al.*, 1981) which does not occur during involuntary submersion. There also appear to be differences in neural efferent control of the heart during fear bradycardia and during the 'diving' bradycardia in the swamp rabbit, *Sylvilagus aquaticus*, where withdrawal of cardiac sympathetic activity contributes to the fear bradycardia but not to the submersion bradycardia (Causby & Smith, 1981; Smith & Tobey, 1983). In addition, Blix & Folkow (1983) have reviewed several cases where the response to submersion is reduced in struggling and stressed animals, but more marked in quiet and calm animals, including man. A comparison of responses to voluntary and involuntary submersion in intact, anaesthetised and decerebrate muskrats, *Ondatra zibethica* (Jones *et al.*, 1982b) supports the contention that fear or stress can reduce rather than enhance the oxygen-conserving response to involuntary submersion by the influence of the conventional defence reaction. Furthermore, it was pointed out by Blix & Folkow (1983) 'that the ["classical diving"] response is present also in decerebrate ducks, which are fairly difficult to scare', and Gabbott & Jones (1986) have shown that transection across the rostral mesencephalon below the level of the hypothalamic defence areas has no effect on the 'diving' bradycardia. In addition, in the domestic duck, denervation of the carotid body chemoreceptors, or breathing pure oxygen before involuntary submersion of naive animals abolishes the cardiac response (Lillo & Jones, 1982; Furilla & Jones, 1986), suggesting that it is largely reflexogenic, though this latter argument is reduced by the finding that carotid body chemoreceptor stimulation in cats anaesthetised with alphaxalone–alphadalone (Althesin, Glaxo) can evoke a simulated defence reaction (see Marshall, 1987).

In favour of hypothesis (b) above is the observation that the bradycardia evoked by involuntary head submersion is susceptible to habituation (Blix & Folkow, 1983; Gabrielsen, 1985; Gabbott & Jones, 1986), even in decerebrate ducks (D. R. Jones, unpublished data). Although the hypothalamic defence areas are not necessary for the development of an oxygen-conserving response, it is possible that the defence-arousal system (perhaps via the mesencephalic/hypothalamic 'area A' in ducks ?) is actively involved in dishabituating the normal response in intact diving animals when exposed to a threatening situation while under water (i.e. each of the two opposing hypotheses may be appropriate under different circumstances). It has recently been demonstrated that freely diving tufted ducks, *Aythya fuligula*, are able to 'switch' to a full bradycardia when they are briefly unable to resurface (Stephenson *et al.*, 1986). Interestingly, the bradycardia only occurs when the ducks apparently become aware of the situation. The onset of this bradycardia is unaffected by chronic carotid body chemoreceptor denervation, though the final reduction in heart rate is less than that in intact ducks (Butler & Stephenson, 1988). It is also interesting to note that the brady-cardia, which is presumably representative of the full oxygen-conserving response, including vasoconstriction in the active muscles, is as intense as that observed in forcibly submerged ducks despite the fact that during the unrestrained dives the animals are continuously active (Fig. 19.6). This indicates that any 'central command' or somatic reflex effect of exercise (even in ischaemic muscles) can be completely suppressed by the oxygen-conserving response, possibly by a mechanism involving the defence-arousal system, though this is purely conjectural at present. Thus, although the role of fear in cardiorespiratory control during voluntary and involuntary submersion is far from resolved, it is clear that the responses are profoundly influenced by the suprabulbar structures of the CNS and the 'psychological state' of the animal.

There are several other lines of evidence which suggest that suprabulbar and possibly cortical influences are effective during voluntary dives in apparently unstressed animals. Recent studies have looked at neural mechanisms of cardiovascular control during unrestrained dives in ducks (Butler & Woakes, 1982a; Furilla & Jones, 1986; Butler & Stephenson, 1988). In contrast to dabbling ducks, diving ducks show a relatively rapidly developing bradycardia upon *involuntary* submersion, about 80% of which occurs as a result of stimulation of receptors in the bill and nares (i.e. chemoreceptor input is relatively unimportant). However, the instantaneous reduction in heart rate from elevated pre-dive levels upon *voluntary* immersion is only inhibited by 10–30% after narial anaesthesia (Furilla & Jones, 1986). Also, it was found that carotid body chemoreceptor stimulation exerts only a slight cardioinhibitory effect during normal voluntary dives, and then only late in the dive (Butler & Woakes, 1982a; Butler & Stephenson, 1988). Breathing gases of varied oxygen concentration between dives has no effect on diving heart rate, though dive duration is positively correlated with oxygen concentration (Furilla & Jones, 1986; Butler & Stephenson, 1988). These data seem to indicate that peripheral influences on heart rate are less important during voluntary dives than during involuntary submersion. The

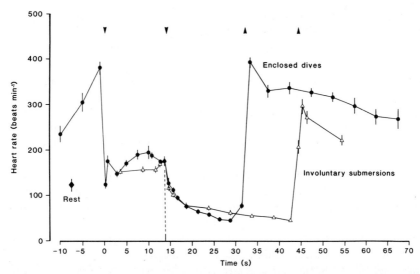

Fig. 19.6.   Mean ($\pm$SE) heart rates in tufted ducks (*Aythya fuligula*) at specific times before, during and after active unrestrained dives in an indoor tank during which the ducks were briefly denied the opportunity to resurface ('enclosed' dives; ●), and before, during and after involuntary submersion (△). Resting heart rate is also illustrated (◆). The descending arrowheads represent the points of head immersion and the ascending arrowheads represent the points of emersion during both enclosed dives and involuntary submersion. The vertical dotted line illustrates the onset of bradycardia which corresponds to the point of head immersion in the case of involuntary submersion and with the point at which the ducks apparently became aware that they were unable to resurface during enclosed dives. The ducks were exercising continuously throughout enclosed dives but were restrained and relatively inactive during involuntary submersions. (Adapted from Stephenson *et al.*, 1986.)

occurrence of cardiorespiratory adjustments in anticipation of immersion or emersion in freely diving birds and mammals also argues in favour of an increased involvement of suprabulbar nervous influences during voluntary dives.

Immediately preceding a voluntary dive there is a preparatory hyperventilation and tachycardia in the tufted duck (Butler & Woakes, 1979) and this is sometimes followed by an increase in cardiac interval before submersion of the nostrils (which may suggest that bradycardia occurs in the absence of apnoea or that apnoea is sometimes initiated prior to nasopharyngeal stimulation) (Butler & Woakes, 1982b). Contrary to the situation at the end of involuntary submersions, expiration may began before the animal reaches the surface during voluntary dives (R. Stephenson, unpublished observations) and heart rate often increases as the animal prepares for surfacing (Casson & Ronald, 1975; Butler & Woakes, 1982b).

It appears that voluntarily diving Weddell seals, *Leptonychotes weddelli*, and tufted ducks can adjust their cardiovascular responses according to an

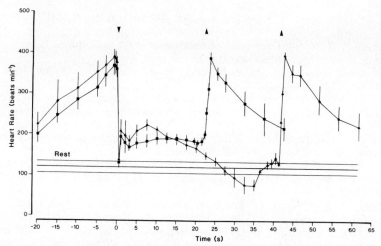

Fig. 19.7. Mean ($\pm$ SE) heart rate at specific times before, during and after normal feeding dives to food at $3\cdot8 \pm 0\cdot22$ m from the water surface (■) and long-duration dives to a horizontal distance of $12\cdot6 \pm 0\cdot07$ m ('extended' dives; ▲) in tufted ducks (*Aythya fuligula*). Horizontal lines represent mean $\pm$ SE resting heart rate. Descending arrowhead and ascending arrowheads represent the points of immersion and emersion respectively. Normal feeding dives, duration $= 22\cdot4 \pm 0\cdot18$ s; $n = 79$, and extend dives duration $= 41\cdot4 \pm 0\cdot32$ s, $n = 55$. (From Stephenson *et al.*, 1986.)

anticipated dive duration or distance, a lower heart rate occurring during longer dives (Kooyman & Campbell, 1972; Hill *et al.*, 1983; Stephenson *et al.*, 1986; Fig. 19.7). The reduction in heart rate during long-distance dives in tufted ducks is only partly suppressed by chronic bilateral denervation of the carotid body chemoreceptors (Butler & Stephenson, 1988). A discussion of the variability of the cardiovascular response to diving in marine mammals and hypothetical models of how the oxygen stores may be managed is presented by Kooyman (1985).

Obviously, the neural control mechanisms involved in cardiorespiratory (and behavioural) control during spontaneous diving activity in unrestrained animals are complex, involving suprabulbar nervous structures, and present a fascinating and challenging area for future research.

## Acknowledgement

The authors' work on this topic is supported by SERC.

## References

Abboud, F. M. & Thames, M. D. (1983). Interaction of cardiovascular reflexes in circulatory control. In *Handbook of Physiology, vol. 3, The Cardiovascular System,* pp. 675–753 (eds J. T. Shepherd & F. M. Abboud). Bethesda, MD: American Physiological Society.

Andersen, H. T. (1959). Depression of metabolism in the duck during experimental diving. *Acta Physiol. Scand.* **46**, 234–9.

Angell-James, J. E. & Daly, M. de B. (1969). Nasal reflexes. *Proc. R. Soc. Med.* **62**, 1287–93.

Angell-James, J. E., Daly, M. de B. & Elsner, R. (1978). Arterial baroreceptor reflexes in the seal and their modification during experimental dives. *Am. J. Physiol.* **234**, H730–9.

Ardell, J. L., Barman, S. M. & Gebber, G. L. (1982). Sympathetic nerve discharge in chronic spinal cat. *Am. J. Physiol.* **243**, H463–70.

Azevedo, A. D., Hilton, S. M. & Timms, R. J. (1981). The influence of hypothalamic stimulation upon skeletal muscle performance in the rabbit. *J. Physiol. Lond.* **313**, 28P–9P.

Bamford, O. S. & Jones, D. R. (1974). On the initiation of apnoea and some cardiovascular responses to submergence in ducks. *Resp. Physiol.* **22**, 199–216.

Bamford, O. S. & Jones, D. R. (1976a). Respiratory and cardiovascular interactions in ducks: the effects of lung denervation on the initiation of and recovery from some cardiovascular responses to submergence. *J. Physiol. Lond.* **259**, 575–96.

Bamford, O. S. & Jones, D. R. (1976b). The effects of asphyxia on afferent activity recorded from the cervical vagus in the duck. *Pflügers Arch.* **366**, 95–9.

Barman, S. M. & Gebber, G. L. (1982). Hypothalamic neurones with activity patterns related to sympathetic nerve discharge. *Am. J. Physiol.* **242**, R34–43.

Barman, S. M. & Gebber, G. L. (1983). Sequence of activation of ventrolateral and dorsal medullary sympathetic neurones. *Am. J. Physiol.* **245**, R438–47.

Belkin, D. A. (1964). Variations in heart rate during voluntary diving in the turtle *Pseudemys concinna*. *Copeia* 321–330.

Bishop, V. S., Malliani, A. & Thoren, P. (1983). Cardiac mechanoreceptors. In *Handbook of Physiology, vol. 3, The Cardiovascular System*, pp. 497–555 (eds J. T. Shepherd & F. M. Abboud). Bethesda, MD: American Physiological Society.

Black, C. P. & Torrance, R. W. (1971). Respiratory oscillations in chemoreceptor discharge in the control of breathing. *Resp. Physiol.* **13**, 221–37.

Blix, A. S. (1986). Diving response of mammals and birds. In *Arctic Underwater Operations*, pp. 73–9 (ed. L. Rey). London: Graham & Trotman.

Blix, A. S. & Folkow, B. (1983). Cardiovascular adjustments to diving in mammals and birds. In *Handbook of Physiology, vol. 3, The Cardiovascular System*, pp. 917–45 (eds J. T. Shepherd & F. M. Abboud). Bethesda, MD: American Physiological Society.

Blix, A. S., Gautvik, E. L. & Refsum, H. (1974). Aspects of the elative roles of peripheral vasoconstriction and vagal bradycardia in the establishment of the 'diving reflex' in ducks. *Acta Physiol. Scand.* **90**, 289–96.

Blix, A. S., Wennergren, G. & Folkow, B. (1976). Cardiac receptors in ducks — a link between vasoconstriction and bradycardia during diving. *Acta Physiol. Scand.* **97**, 13–19.

Blix, A. S., Elsner, R. & Kjekshus, J. K. (1983). Cardiac output and its distribution through capillaries and A–V shunts in diving seals. *Acta Physiol. Scand.* **118**, 109–16.

Butler, P. J. (1982). Respiratory and cardiovascular control during diving in birds and mammals. *J. Exp. Biol.* **100**, 195–221.

Butler, P. J. & Jones, D. R. (1968). Onset of and recovery from diving bradycardia in ducks. *J. Physiol. Lond.* **196**, 255–72.

Butler, P. J. & Jones, D. R. (1971). The effect of variations in heart rate and regional distribution of blood flow on the normal pressor response to diving in ducks. *J. Physiol. Lond.* **214**, 457–79.

Butler, P. J. & Jones, D. R. (1982). The comparative physiology of diving in vertebrates. *Adv. Comp. Physiol. Biochem.* **8**, 179–364.

Butler, P. J. & Stephenson, R. (1988). Chemoreceptor control of heart rate and behaviour during diving in the tufted duck (*Aythya fuligula*). *J. Physiol. Lond.* In press.

Butler, P. J. & Taylor, E. W. (1973). The effects of hypercapnic hypoxia, accompanied by different levels of lung ventilation, on heart rate in the duck. *Resp. Physiol.* **19**, 176–87.

Butler, P. J. & Taylor, E. W. (1983). Factors affecting the respiratory and cardiovascular responses to hypercapnic hypoxia in mallard ducks. *Resp. Physiol.* **53**, 109–27.

Butler, P. J. & Woakes, A. J. (1979). Changes in heart rate and respiratory frequency during natural behaviour of ducks, with particular reference to diving. *J. Exp. Biol.* **79**, 283–300.

Butler, P. J. & Woakes, A. J. (1982a). Control of heart rate by carotid body chemoreceptors during diving in tufted ducks. *J. Appl. Physiol.* **53**, 1405–10.

Butler, P. J. & Woakes, A. J. (1982b). Telemetry of physiological variables from diving and flying birds. *Symp. Zool. Soc. Lond.* **49**, 107–28.

Butler, P. J. & Woakes, A. J. (1984). Heart rate and aerobic metabolism in Humboldt penguins, *Spheniscus humboldti*, during voluntary dives. *J. Exp. Biol.* **108**, 419–428.

Butler, P. J. & Woakes, A. J. (1987). Heart rate in humans during underwater swimming with and without breath-hold. *Resp. Physiol.* **69**, 387–99.

Cabot, J. B. & Cohen, D. H. (1980). Neural control of the avian heart. In *Hearts and Heart-like Organs*, vol. 1, pp. 199–258 (ed. G. H. Bourne). New York: Academic Press.

Casson, D. M. & Ronald, K. (1975). The harp seal, *Pagophilus groenlandicus* (Erxleben, 1777). XIV. Cardiac arrhythmias. *Comp. Biochem. Physiol.* **50A**, 307–14.

Calaresu, F. R., Ciriello, J., Caverson, M. M., Cechetto, D. F. & Krukoff, T. L. (1984). Functional neuroanatomy of central pathways controlling the circulation. In *Hypertension and the Brain*, pp. 3–21 (eds T. A. Kotchen & C. P. Guthrie). New York: Futura Publications.

Causby, L. A. & Smith, E. N. (1981). Control of fear bradycardia in the swamp rabbit, *Sylvilagus aquaticus*. *Comp. Biochem. Physiol.* **69C**, 367–70.

Cohen, M. I. (1964). Respiratory periodicity in the paralyzed, vagotomized cat: hypocapnic polypnea. *Am. J. Physiol.* **206**, 845–54.

Coles, S. K. (1986). Mesencephalic apnoeic regions in the rat. *J. Physiol. Lond.* **382**, 176P.

Coote, J. H., Hilton, S. M. & Perez-Gonzalez, J. F. (1971). The reflex nature of the pressor response to muscular exercise. *J. Physiol. Lond.* **215**, 789–804.

Daly, M. de B. (1983). Peripheral arterial chemoreceptors and the cadiovascular system. In *Physiology of the Peripheral Arterial Chemoreceptors*, pp. 325–393 (eds H. Acker & R. G. O'Regan).

Daly, M. de B. (1986). Interactions between respiration and circulation. In *Handbook of Physiology*, vol. 2 *The Respiratory System*, pp. 529–94 (eds A. P. Fishman & A. B. Fisher. Bethesda, MD: American Physiological Society.

Daly, M. de B., Elsner, R. & Angell-James, J. E. (1977). Cardiorespiratory control by carotid body chemoreceptors during experimental dives in the seal. *Am. J. Physiol.* **232**, H508–16.

Djojosugito, A. M., Folkow, B. & Yonce, L. R. (1969). Neurogenic adjustments of muscle blood flow, cutaneous A–V shunt flow and of venous tone during 'diving' in ducks. *Acta Physiol. Scand.* **75**, 377–86.

Eldridge, F. L., Millhorn, D. E., Kiley, J. P. & Waldrop, T. G. (1985). Stimulation by central command of locomotion, respiration and circulation during exercise. *Resp. Physiol.* **59**, 313–37.

Ellenberger, H., Haselton, J. R., Liskowski, D. R. & Schneiderman, N. (1983). The locations of cardiac chronotropic cardioinhibitory vagal motoneurons in the medulla of the rabbit. *J. Auton. Nerv. Syst.* **9**, 513–29.

Elsner, R., Franklin, D. L., Van Citters, R. L. & Kenney, D. W. (1966). Cardiovascular defense against asphyxia. *Science* **153**, 941–9.

Evans, M. H. & Pepler, P. A. (1974). Respiratory effects mapped by focal stimulation in the rostral brain stem of the anaesthetised rabbit. *Brain Res.* **75**, 41–7.

Fedde, M. R., Gatz, R. N., Slama, H. & Scheid, P. (1974a). Intrapulmonary $CO_2$ receptors in the duck: I. Stimulus specificity. *Resp. Physiol.* **22**, 99–114.

Fedde, M. R., Gatz, R. N., Slama, H. & Scheid, P. (1974b). Intrapulmonary $CO_2$ receptors in the duck: II. Comparison with mechanoreceptors. *Resp. Physiol.* **22**, 115–21.

Feigl, E. & Folkow, B. (1963). Cardiovascular responses in 'diving' and during brain stimulation in ducks. *Acta Physiol. Scand.* **57**, 99–110.

Florin-Christensen, J., Florin-Christensen, M., Corley, E. G., Garcia Samartino, L. & Affani, J. M. (1986). A novel receptive area of key importance for the onset of diving responses in the duck. *Arch. Int. Physiol. Biochim.* **94**, 29–36.

Folkow, B. & Rubinstein, E. H. (1965). Effect of brain stimulation on 'diving' in ducks. *Hvalradets Skr.* **48**, 30–41.

Folkow, B., Fuxe, K. & Sonnenschein, R. R. (1966). Responses of skeletal musculature and its vasculature during 'diving' in the duck: peculiarities of the adrenergic vasoconstrictor innervation. *Acta Physiol. Scand.* **67**, 327–42.

Folkow, B., Nilsson, N. J. & Yonce, L. R. (1967). Effects of 'diving' on cardiac output. *Acta Physiol. Scand.* **70**, 347–61.

Furilla, R. A. & Jones, D. R. (1986). The contribution of nasal receptors to the cardiac response to diving in restrained and unrestrained redhead ducks (*Aythya americana*). *J. Exp. Biol.* **121**, 227–38.

Gabbott, G. R. J. & Jones, D. R. (1986). Psychogenic influences on the cardiac response of the duck (*Anas platyrhynchos*) to forced submersion. *J. Physiol. Lond.* **371**, 71P.

Gabrielsen, G. W. (1985). Free and forced diving in ducks: habituation of the initial dive response. *Acta Physiol. Scand.* **123**, 67–72.

Gabrielsen, G. W. & Smith, E. N. (1985). Physiological responses associated with feigned death in the America opossum. *Acta Physiol. Scand.* **123**, 393–8.

Gallivan, G. J., Kanwisher, J. W. & Best, R. C. (1986). Heart rates and gas exchange in the Amazonian manatee (*Trichechus inunguis*) in relation to diving. *J. Comp. Physiol. B* **156**, 415–23.

Gandevia, S. C., McCloskey, D. I. & Potter, E. K. (1978). Reflex bradycardia occurring in response to diving, nasopharyngeal stimulation and ocular pressure, and its modification by respiration and swallowing. *J. Physiol. Lond.* **276**, 383–94.

Gebber, G. L. & Barman, S. M. (1981). Sympathetic-related activity of brain stem neurones in baroreceptor-denervated cats. *Am. J. Physiol.* **240**, R348–55.

Gooden, B. A. (1980). A comparison *in vitro* of the vasoconstrictor responses of the mesenteric arterial vasculature from the chicken and the duckling to nervous stimulation and to noradrenaline. *Br. J. Pharmacol.* **68**, 263–73.

Goodwin, G. M., McCloskey, D. I. & Mitchell, J. H. (1972). Cardiovascular and respiratory responses to changes in central command during isometric exercise at constant tension. *J. Physiol. Lond.* **226**, 173–90.

Gregory, J. E. (1973). An electrophysiological investigation of the receptor apparatus of the duck's bill. *J. Physiol. Lond.* **229**, 151–64.

Grubb, B., Mills, C. D., Colacino, J. M. & Schmidt-Nielsen, K. (1977). Effect of arterial carbon dioxide on cerebral blood flow in ducks. *Am. J. Physiol.* **232**, H596–601.

Grubb, B., Colacino, J. M. & Schmidt-Nielsen, K. (1978). Cerebral blood flow in birds: effect of hypoxia. *Am. J. Physiol.* **234**, H230–4.

Hance, A. J., Robin, E. D., Halter, J. B., Lewiston, N., Robin, D. A., Cornell, L., Caligiuri, M. & Theodore, J. (1982). Hormonal changes and enforced diving in the harbor seal *Phoca vitulina*. II. Plasma catecholamines. *Am. J. Physiol.* **242**, R528–32.

Hill, R. D., Schneider, R. C., Liggins, G. C., Hochachka, P. W., Schuette, A. H. & Zapol, W. M. (1983). Microprocessor controlled recording of bradycardia during free diving of the Antarctic Weddell seal. *Fed. Proc.* **42**, 470.

Hochachka, P. W. & Somero, G. N. (1984). *Biochemical Adaptation*. Princeton, NJ: Princeton University Press.

Hudson, D. M. & Jones, D. R. (1982). Remarkable blood catecholamine levels in forced diving ducks. *J. Exp. Zool.* **224**, 451–6.

Irving, L. (1934). On the ability of warm-blooded animals to survive without breathing. *Sci. Monogr.* **38**, 422–8.

Irving, L. (1939). Respiration in diving mammals. *Physiol. Rev.* **19**, 112–34.

Irving, L., Scholander, P. F. & Grinnell, S. W. (1942). The regulation of arterial blood pressure in the seal during diving. *Am. J. Physiol.* **135**, 557–66.

Iwamoto, G. A. & Botterman, B. R. (1985). Peripheral factors influencing expression of pressor reflex evoked by muscular contraction. *J. Appl. Physiol.* **58**, 1676–82.

Jones, D. R. (1973). Systemic arterial baroreceptors in ducks and the consequences of their denervation on some cardiovascular responses to diving. *J. Physiol. Lond.* **234**, 499–518.

Jones, D. R. & Bamford, O. S. (1976). Open loop respiratory sensitivity in chickens and ducks. *Am. J. Physiol.* **230**, 861–7.

Jones, D. R. & Holeton, G. F. (1972). Cardiac output of ducks during diving. *Comp. Biochem. Physiol.* **41A**, 639–45.

Jones, D. R. & Johansen, K. (1972). The blood vascular system of birds. In *Avian Biology*, vol. 2, pp. 157–285 (eds D. S. Farner & J. R. King). London: Academic Press.

Jones, D. R., Bryan, R. M., West, N. H., Lord, R. H. & Clark, B. (1979). Regional distribution of blood flow during diving in the duck (*Anas platyrhynchos*). *Can. J. Zool.* **57**, 995–1002.

Jones, D. R., Milsom, W. K. & West, N. H. (1980). Cardiac receptors in ducks: the effect of their stimulation and blockade on diving bradycardia. *Am. J. Physiol.* **238**, R50–6.

Jones, D. R., Milsom, W. K. & Gabbott, G. R. J. (1982a). Role of central and peripheral chemoreceptors in diving responses of ducks. *Am. J. Physiol.* **243**, R537–45.

Jones, D. R., West, N. H., Bamford, O. S., Drummond, P. C. & Lord, R. A. (1982b). The effect of the stress of forcible submergence on the diving response in muskrats (*Ondatra zibethica*). *Can. J. Zool.* **60**, 187–93.

Jones, D. R., Milsom, W. K., Smith, F. M., West, N. H. & Bamford, O. S. (1983). Diving responses in ducks after acute barodenervation. *Am. J. Physiol.* **245**, R222–9.

Jordan, D. & Spyer, K. M. (1987). Central neural mechanisms mediating respiratory–cardiovascular interactions. Chapter 17, this volume.

Kanwisher, J. W. & Gabrielsen, G. W. (1986). The diving response in man. In *Arctic*

*Underwater Operations*, pp. 81–95 (ed. L. Rey). London: Graham & Trotman.

Kanwisher, J. W., Gabrielsen, G. & Kanwisher, N. (1981). Free and forced diving in birds, *Science* **211**, 717–19.

Kjekshus, J. K., Blix, A. S., Elsner, R., Hol, R. & Amundsen, E. (1982). Myocardial blood flow and metabolism in the diving seal. *Am. J. Physiol.* **242**, R97–104.

Klocke, F. J. & Ellis, A. K. (1980). Control of coronary blood flow. *Ann. Rev. Med.* **31**, 489–508.

Kniffki, K.-D., Mense, S. & Schmidt, R. F. (1981). Muscle receptors with fine afferent fibres which may evoke circulatory reflexes. *Circ. Res.* **48**, Suppl. I, 25–31.

Kobinger, W. & Oda, M. (1969). Effects of sympathetic blocking substances on the diving reflex of ducks. *Eur. J. Pharmacol.* **7**, 289–95.

Kooyman, G. L. (1985). Physiology without restraint in diving mammals. *Marine Mammal Science* **1**, 166–78.

Kooyman, G. L. & Campbell, W. B. (1972). Heart rates in freely diving Weddell seals, *Leptonychotes weddelli*. *Comp. Biochem. Physiol.* **43A**, 31–6.

Kooyman, G. L., Kerem, D. H., Campbell, W. B. & Wright, J. J. (1971). Pulmonary function in freely diving Weddell seals, *Leptonychotes weddelli*. *Resp. Physiol.* **12**, 271–82.

Langille, B. L. (1983). Role of venoconstriction in the cardiovascular responses of ducks to head immersion. *Am. J. Physiol.* **244**, R292–8.

Lewis, S. F., Snell, P. G., Taylor, W. F., Hamra, M., Graham, R. M., Pettinger, W. A. & Blomqvist, C. G. (1985). Role of muscle mass and mode of contraction in circulatory responses to exercise. *J. Appl. Physiol.* **58**, 146–51.

Lillo, R. S. & Jones, D. R. (1982). Control of diving responses by carotid bodies and baroreceptors in ducks. *Am. J. Physiol.* **242**, R105–8.

Lin, Y.-C. (1982). Breath-hold diving in terrestrial mammals. In *Exercise and Sports Sciences Reviews*, vol. 10, pp. 270–307 (ed. R. L. Terjung). Philadelphia, PA: Franklin Press.

Lin, Y.-C., Matsuura, D. T. & Whittow, G. C. (1972). Respiratory variation of heart rate in the California sea lion. *Am. J. Physiol.* **222**, 260–4.

McCloskey, D. I. & Mitchell, J. H. (1972). Reflex cardiovascular and respiratory responses originating in exercising muscle. *J. Physiol. Lond.* **224**, 173–86.

Mangalam, H. J. & Jones, D. R. (1984). The effects of breathing different levels of $O_2$ and $CO_2$ on the diving responses of ducks (*Anas platyrhynchos*) and cormorants (*Phalacrocorax auritus*). *J. Comp. Physiol. B.* **154**, 243–7.

Marek, W., Prabhakar, N. R. & Loeschcke, H. H. (1985). Electrical stimulation of arterial and central chemosensory afferents at different times in the respiratory cycle of the cat: I. Ventilatory responses. *Pflügers Arch.* **403**, 415–21.

Marshall, J. M. (1987). Contribution to overall cardiovascular control made by the chemoreceptor-induced alerting/defence response. Chapter 12, this volume.

Milsom, W. K., Jones, D. R. & Gabbott, G. R. J. (1983). Effects of changes in peripheral and central $PCO_2$ on ventilation during recovery from submergence in ducks. *Can. J. Zool.* **61**, 2388–93.

Mitchell, J. H. & Schmidt, R. F. (1983). Cardiovascular reflex control by afferent fibers from skeletal muscle receptors. In *Handbook of Physiology*, vol. 3, *The Cardiovascular System*, pp. 623–58 (eds J. T. Shepherd & F. M. Abboud). Bethesda, MD: American Physiological Society.

Murdaugh, H. V., Cross, C. E., Millen, J. E., Gee, J. B. L. & Robin, E. D. (1968). Dissociation of bradycardia and arterial constriction during diving in the seal *Phoca vitulina*. *Science* **162**, 364–5.

Neubauer, J. A., Feldman, R. S., Huang, J. T., Vinten-Johansen, J. & Weiss, H. R. (1978). Blood flow and relative tissue $PO_2$ of brain and muscle: role of carotid chemoreceptors. *J. Appl. Physiol.* **45**, 419–24.

Pickwell, G. V. (1968). Energy metabolism in ducks during submergence asphyxia: assessment by a direct method. *Comp. Biochem. Physiol.* **27**, 455–85.

Ponte, J. & Purves, M. J. (1974). The role of the carotid body chemoreceptors and carotid sinus baroreceptors in the control of cerebral blood vessels. *J. Physiol. Lond.* **237**, 315–40.

Ronald, K., McCarter, R. & Selley, L. J. (1977) Venous circulation in the harp seal (*Pagophilus groenlandicus*). In *Functional Anatomy of Marine Mammals*, vol. 3, pp. 235–70 (ed. R. J. Harrison). London: Academic Press.

Rybicki, K. J., Waldrop, T. G. & Kaufman, M. P. (1985). Increasing gracilis muscle interstitial potassium concentrations stimulate group III and IV afferents. *J. Appl. Physiol.* **58**, 936–41.

Sawchenko, P. E. (1983). Central connections of the sensory and motor nuclei of the vagus nerve. *J. Auton. Nerv. Syst.* **9**, 13–26.

Scholander, P. F. (1940). Experimental investigations on the respiratory function in diving mammals and birds. *Hvalradets Skr.* **22**, 1–131.

Scremin, O. U., Sonnenschein, R. R. & Rubinstein, E. H. (1983). Cholinergic cerebral vasodilatation: lack of involvement of cranial parasympathetic nerves. *J. Cereb. Blood Flow Metab.* **3**, 362–8.

Smith, E. N. & Tobey, E. W. (1983). Heart-rate response to forced and voluntary diving in swamp rabbits *Sylvilagus aquaticus*. *Physiol. Zool.* **56**, 632–8.

Smith, E. N., Sims, K. & Vich, J. F. (1981). Oxygen consumption of frightened swamp rabbits, *Sylvilagus aquaticus*. *Comp. Biochem. Physiol.* **70A**, 533–6.

Sokolov, E. N. (1963). Higher nervous functions: the orienting reflex. *Ann. Rev. Physiol.* **25**, 545–80.

Stebbins, C. L. & Longhurst, J. C. (1985). Bradykinin-induced chemoreflexes from skeletal muscle: implications for the exercise reflex. *J. Appl. Physiol.* **59**, 56–63.

Stephenson, R., Butler, P. J. & Woakes, A. J. (1986). Diving behaviour and heart rate in tufted ducks (*Aythya fuligula*). *J. Exp. Biol.* **126**, 341–59.

Thimm, F., Carvalho, M., Babka, M. & Meier zu Verl, E. (1984). Reflex increases in heart-rate induced by perfusing the hind leg of the rat with solutions containing lactic acid. *Pflügers Arch.* **400**, 286–93.

Van Citters, R. L., Franklin, D. L., Smith Jr, O. A., Watson, N. W. & Elsner, R. W. (1965). Cardiovascular adaptations to diving in the northern elephant seal *Mirounga angustirostris*. *Comp. Biochem. Physiol.* **16**, 267–76.

Wennergren, G., Little, R. & Oberg, B. (1976). Studies on the central integration of excitatory chemoreceptor influences and inhibitory baroreceptor and cardiac receptor influences. *Acta Physiol. Scand.* **96**, 1–18.

Wilson, J. X. & West, N. H. (1986). Cardiovascular responses to neurohormones in conscious chickens and ducks. *Gen. Comp. Endocrinol.* **62**, 268–80.

Woakes, A. J. & Butler, P. J. (1983). Swimming and diving in tufted ducks, *Aythya fuligula*, with particular reference to heart rate and gas exchange. *J. Exp. Biol.* **107**, 311–29.

Zapol, W. M., Liggins, G. C., Schneider, R. C., Qvist, J., Snider, M. T., Creasy, R. K. & Hochachka, P. W. (1979). Regional blood flow during simulated diving in the conscious Weddell seal. *J. Appl. Physiol.* **47**, 968–73.

Zweers, G. A. (1971). A stereotactic atlas of the brainstem of the mallard (*Anas platyrhynchos* L.). Assen: Koninklijke van Gorcum N. V.

# 20

# Phylogeny of renal, cardiovascular and endocrine activity of the renin–angiotensin system

## I. W. Henderson

*Department of Zoology, University of Sheffield, Sheffield S10 2TN, UK*

## 20.1. Introduction

In physiological and biochemical terms the vertebrates form a remarkably coherent grouping that maintains an extracellular fluid at or around 300 mosmolal, contained within a volume that occupies the equivalent of approximately 25% of the body weight. There are some curious exceptions in osmotic terms (marine elasmobranch or cartilaginous fishes, certain cyclostomes and under some circumstances certain anuran amphibians are examples), but even in these animals there are clear volume- and ionic-regulatory mechanisms. Thus although the elasmobranch fishes maintain their extracellular fluid hyperosomotic to sea water, by virtue of what has been termed 'physiological uraemia', the vertebrate imprint of sodium concentrations being regulated below that of sea water is apparent.

The 'normal' values for the homeostatic state of extracellular fluid with respect to its overall volume, osmolality and ionic species are sustained often in the face of widely disparate environmental availabilities of water and individual solutes. To achieve this state of dynamic homeostatic equilibrium between the organism and its habitat, vertebrates have refined a wide range of structures, from specialised solute-absorbing and excreting glands, to the gut and the integument. Throughout the series, however, the kidney is a constant feature, existing, and defined in embryological terms, as pro-, meso- and metanephros.

The external morphology of the kidney varies considerably but its component parts, again with relatively minor variations, are the renal tubules or nephroi and these remain remarkably invariant. Progenitorially, the tubule comprised an ultrafiltering device — the glomerulus — and a conduit to the outside or to the urinary bladder — the renal tubule itself. The latter subsequently accrued the abilities both to tranfer unwanted materials from the blood side into the tubular lumen for elimination, and to reabsorb useful materials that had been filtered. Clearly a battery of specific transport systems were obligatory accompaniments to this evolution. Moreover, given the ultimate source of energy for the preparation of urine — hydrostatic pressure from the heart transferred within the closed vasculature applied to the glomerulus — there was clearly a need for mechanisms that regulated both the pressure and volume relationships of blood flow to the kidney. Early homeostatic links will thus have been established between blood pressure regulation, the selective distribution of cardiac output to different vascular beds and the maintenance of fluid and electrolyte composition.

This relatively uncontroversial introduction to the kidney and its central position in vertebrate body fluid homeostasis belies the huge variation and plasticity of function that kidney function displays. The enormous functional range is clearly the result of the fluid and electrolyte economy imposed by the environmental availability of water and solutes. One may highlight some examples. In certain marine teleosts there has been a secondary loss of glomeruli which has been interpreted as an adaptive response to the hyperosmotic environment with the concomitant passive efflux of water; glomerular filtration in a sense placed added strain upon volume regulation. Secondly, many desert rodents, producing urines which are some 20 or 30 times more concentrated than their plasmas, can be contrasted with the extraordinary diluting capacity of many fresh-water fishes and amphibia whose urines are more than ten times more dilute than their respective plasmas. There are of course specific structural modifications for some of these abilities (the long loops of Henle in the rodent example), but nevertheless the basic unit is similar in all vertebrates (Fig. 20.1).

The kidney has thus been placed as a key and universal structure that, alongside the various extrarenal osmoregulatory effector systems, maintains homeostasis in the face of varying environmental characteristics both acute and chronic. Alongside these regulatory structures the vertebrates possesses a spectrum of hormones that act locally within the organ, in a paracrine fashion, whereas others may be released at a distance from their target organ in response to a specific stimulus (plasma volume or osmolality, for example) and are carried in the circulation to induce the appropriate homeostatic response in a classical endocrine manner.

With a few exceptions, the vertebrate endocrine system again shows a remarkable homogeneity of organisation, and indeed the chemical natures of the secretions show more resemblances than differences. Perhaps the most intriguing aspects of vertebrate endocrinology are that although a similar chemical may be produced from a genuinely homologous gland, the biological effects may differ, and of course the target cell or tissue will vary. In other words the same hormone may occur in divergent species but its site(s) of action and elicited responses contrast markedly. It has been noted that there is some uniformity within the vertebrate endocrine system but the curious differences include the Corpuscles of Stannius of teleost fishes, the apparent restriction of the parathyroid glands to tetrapod vertebrates, and

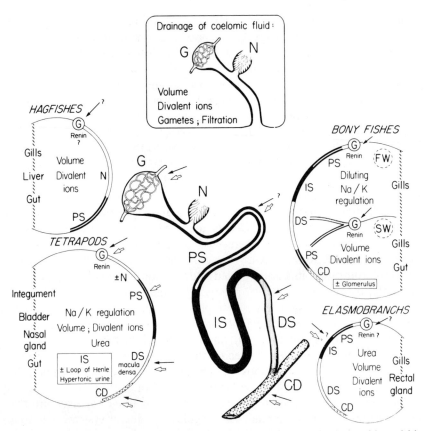

Fig. 20.1.   The basic nephron unit of the vertebrate kidney and relationships within hormones. The original coelomoduct (inset) is postulated to have given rise to glomerulus (G), proximal segment (PS), intermediate segment (IS), distal segment (DS) and collecting duct (CD). A ciliated nephrostome (N) may or may not be retained in the adult. General sites of peptide ($\checkmark$) and steroid hormones ($\circlearrowright$) are indicated. The functional relationships between hagfishes, bony fishes in fresh-water and sea-water elasmobranchs and tetrapods are illustrated. (From Balment *et al.*, 1980.)

most relevant to the present chapter the *possible* spasmodic occurrence of the renin–angiotensin system.

## 20.2.  The renin-angiotensin system

It has been argued above that the kidney is central to the regulation of both the volume and composition of the extracellular fluid. Given its uniform presence, albeit at different levels of organisation, it is perhaps not altogether surprising that the kidney has adopted, alongside its exocrine functions, major endocrine ones. In addition, specific intrarenal receptors monitor both the volume and composition of extracellular fluid to elicit appropriate neuroendocrine responses to perturbations. Many of the substances produced verify that the associations between renal exocrine function and cardiovascular regulation are well entrenched — an aspect that will be emphasised later with regard to at least one of the active hormones produced, angiotensin II. The renal endocrine system encompasses trophic functions on other tissues including endocrine glands as well as its paracrine functions (Fig. 20.2). Thus the mammalian kidney, at least, participates in the cholecalciferol cascade to generate active metabolites of vitamin $D_3$, and produces prostaglandins, kallikrein, erythropoeitin and renin, the subject of this chapter.

The renin–angiotensin system has a history that begins with the observations of Tigerstedt & Bergman in 1898 who observed that saline extracts of rabbits injected into anaesthetised rabbits produced a sustained increase in arterial blood pressure. These observations were controversial, and considerable debate surrounded them. Studies both confirmed and refuted the observations, and much emotion was spent discussing them (see Gibbons *et al.*, 1984). In 1934, the pathophysiological significance became apparent when Goldblatt and colleagues demonstrated that induction of renal ischaemia by partial constriction of a renal artery produced a sustained increase in arterial blood pressure leading to malignant hypertension; the syndrome could be alleviated by removal of the affected kidney. Subsequent studies showed that a variety of manoeuvres, all of which produced degrees of renal ischaemia or a reduced renal perfusion, produced hypertension. There had been a long association, often somewhat anecdotal, between the kidney and cardiovascular disease, and it was these observations that initiated the hunt for a humoral factor from the kidney that affected arterial blood pressure. Several classic studies appeared after these seminal observations to identify the/a renal humor that was associated with arterial disease (Pickering & Prinzmetal, 1938; Page & Helmer, 1940; Braun-Menendez *et al.*, 1940, 1943). The substance was termed 'angiotonin' by some and 'hypertensin' by others, but eventually a compromise term, angiotensin, was accepted.

The kidney had thus been identified as an element in the etiology of hypertension and by implication in normal blood-pressure homeostasis. There were, however, a number of inconsistencies. For example, oedema and hypokalaemia, often associated with certain types of hypertension, were not readily reconciled on the basis of a simple vasoconstrictor substance of renal origin. Some years later the matter was resolved — at least in part — when several laboratories, both experimental and clinical, came to the conclusion that angiotensin, in addition to affecting arterial blood pressure directly, also had secondary effects upon many other physiological functions. Most notably, it had a potent stimulatory action upon the adrenal cortical

## SOME FUNCTIONS OF THE VERTEBRATE KIDNEY

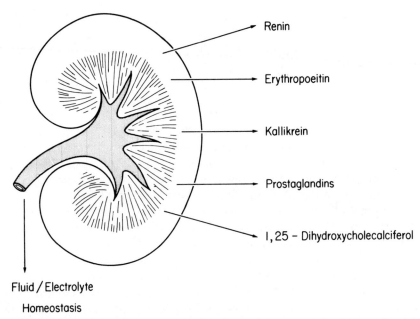

Fig. 20.2.   The endocrine and exocrine functions of the mammalian kidney. Some of the endocrine functions are almost certainly paracrine, and others have systemic actions.

production of aldosterone in the dog, man and sheep and, although less easily demonstrable, in the laboratory rat (see Davis, 1963; Laragh *et al.*, 1963; Ganong *et al.*, 1966).

   The renin–angiotensin system has now been further defined and consists of the substrate (*angiotensinogen*), almost certainly of hepatic origin; *renin* itself, which generates the decapeptide; *angiotensin I*, which lacks significant known biological activity; and *angiotensin II*, the biologically active octapeptide. A further product of the system, *angiotensin III*, is a heptapeptide derived either from angiotensin II or possibly directly from angiotensin I (Fig. 20.3). Other important rate-limiting components of the system are

Fig. 20.3.   General scheme of the renin–angiotensin system. The amino acid sequences are those known for man ⟳ indicate known routes of transformations and the broken arrows ⟳ postulated routes.

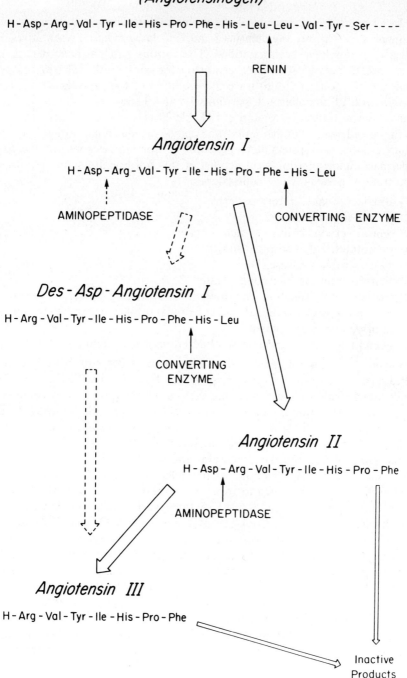

Renin Substrate
(Angiotensinogen)

H - Asp - Arg - Val - Tyr - Ile - His - Pro - Phe - His - Leu - Leu - Val - Tyr - Ser - - - -

RENIN

Angiotensin I

H - Asp - Arg - Val - Tyr - Ile - His - Pro - Phe - His - Leu

AMINOPEPTIDASE

CONVERTING ENZYME

Des - Asp - Angiotensin I

H - Arg - Val - Tyr - Ile - His - Pro - Phe - His - Leu

CONVERTING ENZYME

Angiotensin II

H - Asp - Arg - Val - Tyr - Ile - His - Pro - Phe

AMINOPEPTIDASE

Angiotensin III

H - Arg - Val - Tyr - Ile - His - Pro - Phe

Inactive Products

kininase-II, (*angiotensin-I-converting enzyme*) and the *angiotensinases*, which may be non-specific but destroy the biologically active peptides (see Davis, 1975; Keeton & Campbell, 1980).

In terms of the phylogeny of the renin–angiotensin system, amino acid sequences for various angiotensins I and II isolated from representatives of diverse groups have been described. The various patterns have particular relevance to biological activity, especially the comparative pharmacology, and of course our ability to trace the evolution of the peptides. Of the ten amino acids of angiotensin I, positions 1,5 and 9 seem to be the sites where varying substitutions have occurred (Table 20.1).

In considering the evolution and phylogenetic relationships of the renin–angiotensin system it is pertinent to summarise some of the key pharmacological/physiological actions of this hormonal system. The wide spectrum of effects include actions upon:

(1) adrenocortical secretory patterns;
(2) arterial blood pressure;
(3) central nervous control of fluid intake;
(4) gastrointestinal absorptive activity;
(5) gonadotrophin release;
(6) neurohypophysial hormone release;
(7) renal excretory function, both in terms of regulating glomerular filtration rate and possibly by directly affecting renal tubular transport of sodium, chloride and even potassium;
(8) sympathetic 'tone' and release of adrenomedullary amines.

Given this range of biological actions, it is hardly surprising that the release of renin from the kidney is governed by a multitude of factors. To understand some of the controlling factors, it is relevant to examine the source of renin within the kidney and its relationships with the juxtaglomerular apparatus. The latter consists of *granular epithelioid* (or *juxtaglomerular*) *cells* lying in the afferent glomerular arteriole, with *extraglomerular mesangial cells* between the glomerulus and the distal convoluted tubule of the same nephron. At this point of the distal tubule, specialised columnar epithelial cells are arranged to form the *macula densa*. A variety of terms have been applied over the years to these various components and are summarised in Fig. 20.4. Cook (1963) and Sokabe & Ogawa (1974) give a detailed analysis of the various alternative terms used to describe the component parts of the mammalian juxtaglomerular apparatus and their possible homologies. It should be emphasised that this arrangement is probably unique to mammals, and although homologous structures *may* exist in non-mammalian vertebrates, the anatomical juxtapositioning does not. For example a macula densa has not been clearly defined in fishes; indeed it may be a structure acquired by amniotic vertebrates. In addition, juxtaglomerular-like cells may appear at some distance from the glomerulus,

Table 20.1. Amino acid compositions and sequences of several vertebrate angiotensins

| *Amino acid and number* | | | | | | | | | | *Species* |
|---|---|---|---|---|---|---|---|---|---|---|
| 1 | 2 | 3 | 4 | 5 | 6 | 7 | 8 | 9 | 10 | |
| Asp | Arg | Val | Tyr | Val | His | Pro | Phe | His | Leu | Ox, turtle (1, 2) |
| Asp | — | — | — | Ile | — | — | — | His | — | Man, horse, rat, rat, rabbit, pig (3, 4, 5) |
| Asp | — | — | — | Val | — | — | — | Ser | — | Fowl (6) |
| Asp | — | — | — | Val | — | — | — | Tyr | — | Snake (7) |
| Asp | — | — | — | Val | — | — | — | Asn | — | Bullfrog (8) |
| Asp or Asn | — | — | — | Val | — | — | — | Asn | — | Salmon (9) |
| Asn | — | — | — | Val | — | — | — | His | — | Japanese goosefish (10) |
| Asp or Asn | — | — | — | Val | — | — | — | Gly | — | Eel (11, 12) |

*References.* 1: Elliott & Peart (1956); 2: Hasegawa *et al.* (1984); 3: Arakawa *et al.* (1967); 4: Skeggs *et al.* (1957); 5: Sokabe & Nakajima (1972); 6: Nakayama *et al.* (1973); 7: Nakayama *et al.* (1977); 8: Hasegawa *et al.* (1983a); 9: Takemoto *et al.* (1983); 10: Hayashi *et al.* (1978); 11: Hasegawa *et al.* (1983b); 12: Khosla *et al.* (1985).

reaching the renal arteries themselves in some species, and are also present in aglomerular teleosts. The better term for these structures is therefore 'granular epithelioid cells' (Sokabe, 1974).

The anatomical arrangement of the mammalian juxtaglomerular apparatus generated early speculation as to how renin release was governed. Many incisive but regrettably not always definitive experiments were executed to assess, for example, the relationships between the macula densa and the granular epithelioid cells and the role of renal baroreceptors in regulating renin release. Very generally there appears to be an inverse relationship between renin secretion and sodium load at the macula densa as well as with the degree of 'stretch' on the afferent arteriole; the latter mechanism probably involves a paracrine system involving prostaglandins. Among other endogenous, probably not all physiological, influences upon the release of renin from the mammalian kidney are: antidiuretic hormone, angiotensin II, prostaglandins, the sympathetic nervous system, serotonin, corticosteroids and other hormones such as growth hormone, somatostatin, parathormone and adrenocorticotrophic hormone, as well as calcium, magnesium and potassium ions. Davis & Freeman (1976) and Keeton & Campbell (1980) comprehensively and critically review these and other controlling influences upon renin release.

The pharmacological/physiological effects of angiotensin given above, together with the factors that control the release of renin, have for the most part been described for a few mammalian species. It is only relatively recently that some insight has been gained into the comparative physiology and

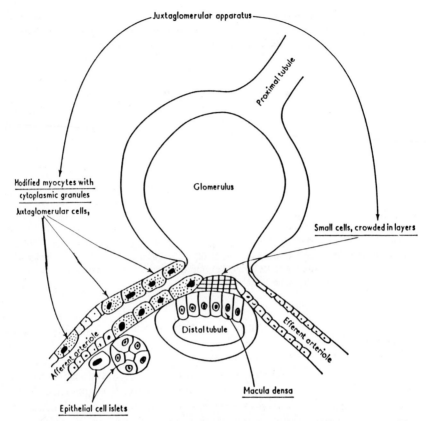

Fig. 20.4.  Component parts of the mammalian juxtaglomerular apparatus. (From Cook, 1963.)

endocrinology of the renin–angiotensin system of vertebrates as a whole. Several comprehensive reviews have discussed specific aspects of possible evolutionary relationships of the system among non-mammalian vertebrates (Taylor, 1977; Nishimura, 1978, 1980ab; Henderson *et al.*, 1981); a detailed analysis of all the experimental evidence need not therefore be attempted in this chapter. Instead, individual vertebrate groups will be discussed with respect to the occurrence of the different components of the system, and some reference will be made to possible physiological roles.

### 20.3.1. *Agnatha*

As with most other aspects of cyclostome endocrinology, information is sparse and few definitive observations have been made on the renin–angiotensin system. Granular epithelioid cells have not been described (Sokabe & Ogawa, 1974), and homologous renal and plasma incubations do not generate active pressor material in the standard rat bioassay (Nishimura *et al.*, 1970). Tentative evidence has, however, been produced to indicate that incubation of crude lamprey (*Lampetra fluviatilis*) renal extracts with a canine renin-substrate preparation generate an angiotensin-like vasoactive material (Henderson *et al.*, 1981). This material would obviously be dog angiotensin I so that its activity may be more easily recognised by the rat vascular receptor than perhaps a cyclostome angiotensin, whose peptide sequence is likely to differ. Of interest with respect to the possible presence of angiotensin in this group are the observations that mammalian angiotensin is pressor, although the effect was considered to result from activation of the sympathetic nervous system (Carroll & Opdyke, 1982).

### 20.3.2. *Chondrichthyes*

This group of fishes is perhaps the most ancient vertebrate group, in that they have remained little changed over millennia and apparently retain many of the characteristics of the 'stem' vertebrate stock. There is a degree of controversy as to whether they possess a true renin–angiotensin system. Thus granular epithelioid cells have not been demonstrated (Sokabe & Ogawa, 1974), and homologous incubations of renal extracts with plasma failed to generate material that was pressor in the rat bioassay (Nishimura *et al.*, 1970). However, there is tentative evidence to suggest the presence of renal materials that react with canine angiotensinogen to generate vasoactive substances (Henderson *et al.*, 1981). More recently, purer renal extracts from the dogfish incubated with partially purified 'renin-substrate' from the dogfish gave potent pressor responses in dogfish;this material was weakly active in the rat pressor bioassay (L. B. O'Toole, I. W. Henderson, B. M. Uva, P. Ghiani, M. A. Masini & N. Hazon, unpublished observations). These observations emphasise earlier remarks regarding the structure/ activity relationships of the angiotensin molecule and the changing amino acid sequence that will inevitably influence interaction of receptors in hetero-logous bioassays.

There is other, also tenuous, evidence for an elasmobranch renal pressor system although its character may differ in detail. The presence of an angiotensin I converting enzyme, for example, has been identified (Opdyke & Holcombe, 1976), and mammalian angiotensin II may increase dogfish arterial blood pressure via the sympathetic nervous system (Opdyke *et al.*, 1981), an effect that may also occur in mammals (see above). Furthermore it has also been shown that renal extracts of the dogfish and mammalian angiotensin II increase plasma concentrations of an endogenous corticoster-oid, 1-*a*-hydroxycorticosterone (Hazon & Henderson, 1985). Thus, although the evidence remains scanty, the presence of angiotensin receptors for activating adrenocortical secretion and the sympathetic nervous system as well as for vasconstriction has been indicated. Set against these more positive findings must be the observations of Churchill *et al.* (1985) who were unable to detect changes in arterial blood pressure, glomerular filtration rate, urine flow and sodium excretion following intravenous infusions of mammalian angiotensin II (18 to 36 ng kg$^{-1}$ body wt/min). Clearly there are insufficient data to speculate upon the physiological relevance of these observations.

It is of course always difficult to make definitive assertions about the absence of a hormone or hormonal system. With respect to the elasmo-branchs, it is important to note that a phosphoglyceride with potent renin inhibitory activity is present in large quantities in renal extracts of the Mako shark, *Isurus oxyrinchus* (Turcotte *et al.*, 1973). This inhibitor of the renin–angiotensinogen reaction is akin to that described for hog kidney, and may well partially explain the failures to identify positively an endogenous renin–angiotensin system in cartilaginous fishes.

### 20.3.3. *Actinopterygii*

Among the ray-finned fishes one begins to identify with greater certainty components of the renin–angiotensin system. Thus granular epithelioid cells have been observed in representative teleost and holostean, but surprisingly not chondrostean, fishes. The actual location of these cells, present even in the absence of a glomerulus, varies enormously (Sokabe, 1974). Among dipnoan fishes granular epithelioid cells have been described (Nishimura *et al.*, 1973). The presence of a macula densa and associated accompaniments of the juxtaglomerular apparatus have not been unequivocally demonstrated in any of the fish types mentioned above.

In spite of some earlier doubts about the presence of renin-like materials in the kidneys of certain teleosts, there is now a wealth of evidence suggesting its presence, and several piscine angiotensins have been sequenced (see Table 20.1). In addition various bioassays and radioimmunoassays have been applied to assess renin activity and angiotensins I and II in plasma of stenohaline marine and fresh-water teleosts as well as euryhaline species adapting to either enviroment. The changes that take place when euryhaline teleosts are transferred from fresh water to sea water suggest that renin is released on entering the hyperosmotic milieu and the opposite change takes place on back transfer, although there are recorded exceptions (cf. Malvin & Vander, 1967; Sokabe *et al.*, 1973; Nishimura *et al.*, 1976; Henderson *et al.*, 1976). Histologically the granular epithelioid cells appear more active in fish in marine or brackish-water environments.

Considering some of the general effects of angiotensin II listed earlier, it may or may not be coincidence that in sea-water adapted euryhaline species there appears to be increased adrenocortical activity, a relative polydipsia and a glomerular antidiuresis (see Henderson & Garland, 1980). These coincident changes have their parallels pharmacologically in that exogenous angiotensins may be antidiuretic in sea-water teleost representatives (Brown *et al.*, 1980), certainly are dipsogenic (Hirano *et al.*, 1978; Malvin *et al.*, 1980; Hirano & Masegawa, 1984) and also increase the secretory rates of cortisol (Henderson *et al.*, 1974, 1976). This quite plausible role for the renin-angiotensin system in assisting the adaptation to hyperosmotic environments must, however, be viewed alongside a number of other studies which demonstrate less readily such a role, including a number employing angiotensin converting enzyme inhibitors and angiotensin antagonists (Nishimura *et al.*, 1978; Kenyon *et al.*, 1985).

Moreover Nishimura (1978) has argued cogently that the renin–angiotensin system primarily has more of a cardiovascular role rather than one related to renal regulation of fluid and electrolytes, or indeed modulation of adrenocortical function. Evidence in favour of this comes from studies of the renin responses to hypotension, blockade of angiotensin I converting enzyme, and the use of adrenergic blockers (Nishimura & Sawyer, 1976; Nishimura *et al.*, 1978; Zucker & Nishimura, 1981). In other bony fish, mention should be made briefly of some studies that have been carried out on dipnoan representatives. Thus renin is present in species of lungfish (Nishimura *et al.*, 1973; Blair-West *et al.*, 1977) and exogenous angiotensin II is diuretic, natriuretic and pressor, but interestingly does not apparently affect corticosteroid concentrations in plasma (Sawyer *et al.*, 1976; Blair-West *et al.*, 1977).

Thus in actinopterygian fishes there is considerable circumstantial evidence for physiological roles of the renin–angiotensin system in the regulation of renal function, voluntary fluid intake, cardiovascular function and adrenocortical secretory patterns. More definitive data are, however, required to delineate exact functions. Moreover, the relationships between renin and other hormonal systems, adrenal cortex apart, are poorly understood although recent data suggest that a feedback system is present between angiotensin and the neurohypophysial peptide, arginine vasotocin (Henderson *et al.*, 1985: see Fig. 20.5), which is dependent upon environmental salinity.

### 20.3.4. *Amphibia*

In the Amphibia one begins to recognise more truly a juxtaglomerular apparatus, with distinct granular epithelioid cells adjacent to the glomerulus and a nephron arrangement that at least in part resembles a macula densa (see Lamers *et al.*, 1974; Sokabe & Ogawa, 1974). It is of interest here that in the Amphibia interrenal cells are often juxtaposed to these elements so that within a few cubic micrometres there is the sodium(?) sensor of the macula densa, the source of renin and one of angiotensin's target glands — the aldosterone-secreting adrenocortical cell — whose own target may be the distal nephron.

Renin has been detected in both the plasma and kidney of anuran and urodele amphibians (Grill *et al.*, 1972; Worley *et al.*, 1978) and an angiotensin

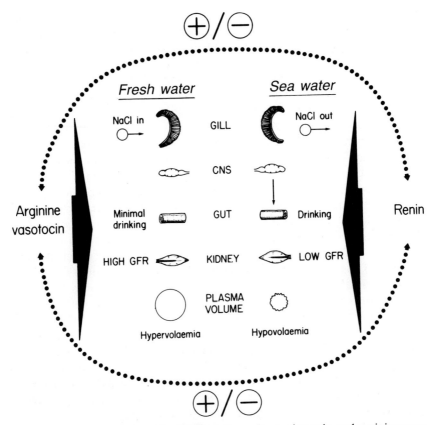

Fig. 20.5.  Possible relationships between the renin–angiotensin and arginine vasotocin in euryhaline teleosts with respect to their feedback control one with another
and with respect to their sites of action.

has been sequenced (Table 20.1). The physiological relationships of the
renin–angiotensin system are not clear, however. Thus distinct changes in the
system have not consistently resulted from sodium overload, sodium depletion, dehydration or haemorrhage (Davis *et al.*, 1970; Capelli *et al.*, 1970;
Nolly & Fasciolo, 1971; Sokabe *et al.*, 1972; Garland & Henderson, 1975).
There are, however, distinct adrenocorticosteroidogenic responses to homologous renin and heterologous angiotensin injections (Johnston *et al.*, 1967;
Ulick & Feinholtz, 1968; Taylor *et al.*, 1972; Dupont *et al.*, 1976). Dipsogenic
responses in amphibians have not been recorded (Hirano *et al.*, 1978;
Kobayashi *et al.*, 1979), and direct actions (that is, without affecting
sympathetic nervous activity) upon the vasculature have been doubted
(Carroll & Opdyke, 1982).

## 20.3.5. *Reptilia*

It is perhaps surprising that the kidney of reptiles does not apparently contain a macula densa, although granular epithelioid cells and renal renin activity have been noted (Sokabe *et al.*, 1969; Uva & Vallarino, 1982). An angiotensin from a reptilian representative has also been sequenced (Table 20.1).

There have been limited pharmacological and physiological studies upon the renin-angiotensin system of reptiles. Thus there is doubt about an angiotensin action upon the adrenocortical homologue (Nothstine *et al.*, 1971; Callard, 1975). Of the other aspects of renin–angiotensin's pharmacology, dipsogenicity has been shown (Fitzsimons & Kaufman, 1977; Kobayashi *et al.*, 1979), but its actions on the cardiovasculature are uncertain in the sense of being either direct or via the sympathetic nervous system (Stephens, 1981).

## 20.3.6. *Aves*

The birds present several curious specialisations of the renin–angiotensin system, some of which seem likely to be refinements (or more arguably dichotomies from proto-reptilian stock) of the general mammalian scheme presented earlier, and others have taken on quite unique characters (Wilson, 1984a). Wilson (1984a) gives comprehensive treatment in his review to the avian system and aptly concludes with respect to the renin–angiotensin systems, 'Similar features in mammals and birds ... differ from those in reptiles ... [and] may have evolved independently ... and ... not be ... derived from a common ancestry'. In other words one must be cautious with respect to the avian system about drawing exact parallels with other vertebrates, since in a number of publications cited by Wilson (1984b), cardiovascular, adrenocortical, adrenergic and renal responses to exogenous angiotensin II show a unique character.

Renal granular epithelioid cells and a macula densa have been demonstrated, and the general topography resembles that of mammals. A number of reports have, however, indicated a different character with respect to general histology, ultrastructure and topography of the avian system compared with mammals (e.g. Ogawa & Sokabe, 1971; Wideman *et al.*, 1981). Renin has been extracted from a number of avian kidneys and generates pressor substances from both homologous plasma and from heterologous renin substrates. An avian angiotensin has been sequenced (Table 20.1).

Release of renin may be influenced by sodium status and by extracellular or plasma volume (Nishimura & Bailey, 1982; Taylor *et al.*, 1970; Chan & Holmes, 1971), and exogenous angiotensin produces diuretic with inconsistent natriuretic responses (Langford & Fallis, 1966; Cuypers, 1965) and an increase in drinking (Kaufman & Peters, 1980; Fitzsimons *et al.*, 1982). The latter response may vary, and it has been suggested that the particular bird's ecological history, in terms of water availability, influences the dipsogenic reaction (Kobayashi *et al.*, 1979). The adrenal cortical secretory patterns are stimulated by exogenous angiotensin as well as by endogenous renin, although again there are inconsistencies (De Roos, and De Roos, 1963; Taylor *et al.*, 1970).

It is perhaps within the area of blood-pressure regulation and control of sympathetic nervous function that the avian renin–angiotensin system appears to differ most significantly from other vertebrate types. Although there remain some unresolved features of the interactions in these areas, it has been stated (Wilson, 1984b) that the entire avian pressor response to angiotensin may rely upon release of catecholamines. Indeed Nishimura *et al.* (1982) observed, under particular circumstances, a significant vasodepressor response to angiotensin II. It may, however, be that the systems interact in a similar fashion to mammals, but primacy has been given during evolution to different components in the closely intermingling series of tissue reactions.

### 20.4. Conclusion

In conclusion, this brief review has attempted to highlight certain key characteristics of the renin–angiotensin system among vertebrates. Particular emphasis has been placed on non-mammalian vertebrates, since by understanding mechanisms in these groups the comparative endocrinologist aims to assess common features and also to identify differences, either in absolute terms or in terms of degree of emphasis. Nishimura (1980a), in a critical review, posed a number of key questions related to the evolution of this system and the possible uniformity of its actions. In general terms the questions addressed the possible universality of renin to participate in: blood volume/pressure regulation; adrenergic activity; renal function; and adrenocortical control. Scanning the published literature it is not possible to affirm with confidence that there is indeed uniformity in all the groups:

(1) The component parts of the cascade starting with the generation of angiotensinogen and prorenin have not been defined in all types.
(2) Tissue receptors, albeit mostly to heterologous angiotensins, clearly differ with respect to distribution as between vascular, renal, adrenocortical, etc., and such differences are obviously reflected in the varying overall responses.
(3) The vascular responses among vertebrates contain a varying degree of reliance upon the adrenergic nervous system, a feature that is currently quite controversial.
(4) With regard to extracellular fluid volume regulation, different vertebrates

vary very much with regard to the renal and the central nervous dipsogenic reactions, features which one must presume depend on the imposed environmental regimes and the homeostatic adaptations thereto.

This chapter has exclusively considered the renal enzyme, renin, and has not made reference to extrarenal renins which occur in tissues that include in mammals at least blood vessels, the pregnant uterus, the adrenal gland, salivary glands and of course the brain wherein a complete renin–angiotensin system exists (see Ganong, 1977, and the account by Suter in Chapter 8). The functions of these systems are beginning to come under study, largely as paracrine regulators. The exact nature of their actions and control are uncertain. They certainly cannot be discussed in terms of vertebrate endocrine phylogeny, since to date sources of non-mammalian extrarenal renin-like or angiotensin-like materials have not been extensively sought and may include such sources as the corpuscles of Stannius of teleost fishes (Hasegawa *et al.*, 1982), and the myocardium (Yunge *et al.*, 1980) and integument (Erspamer *et al.*, 1979) of frogs.

If there is such widespread distribution of renins and angiotensins in non-mammalian vertebrates as in mammals, then a whole new avenue of study appears. In addition it raises the matter of why renin has become so concentrated in the kidney, since few would doubt that renal renin is the major material that is in the circulation. It was argued earlier that, to execute its exocrine role as a body fluid homeostat with efficiency, it necessarily had to have interfaces with the cardiovasculature and with other systemic hormones that affected excretory patterns. The anatomical arrangements of the nephron also demanded communication between glomerulus, proximal and distal segments, hence the paracrine nature of the intrarenal systems.

## References

Arakawa, K., Nakatani, M., Minohara, A. & Nakamura, M. (1967). Isolation and amino acid composition of human angiotensin I. *Biochem. J.* **104**, 900–6.

Balment, R. J., Henderson, I. W. & Chester Jones, I. (1980) The adrenal cortex and its homologues: evolutionary considerations. In *General, Comparative and Clinical Endocrinology of the Adrenal Cortex*, vol. 3, pp 525–62 (eds I. Chester Jones & I. W. Henderson). New York: Academic Press.

Blair-West, J. R., Coghlan, J. P., Denton, D. A., Gibson, A. P., Oddie, C. J., Sawyer, W. H. & Scoggins, B. A. (1977). Plasma renin activity and blood corticosteroids in the australian lungfish, *Neoceratodus forsteri. J. Endocrinol.* **73**, 137–42.

Braun-Menendez, E., Fasciolo, J. C., Leloir, C. F. & Munoz, J. M. (1940). The substance causing renal hypertension. *J. Physiol.* **98**, 283–98.

Braun-Menendez, E., Fasciolo, J. C., Leloir, L. F., Munoz, J. M. & Taquini, A. C. (1943). *Hipertension arterial nefrogena*. Buenos Aires: Libreria Y Editorial El Ateneo.

Brown, J. A., Oliver, J. A., Henderson, I. W. & Jackson, B. A. (1980), Angiotensin and single nephron glomerular function in the trout, *Salmo gairdneri. Am. J. Physiol.* **245**, R509–14.

Callard, G. V. (1975). Corticotropic effects on isolated interrenal cells of the turtle (*Chrysemys picta*). *Gen. Comp. Endocrinol.* **26**, 301–9.

Capelli, J. P., Wesson, L. G.& Aponte, G. E. (1970). A phylogenetic study of the renin–angiotensin system. *Am. J. Physiol.* **218**, 1171–8.

Carroll, R. G. & Opdyke, D. F. (1982). Evolution of angiotensin II-induced catecholamine release. *Am. J. Physiology.* **243**, R65–9.

Chan, M. Y. & Holmes, W. N. (1971). Studies on a 'renin–angiotensin' system in the normal and hypophysectomized pigeon (*Columba livia*). *Gen. Comp. Endocrinol.* **16**, 304–11.

Churchill, P. C., Malvin, R. L., & Churchill, M. C. (1985). Lack of renal effects of DOCA, ACTH, spironolactone and angiotensin II in *Squalus acanthias. J. Exp. Zool.* **234**, 17–22.

Cook, W. F. (1963). Renin and the juxtaglomerular apparatus. *Mem. Soc. Endocrinol.* **13**, 247–54.

Cuypers, Y. (1965). L'action tubulaire renale de l'angiotensine II amide chez le coq. *Arch. Int. Pharmacodyn. Thér.* **155**, 495–6.

Davis, J. O. (1963). Importance of the renin–angiotensin system in the control of aldosterone secretion. *Mem. Soc. Endocrinol.* **13**, 325–39.

Davis, J. O. (1975). The use of blocking agents to define the functions of the renin–angiotensin system. *Clin. Sci. Mol. Med.* **48**, 3s–14s.

Davis, J. O. & Freeman, R. F. (1976). Mechanisms controlling renin release. *Physiol. Rev.* **56**, 1–56.

Davis, J. O., Copeland, D. L., Taylor, A. A. & Baumber, J. S. (1970). Plasma electrolyte concentrations and steroid secretion in the bullfrog and opossum. *Am. J. Physiol.* **219**, 555–9.

De Roos, R. M. & De Roos, C. C. (1963). Angiotensin II: its effects on corticoid production by chicken adrenals *in vitro. Science.* **141**, 1284.

Dupont, W., LeBoulanger, F., Vaudry, H. & Vaillant, R. (1976). Regulation of the aldosterone secretion in the frog, *Rana esculenta* L. *Gen. Comp. Endocrinol.* **29**, 51–60.

Elliott, D. F. & Peart, W. S. (1956). Amino acid sequence in a hypertensin. *Nature, London.* **177**, 527–8.

Erspamer, V., Melchiorri, P., Nakajima, T., Yasuhara, T. & Endean, R. (1979). Amino acid composition and sequence of crinia-angiotensin, an angiotensin II-like undecapeptide from the skin of the australian frog, *Crinia georgiana. Experientia* **35**, 1132–5.

Fitzsimons, J. T. & Kaufman, S. (1977). Cellular and extracellular dehydration and angiotensin as stimuli to drinking in the common iguana, *Iguana iguana. J. Physiol. London* **265**, 443–63.

Fitzsimons, J. T., Massi, M. & Thornton, S. N. (1982). The effects of changes in osmolality and sodium concentrations on angiotensin induced drinking in the pigeon. *J. Physiol. London* **330**, 1–14.

Ganong, W. F. (1977). The renin-angiotensin system and the central nervous system. *Fed. Proc.* **36**, 1771–5.

Ganong, W. F., Biglieri, E. G. & Mulrow, P. H. (1966). Mechanisms regulating adrenocortical secretion of aldosterone and glucocorticoids. *Recent Prog. Hormone Res.* **22**, 381–430.

Garland, H. O. & Henderson, I. W. (1975). Influence of environmental salinity on renal and adrenocortical function in the toad, *Bufo marinus. Gen. Comp. Endocrinol.* **27**, 136–43.

Gibbons, G. H., Dzau, V. J., Farhi, E. R. & Barger, A. C. (1984). Interaction of signals influencing renin release. *Ann. Rev. Physiol.* **46**, 291–308.

Goldblatt, H., Lynch, J., Hanzal, R. F. & Summerville, W. (1934). Studies on experimental hypertension. I. Production of persistent elevation of systolic pressure by means of renal ischemia. *J. Exp. Med.* **59**, 347–79.

Grill, G., Granger, P. & Thurau, K. (1972). The renin–angiotensin system of amphibians. I. Determination of the renin content of the amphibian kidney. *Pflügers Arch.* **331**, 1–12.

Hazon, N. & Henderson, I. W. (1985). Factors affecting the secretory dynamics of 1-α-hydroxy-corticosterone in the dogfish, *Scyliorhinus canicula. Gen. Comp. Endocrinol.* **59**, 50–5.

Hasegawa, Y., Watanabe, T. X., Sokabe, H., Takemoto, Y., Nakajima, T., Kumagae, S. & Sakakibara, S. (1982). Chemical structure of angiotensins originated from the corpuscles of Stannius in the salmon, *Oncorhynchus keta*. In. *Comparative Endocrinology of Calcium Regulation*, pp. 155–9. (eds C. Oguro & P. K. T. Pang). Japan Scientific Societies Press.

Hasegawa, Y., Watanabe, T. X., Sokabe, H. & Nakajima, T. (1983a). Chemical structure of angiotensin in the bullfrog, *Rana catesbeiana. Gen. Comp. Endocrinol.* **50**, 75–80.

Hasegawa, Y., Nakajima, T. and Sokabe, H. (1983b) Chemical structure of angiotensin formed with kidney renin in the Japanese eel, *Anguilla japonica. Biomed. Res.* **4**, 417–20.

Hasegawa, Y., Cipolle, M., Watanabe, T. X., Nakajima, A. T., Sokabe, H. & Zehr, J. E. (1984). Chemical structure of angiotensin in the turtle, *Pseudemys scripta. Gen. Comp. Endocrinol.* **53**, 159–62.

Hayashi, T., Nakayama, T., Nakajima, T. & Sokabe, H. (1978). Structure of angiotensin formed by the kidney of Japanese goosefish and its identification by Dansyl method. *Chem. Pharm. Bull.* **26**, 215–19.

Henderson, I. W. & Garland, H. O. (1980). The interrenal gland of Pisces: Part 2 — Physiology. In *General, Comparative and Clinical Endocrinology of the Adrenal Cortex*, vol. 3, pp. 471–523 (eds I. Chester Jones & I. W. Henderson). New York: Academic Press.

Henderson, I. W., Sa'di, M. N. and Hargreaves, G. (1974). Studies on the production and metabolic clearance rates of cortisol in the European eel, *Anguilla anguilla* L. *J. Steroid Biochem.* **5**, 701–7.

Henderson, I. W., Jotisankasa, V., Mosley, W. & Oguri, M. (1976). Endocrine and environmental influences upon plasma cortisol and plasma renin activity of the eel, *Anguilla anguilla* L. *J. Endocrinol.* **70**, 81–95.

Henderson, I. W., Oliver, J. A., McKeever, A. & Hazon, N. (1981). Phylogenetic aspects of the renin–angiotensin system. In *Advances in Animal and Comparative Physiology*, pp. 355–63 (eds G. Pethes & V. L. Frenyo). Oxford: Pergamon Press.

Henderson, I. W., Hazon, N. & Hughes, K. (1985). Hormones, ionic regulation and kidney function in fishes. In *Physiological Adaptations of Marine Animals* (ed. M. Laverack) *Symp. Soc. Exp. Biol.* **XXXIX**, 245–65.

Hirano, T. & Hasegawa, S. (1984). Effects of angiotensins and other vasoactive substances on drinking in the eel, *Anguilla japonica. Zool. Sci.* **1**, 106–13.

Hirano, T., Takei, Y. & Kobayashi, H. (1978). Angiotensin and drinking in the eel and the frog. In *Osmotic and Volume Regulation*, pp. 123–34 (eds C. B. Jorgensen & E. Skadhauge). Alfred Benzon Symposium XI. Copenhagen: Munksgaard.

Johnston, C. I., Davis, J. O., Wright, F. S. & Howards, S. S. (1967). Effects of renin and ACTH on adrenal steroid secretion in the American bullfrog. *Am. J. Physiol.* **213**, 393–9.

Kaufman, S. & Peters, G. (1980). Regulatory drinking in the pigeon, *Columba livia Am. J. Physiol.* **239**, R219–25.

Keeton, T. K. & Campbell, W. B. (1980). The pharmacologic alteration of renin release. *Pharmacol. Rev.* **32**, 81–227.

Kenyon, C. J., McKeever, A., Oliver, J. A. & Henderson, I. W. (1985). Control of renal and adrenocortical function by the renin-angiotensin system in two euryhaline teleost fishes. *Gen. Comp. Endocrinol.* **58**, 93–100.

Khosla, M. C., Nishimura, H., Hasegawa, Y. & Bumpus, F. M. (1985). Identification and synthesis of [1-asparagine, 5-valine, 9-glycine] angiotensin I produced from plasma of the American eel, *Anguilla rostrata. Gen. Comp. Endocrinol.* **57**, 223–33.

Kobayashi, H., Uemura, H., Wada, M. & Takei, Y. (1979). Ecological adaptations of angiotensin-induced thirst mechanism in tetrapods. *Gen. Comp. Endocrinol.* **38**, 93–104.

Lamers, A. P. M., van Dongen, W. J. & van Kemenade, J. A. M. (1974). An ultrastructural study of the juxtaglomerular apparatus in the toad, *Bufo bufo. Cell Tiss. Res.* **153**, 449–64.

Langford, H. G. & Fallis, N. (1966). Diuretic effect of angiotensin in the chicken. *Proc. Soc. Exp. Biol. Med.* **123**, 317–21.

Laragh, J. H., Cannon, P. J., Ames, R. P., Sicinski, A. M. & Borkowski, A. J. (1963). Aldosteronism in man: mechanisms controlling secretion of the hormone, role of angiotensin. *Men. Soc. Endocrinol.* **13**, 363–78.

Malvin, R. L. & Vander, A. J. (1967). Plasma renin activity in marine teleosts and Cetacea. *Am. J. Physiol.* **213**, 1582–4.

Malvin, R. L., Schiff, D. & Eiger, S. (1980). Angiotensin and drinking rates in the euryhaline killifish. *Am. J. Physiol.* **239**, R31–4.

Nakayama, T., Nakajima, T. & Sokabe, H. (1973). Structure of fowl angiotensin and its identification by D. N. S. method. *Chem. Pharm. Bull.* **21**, 2085–7.

Nakayama, T., Nakajima, T. & Sokabe, H. (1977). Structure of snake (*Elaphe climocophora*) angiotensin. *Chem. Pharm. Bull.* **25**, 3255–60.

Nishimura, H. (1978). Physiological evolution of the renin–angiotensin system. *Jpn. Heart J.* **19**, 806–22.

Nishimura, H. (1980a). Comparative endocrinology of renin and angiotensin. In *The Renin–Angiotensin System*, pp. 29–77 (eds: J. A. Johnson & R. R. Anderson). New York: Plenum.

Nishimura, H. (1980b). Evolution of the renin–angiotensin system. In *Evolution of Vertebrate Endocrine Systems*, pp. 373–404 (eds P. K. T. Pang & A. Epple). Lubbock, Texas: Graduate Studies No. 21, Texas Tech University.

Nishimura, H. & Sawyer, W. H. (1976). Vasopressor, diuretic and natriuretic responses to angiotensins by the american eel, *Anguilla rostrata. Gen. Comp. Endocrinol.* **29**, 337–48.

Nishimura, J. & Bailey, J. R. (1982). Intra-renal renin–angiotensin system in primitive vertebrates. *Kidney Int.* **22**, Suppl. 12, S185–92.

Nishimura, H., Oguri, M., Ogawa, M., Sokabe, H. & Imai, M. (1970). Absence of renin in kidneys of elasmobranchs and cyclostomes. *Am. J. Physiol.* **218**, 911–15.

Nishimura, H., Ogawa, M. & Sawyer, W. H. (1973). Renin–angiotensin system in primitive bony fishes and a holocephalan. *Am. J. Physiol.* **224**, 950–6.

Nishimura, H., Sawyer, W. H. & Nigrelli, R. F. (1976). Renin, cortisol and plasma volume in marine teleost fishes adapted to dilute media. *J. Endocrinol.* **70**, 47–59.

Nishimura, H., Norton, V. M. & Bumpus, F. M. (1978). Lack of specific inhibition of angiotensin II in eels by angiotensin antagonists. *Am. J. Physiol.* **235**, H95–103.

Nishimura, H., Nakamura, Y., Sumner, R. P. & Khosla, M. C. (1982). Vasopressor and depressor actions of angiotensin in the anesthetized fowl. *Am. J. Physiol.* **242**, H314–24.

Nolly, H. L. & Fasciolo, J. C. (1971). Renin–angiotensin system and homeostasis in *Bufo arenarum. Comp. Biochem. Physiol.* **39A**, 833–41.

Nothstine, S. A., Davis, J. O. & De Roos, R. M. (1971). Kidney extracts and ACTH on adrenal secretion in a turtle and a crocodilian. *Am. J. Physiol.* **221**, 726–32.

Ogawa, M. & Sokabe, H. (1971). The macula densa site of avian kidney. *Z. Zellforsch. Mikroskop. Anat.* **120**, 29–36.

Opdyke, D. F. & Holcombe, R. (1976). Response to angiotensin I and II and to A-I converting enzyme inhibitor in a shark. *Am. J. Physiol.* **231**, 1750–3.

Opdyke, D. F., Carroll, R. G., Keller, N. E. & Taylor, A. A. (1981). Angiotensin II releases catecholamines in dogfish. *Comp. Biochem. Physiol.* **70C**, 131–4.

Page, I. H. & Helmer, O. M. (1940). A crystalline pressor substance, angiotonin, resulting from the reaction between renin and renin activator. *J. Exp. Med.* **71**, 29–42.

Pickering, G. W. & Prinzmetal, M. (1938). Some observations on renin, a pressor substance contained in normal kidney, together with a method for its biological assay. *Clin. Sci.* **3**, 211.

Sawyer, W. H., Blair-West, J. R., Simpson, P. A. & Sawyer, M. K. (1976). Renal responses of Australian lungfish to vasotocin, angiotensin II and NaCl infusion. *Am. J. Physiol.* **231**, 593–602.

Skeggs, L. T., Lentz, K. E., Kahn, J. R. Shumway, N. P. & Woods, K. R. (1957). Amino acid sequence of hypertensin II. *J. Exp. Med.* **104**, 193–7.

Sokabe, H. (1974). Phylogeny of the renal effects of angiotensin. *Kidney Int.* **6**, 263–71.

Sokabe, H. & Nakajima, T. (1972). Chemical structure and role of angiotensins in vertebrates. *Gen. Comp. Endocrinol.* Suppl. **3**, 382–92.

Sokabe, H. & Ogawa, M. (1974). Comparative studies of the juxtaglomerular apparatus. *Int. Rev. Cytol.* **37**, 271–327.

Sokabe, H., Ogawa, M., Oguri, M. & Nishimura, H. (1969). Evolution of the juxtaglomerular apparatus in the vertebrate kidneys. *Texas Rep. Biol. Med.* **27**, 867–85.

Sokabe, H., Nishimura, H., Kawabe, K., Tenmoki, S. & Arai, T. (1972). Plasma renin activity in varying hydrated states in the bullfrog. *Am. J. Physiol.* **222**, 142–6.

Sokabe, H., Oide, H., Ogawa, M. & Utida, S. (1973). Plasma renin activity in Japanese eels (*Anguilla japonica*) adapted to sea water or in dehydration. *Gen. Comp. Endocrinol.* **21**, 160–7.

Stephens, G. A. (1981). Blockade of angiotensin pressor activity in the fresh water turtle. *Gen. Comp. Endocrinol.* **45**, 364–71.

Takemoto, Y., Nakajima, T., Hasegawa, Y., Watanabe, T. X., Sokabe, H. Kumagae, S. I. & Sakakibara, S. (1983). Chemical structure of angiotensins formed by incubating plasma with kidney and the corpuscles of Stannius in the chum salmon. *Gen. Comp. Endocrinol.* **51**, 219–27.

Taylor, A. A. (1977). Comparative physiology of the renin–angiotensin system. *Fed. Proc.* **36**, 1776–80.

Taylor, A. A., Davis, J. O. & Braverman, b. (1972). Deoxycorticosterone secretion in the bullfrog: effects of ACTH, hypophysectomy and renin. *Am. J. Physiol.* **233**, 858–63.

Taylor, A. A., Davis, J. O., Breitenbach, R. P. & Hartroft, P. M. (1970) Adrenal steroid secretion and a renal pressor system in the chicken (*Gallus domesticus*). *Gen. Comp. Endocrinol.* **14**, 321–33.

Tigerstedt, R. & Bergman, R. (1898). Niere und kreislauf. *Skand. Arch. Physiol.* **8**, 223–71.

Turcotte, J. G., Boyad, R. E., Quinn, J. G. & Smeby, R. R. (1973). Isolation and renin-inhibitory activity of phosphoglyceride from shark kidney. *J. Med. Chem.* **16**, 166–8.

Ulick, S. & Feinholtz, E. (1968). Metabolism and rate of secretion of aldosterone in the bullfrog. *J. Clin. Invest.* **47**, 2523–30.

Uva, B. M. & Vallarino, M. (1982). Renin–angiotensin system and osmoregulation in the terrestial chelonian, *Testudo hermanni* Gmelin. *Comp. Biochem. Physiol.* **71A**, 449–51.

Wideman, R. F., Braun, E. J. & Anderson, G. L. (1981). Microanatomy of the renal cortex in the domestic fowl. *J. Morphol.* **168**, 249–67.

Wilson, J. X. (1984a). Coevolution of the renin–angiotensin system and the nervous control of blood circulation. *Can. J. Zool.* **62**, 137–47.

Wilson, J. X. (1984b). The renin–angiotensin system in non-mammalian vertebrates. *Endocrine Rev.* **5**, 45–61.

Worley, R. T. S., Rich, G. T. & Prior, J. S. (1978). Effects of calcium ionophore Br-X537A on renin synthesis and release in *Amphiuma means* kidney culture. *Nature, London* **271**, 174–6.

Yunge, L., Ballak, M., Beuzeron, J., Lacasse, J. & Cantin, M. (1980). Ultrastructural cytochemistry of atrial and ventricular cardiocytes of the bullfrog (*Rana catesbeiana*). Relationship of specific granules with renin-like activity of the myocardium. *Can. J. Physiol. Pharmacol.* **58**, 1463–72.

Zucker, A. & Nishimura, H. (1981). Renal respones to vasoactive homones in the aglomeoular toadfish, *Opsanus tau. Gen. Comp.* Endocrinol. **43**, 1–9.

# Index

# Index of animals

Animals mentioned in the text are listed by their common or specific names, according to the mode of reference of each author, in alphabetic order under the broad taxonomic headings of invertebrates, fish, amphibians, reptiles, birds and mammals.

**Invertebrates**
*Crustacea*
  *Astacus leptodactylus*, crayfish 291
  *Birgus latro*, coconut crab 284
  *Cancer magister* 296
  *Carcinus maenas* 81, 82, 278, 283, 295, 296, 297
  *Cardisoma* 292
  crabs 80
  crayfish 279, 283, 284
  decapodan crustaceans 80–109, 277–9, 282–4, 290–2, 294–7
  hermit crabs 88
  *Homarus gammarus*, lobster 81, 99
  land crabs 284
  *Libinia* 291
  lobster 80, 88, 101, 104, 280, 286
  *Nephrops norvegicus* 296
  *Panulirus interruptus* 290
  *Portunus* 296
  *Procambarus simulans*, crayfish 294

*Chelicerata*
  *Limulus polyphemus* 284

*Insecta*
  *Rhodnius prolixus* 217

*Mollusca*
  *Aplysia* 241
  *Helix albolabris* 241

**Fish**
*Cyclostomata* 39, 117, 118

*Eptatretus stouti* 126
hagfish 118
*Lampetra*, lamprey 305
*L. fluviatilis* 403
lampetroids 119
*Myxine*, hagfish 119, 305
*M. glutinosa* 126
myxinoids 118

*Chondrichthyes*
  cartilaginous fishes
  **Holocephali** 306
  **Elasmobranch fishes** 115, 117, 119, 120, 278, 281, 284, 304, 394
  *Cetorhinus* 306
  dogfish 280, 281, 285, 286, 288, 403
  *Heterodontus portusjacksoni* Port Jackson shark 285
  *Hydrologus collei* 306, 308
  *Isurus oxyrinchus* mako shark 404
  *Raja clavata* 306, 308
  *Selache maxima* 306
  selachians 120
  *Squalus acanthius*, spiny dogfish 125, 128, 306. 308
  *Squalus suckleyi* 124
  *Scyliorhinus canicula* 280, 282, 304, 306–8, 310, 311
  *Scyliorhinus stellaris* 123, 125
  shark 20
  *Torpedo marmorata* 292

*Osteichthyes*, bony fishes
  **Actinopterygii** 117, 120, 404